OUTLINES
IN PATHOLOGY

OUTLINES IN PATHOLOGY

JOHN H. SINARD, MD, PhD

Assistant Professor
Department of Pathology
Yale University School of Medicine
New Haven, Connecticut

W.B. SAUNDERS COMPANY
A Division of Harcourt Brace & Company
Philadelphia London Toronto Montreal Sydney Tokyo

W.B. SAUNDERS COMPANY
A Division of Harcourt Brace & Company

The Curtis Center
Independence Square West
Philadelphia, Pennsylvania 19106

Library of Congress Cataloging-in-Publication Data

Sinard, John H.
Outlines in pathology / John H. Sinard.—1st ed.

p.   cm.

Includes bibliographical references.

ISBN 0-7216-6341-9

1. Pathology—Outlines, syllabi, etc.   I. Title.
    [DNLM: 1. Pathology—outlines.   QZ 18.2 S615o 1996]

RB32.S56 1996

616.07–dc20

DNLM/DLC   95-24406

OUTLINES IN PATHOLOGY   ISBN 0-7216-6341-9

Printed in the United States of America.

Last digit is the print number: 9   8   7   6   5   4   3   2

To my parents and brothers,
for their continuous support
and encouragement

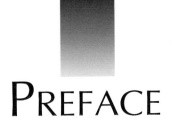

PREFACE

There are a lot of excellent pathology texts available. When I began my formal training in pathology, I was at first glad to discover this was the case, and then later somewhat overwhelmed by the large volume of material that needed to be digested. To help me in assimilating this large amount of information, I began early in my residency (and later with much greater fervor as my boards approached) to assemble a set of comprehensive outlines that discussed all of the major, and at least mentioned most of the minor, non-neoplastic and neoplastic disease processes. In assembling these outlines, I drew on material from multiple general and specialty textbooks of pathology. Into this framework, I inserted notes from numerous lectures, seminars, journal articles, and many informal discussions with attendings, often over the sign-out microscope. Where they contributed to an understanding of disease processes, I added discussions of anatomy, embryology, cell biology, and physiology. The result of this effort is seen in the pages that follow.

When I first started to make these outlines, it was certainly not with any plans of having them published. However, colleagues of mine who have seen them (and used them) have found them very helpful, and it was consistently suggested that I look into getting them published. Obviously, because you are reading this, the W.B. Saunders Company also thought others might find this helpful. Because of the outline format used, this work is not intended to replace any existing pathology text. Rather, it is intended as a study guide for pathologists in training, especially those preparing for the anatomic pathology boards, as a quick reference guide for pathologists in practice, and as a concise yet comprehensive summary for medical students interested in pathology. Only time will tell how successfully this work fulfills these goals. Every effort has been extended to ensure both the accuracy and completeness of this material. However, as our understanding of disease processes evolves, the framework in which we view these processes must shift to accommodate. I would certainly welcome any comments from readers, especially as pertains to errors that may have made their way into this text, omissions, or any other suggestions as to how these outlines might be improved.

Although the task of assimilating the information from various sources into a consistent outline format was largely my effort, I would like to extend special thanks to a few of the individuals who have indirectly made this text possible. I particularly acknowledge the influence of Juan Rosai, the director of the pathology residency training program during my first year at the Yale–New Haven Hospital. The framework of my approach to pathology was developed largely in line with his instruction, and his dedication to resident teaching has in a large way shaped my philosophy of pathology training. I would also like to thank Jon Morrow and Stuart Flynn, each of whom also served a year as program director during my training and contributed to my approach to this subject. I also acknowledge the much appreciated mentorship of Stuart Flynn and the instruction of many of the other senior faculty in the Department of Pathology at Yale during my early "formative" years as a pathologist, including Maria Luisa Carcangiu, Darryl Carter, Richard Eisen, Walker Smith, Brian West, Raymond Yesner, and others. I can only hope that some of their wisdom has made its way into my head and thus into these outlines. Equally important have been the contributions of my colleagues in training, both in a direct way to the text of this work and in an indirect way to my understanding of pathology. I thank, in particular, Vinita Parkash, David Rimm, and Harold Sánchez. Finally, I thank Chris Gilligan for convincing me to have these outlines published.

John H. Sinard, MD, PhD

CONTENTS

xii *Contents*

Benign Neoplasms
    Condyloma, Melanocytic Nevi, Hidradenoma
    Papilliferum (Papillary Hidradenoma),
    Angiomyofibroblastoma, Ectopic Mammary
    Tissue, Other Benign Lesions
Bowenoid Papulosis
Vulvar Intraepithelial Neoplasia (VIN)
Bowen's Disease

Squamous Cell Carcinoma
Other Carcinomas
    Verrucous, Basal Cell
Paget's Disease
Malignant Melanoma
Aggressive Angiomyxoma
Bartholin Gland Carcinoma

Normal Anatomy/Physiology
Inflammatory and Related Disorders
    Duct Ectasia, Fat Necrosis, Calcifications,
    Others
Fibrocystic Disease
Adenosis
    Sclerosing Adenosis, Radial Scar, Blunt Duct,
    Nodular, Microglandular, Adenomyoepithelial
    (Apocrine), Atypical Apocrine Sclerosing
    Lesion, Virginal Hypertrophy

Adenoma
    Lactating, Tubular, Intraductal Papilloma,
    Nipple Adenoma
Fibroadenoma
    Juvenile (Giant, Massive, Fetal, Cellular)
    Fibroadenoma, Malignant Transformation
Hyperplasia, Ductal and Lobular
    Atypical Hyperplasia, Ductal and Lobular

General
    Risk Factors, Diagnosis, Molecular Biology,
    Spread, Grading, Staging, Therapy, Prognosis
Ductal Carcinoma in Situ
    Comedocarcinoma, Solid, Cribriform,
    Papillary, Micropapillary, Cystic
    Hypersecretory, Clinging, Lobular
    Cancerization
Infiltrating Ductal Carcinoma
    Classic, Tubular, Cribriform, Mucinous,
    Juvenile (secretory), Medullary, Invasive

Papillary, Apocrine, Carcinoid, Metaplastic,
    Inflammatory, Paget's Disease
Lobular Carcinoma in Situ
Invasive Lobular Carcinoma
    Classic Type, Signet Ring, Others
Sweat-Gland Type Carcinomas
    Benign, Adenoid Cystic Carcinoma, Other
    Malignant
Myoepithelial Malignancies
    Adenomyoepithelioma, Clear Cell Carcinoma,
    Spindle Cell Myoepithelioma

Phylloides Tumor
Vascular Tumors
    Pseudoangiomatous Hyperplasia,
    Angiosarcoma, Hemangioma, Angiolipoma

Miscellaneous ''Tumors''
    Stromal Sarcoma, Granular Cell Tumor,
    Fibromatosis, Nodular Fasciitis, Malignant
    Lymphoma, Granulocytic Sarcoma

Gynecomastia
Other Benign Lesions

Carcinoma

Normal Anatomy
Embryology
    Thyroglossal Duct Cyst, Heterotopia

Clinical Syndromes
    Goiter, Hyperthyroidism, Hypothyroidism

Acute Thyroiditis
Granulomatous Thyroiditis
    de Quervain's, Palpation, Other
    Granulomatous

Autoimmune Thyroiditis
    Lymphocytic, Hashimoto's Thyroiditis
Riedel's Thyroiditis
Other Nonproliferative Lesions

Dyshormonogenetic Goiter
Diffuse Hyperplasia (Graves' Disease)

Nodular Hyperplasia
    Endemic Goiter, Sporadic Nodular Goiter,
    Sequestered Thyroid Nodule
C-Cell Hyperplasia

GENERAL TOPICS

1

INFLAMMATION AND IMMUNOLOGY

INFLAMMATION

Cell Injury

REVERSIBLE
Cell swelling (depletion of ATP, Na leak, water enters)
Cytoplasmic fatty change (altered lipid metabolism)
Blebs on cell surface with loss of microvilli
Nuclear chromatin clumping
Endoplasmic reticulum (ER) swelling/detachment of ribosomes
Small densities in mitochondria

IRREVERSIBLE
Cytoplasmic eosinophilia (loss of ribonucleoproteins)
Nuclear shrinkage/pyknosis/karyolysis/karyorrhexis
Cell membrane defects and myelin figures
Large mitochondrial deposits/swelling of mitochondria
Swelling of lysosomes, lysis of ER
Loss of coenzymes and RNA
If reperfused, influx of calcium; calcification

APOPTOSIS
AKA: programmed cell death
Physiologic process that occurs in the *absence* of inflammation
Affects single cells (unlike necrosis or inflammatory injury, which usually affects regions)
Pyknosis, chromatin clumping
DNA digestion is internucleosomal, resulting in a ladder pattern on gel electrophoresis (unlike the diffuse smear seen in nonphysiologic necrosis)

Acute Inflammation

OVERVIEW
Reaction of tissue (not simply cells) to injury; involves soluble factors, inflammatory cells, fibroblasts, vessels
Can be initiated by physical injury, bacteria, immune complexes, neurotoxins, endotoxin, etc.
Occurs in viable tissue—if tissue is dead, inflammation will occur at periphery
Inflammation is a process, not an event

HISTORY
Cornelius Celsus (1st century): tumor, rubor, calor, dolor (swelling, redness, heat, pain); loss of function later added as another sign of inflammation
John Hunter (1793): noted that inflammation is nonspecific host response with "salutary" effect
Julius Cohnheim (1888): detailed microscopic descriptions of inflammation in frog mesentery; stressed the importance of the vasculature

Elie Metchnikoff (1882): phagocytosis and the cellular component of inflammation

VASCULAR CHANGES
Transient vasoconstriction (seconds to minutes)
Vasodilation of arterioles; increased blood flow produces redness and heat
Increased permeability (transudate initially [low protein content, specific gravity <1.012], then exudate); produces swelling and pain
Local decreased blood of circulation (partial stasis)
Margination, emigration, and chemotaxis of leukocytes

SOLUBLE INFLAMMATORY MEDIATORS (BY ACTION)
- Increased vascular permeability

Histamine	*PAF*	*Leukotrienes C,D,E*
Serotonin	C3a	Bradykinin

- Vasodilatation

  Prostaglandins E,D,I Serotonin Bradykinin

- Vasoconstriction

  Thromboxane A_2 Leukotrienes C,D,E

- Chemotaxis

C5a	Interleukin-1 (indirectly)
C3a	*Leukotriene B_4* Endotoxin

- Opsinization

  Fc fragment of IgG   C3b

- Smooth muscle contraction

  Bradykinin Leukotrienes

- Platelet aggregation

  Thromboxane A_2 promotes   Prostacyclin inhibits

- Pain

  Bradykinin PGE_2

- Fever

  Interleukin-1 TNF Prostaglandins

SOLUBLE INFLAMMATORY MEDIATORS (BY AGENT)
Histamine (mast cells, basophils): β-imadazolylethylamine (decarboxylated histidine); vasodilation and increased vascular permeability, mucus production
Serotonin (mast cells): 5-hydroxytryptamine; vasodilation and increased vascular permeability
Platelet activating factor (PAF) (basophils): acetylated glycerol ether phosphocholine; platelet aggregation, vasodilation, and increased permeability ($100—10,000 \times$ more potent than histamine)
Interleukin-1 (IL-1) (all cell types): stimulated by immune complexes; promotes chemotaxis by endothelial effects; systemically; causes fever, sleepiness, leukocytosis
Tumor necrosis factor (TNF) (stimulated macrophages): AKA: cachectin; effects similar to IL-1
Anaphylatoxins: C3a and C5a
- Complement system (plasma factors)

  C5a: chemotaxis, some increase in vascular permeability

  C3a: increase vascular permeability, chemotaxis

  C3b: opsinization—activation of leukocyte needed

  C5b-9: membrane attack complex

Fc: opsinization—no activation needed
- Kinin system (plasma factors)

Bradykinin: nonapeptide; increased vascular permeability, dilated blood vessels, pain, smooth muscle contraction

Kallikrein: enzyme that cleaves kininogens to form bradykinin; chemotactic, causes platelet aggregation

Hageman factor (factor XIIa): initiates clotting, fibrinolytic, kinin, and complement systems
- Arachidonic acid metabolism (leukocytes)

Inhibited by corticosteroids

Two arms: lipoxygenase and cyclooxygenase

Lipoxygenase: production of leukotrienes: B, chemotaxis; C,D,E: vasoconstriction, bronchoconstriction, vascular permeability

Cyclooxygenase: production of thromboxane A_2 (vaso-constriction, platelet aggregation), prostacyclin (PGI_2; vasodilation, decreased platelet aggregation), and prostaglandins (PGD_2: vasodilatation and edema; PGE_2: pain, fever); this pathway inhibited by aspirin and by indomethacin

ADHESION OF LEUKOCYTES TO VASCULAR ENDOTHELIUM (MARGINATION)

On leukocytes
- LFA-1, MAC-1, CD11/CD18: heterodimers with different alpha subunits (150–180 kD) but the same beta subunit (95 kD); belong to integrin family (see later)
- When stimulated by chemotactic factors (C5a, TNF), receptors in the intracellular vesicles move to the surface

On endothelial cells
- ICAM-1: intercellular adhesion molecule (polys, lymphocytes)
- ELAM-1: endothelial leukocyte adhesion molecule (polys)
- VCAM-1: vascular cell adhesion molecule (lymphocytes, monocytes)
- Expression increased by IL-1 and TNF

CELLULAR COMPONENTS

Initially, neutrophils predominate (24–48 hr); life expectancy in tissue of 4 days

Later, monocytes and lymphocytes predominate (chemotactic signals for monocytes persist longer)

When monocytes enter tissue, undergo conversion to tissue macrophages—long half-life

MODULATORS OF THE INFLAMMATORY RESPONSE

Persistence of initiating/complicating agent (microorganisms, either initial agent or secondary infection; devitalized tissue, foreign bodies)

Immunologic function/access [leukocyte function, immunosuppression (steroids), vascularity of tissue]

Systemic factors (nutritional states, diseases, e.g., diabetes)

Extent/degree of tissue injury

ORGANIZATION

Process by which coagulated blood is converted to granulation tissue, a loose collection of numerous inflammatory cells and debris in a matrix of fibrin, newly formed blood vessels, and fibroblasts/myofibroblasts

Myofibroblasts mediate wound contraction

With increasing "organization," debris is removed, cellularity decreases; fibrosis and scarring can occur

Chronic Inflammation

In contrast to acute inflammation (which is predominantly exudative), chronic inflammation is proliferative

Chronic inflammation develops when stimulus persists

Macrophages and giant cells: central actors

Plasma cells, lymphocytes

Eosinophils: granules contain major basic protein (highly cationic, MW 14 kD, toxic to parasites)

Fibroblasts and myofibroblasts

Patterns of Chronic Inflammation

SEROUS

Exudate of predominantly serum, e.g., burn blister

FIBRINOUS

Fibrin and inflammatory cells, e.g., pericarditis

SUPPURATIVE

Neutrophils, often walled off, e.g., abscess

GRANULOMATOUS

Induced by the presence of indigestible foreign bodies or by large excess of antibody over antigen

Epithelioid histiocytes: less phagocytic than macrophages, highly active protein synthesis machinery

Central caseous necrosis may be present

Giant cells:
- Langhans': nuclei arranged in horseshoe pattern around periphery; more common with infectious causes
- Touton: nuclei aggregate in center of cell; more common in foreign body reactions

Causes: infectious (tuberculosis, leprosy, syphilis, actinomycosis, cat scratch, fungi, parasites), foreign bodies (sutures, splinters, silicosis, berylliosis), antibody mediated (rheumatic fever, rheumatoid disease), idiopathic (sarcoidosis)

ULCER

Necrosis, granulation tissue, loss of epithelium, e.g., peptic ulcer

OUTCOMES OF INFLAMMATION

Depends on degree of tissue injury and persistence of initiating agent(s)

Resolution: restoration of the site to normal

Regeneration: replacement of lost specialized cells by similarly differentiated cells, with or without restoration of normal tissue architecture

Repair/scarring: replacement of lost tissue by granulation tissue and fibrosis

Metaplasia: replacement of one type of tissue (usually epithelium) with another type of tissue

Repair

WOUND HEALING

Primary intention (small wounds): ends of wound sutured together

Secondary intention (larger wounds): tissue must grow in from edges

GROWTH FACTORS

Epidermal growth factor (EGF): 6 kD peptide; binds to tyrosine kinase receptors, mitogenic

Platelet derived growth factor (PDGF): 30 kD highly cationic heterodimer; produced by macrophages, endothelium, and smooth muscle cells as well as platelets; competence factor, but requires a progression factor for mitogenesis

Fibroblast growth factor (FGF): potent angiogenic agent

Transforming growth factor (TGF): α: similar to EGF; β: growth inhibitor (ceases liver regeneration following partial hepatectomy), fibroblast chemotaxis

[handwritten top margin: 1 skin, bone / 2 cartilage / 3 Bl. vessels /ut / 4 BM]

[handwritten top right: Ig heavy chain on 14]

Alpha interferon: growth inhibitor
Prostaglandin E$_2$: growth inhibitor

COLLAGEN

Ten types: I in skin and bone; II in cartilage; III in blood vessels and uterus; IV in basement membranes; I–III are fibrillar, rest are amorphous

Synthesis: Three tropocollagen alpha chains form left-handed helix (Gly every third position); alpha-hydroxylation of proline, secreted as procollagen, ends cleaved, forms filaments, crosslinked via lysine oxidation

As wound heals, type III collagen replaced by type I; maximum strength at 3 months

CELL–CELL INTERACTIONS

Integrins: families of heterodimeric cell surface receptors; many bind matrix proteins by recognizing the tripeptide Arg-Gly-Asp (RGD); include fibronectin receptor

All members of an integrin family share the same beta subunit

CELL MATRIX COMPONENTS

Elastin: 70 kD, covalently crosslinked chains, long half-life

Laminin: most abundant glycoprotein in basement membrane, 850 kD cross-shaped tripeptide; spans basement membrane, binding to cell surface and other matrix components; center of cross contains binding site for cell surface laminin receptors; ends of short arms bind collagen IV; end of long arm binds heparin

Proteoglycans: glycosaminoglycans (long, nonbranching polysaccharide chains of repeating disaccharide units, 4–50 kD: e.g., heparan sulfate, heparin, hyaluronic acid, chondroitin sulfate, etc.) linked to protein core (protein usually ~5% total mass of 3–5 megadaltons)

Fibronectin: major adhesion molecule of the interstitial tissue; 440 kD disulfide linked dimer; binds to cell surface, fibrin, collagen, and heparin; cells bind to fibronectin by a receptor that recognizes RGD sequence (Arg-Gly-Asp) on fibronectin; in addition to cell adhesion, also directs cell migration during embryogenesis

IMMUNOLOGY

[handwritten: constant class / variable specificity / constant = class]

ANTIBODIES

Constant region determines antibody class; variable region determines antigen specificity

Composed of heavy and light chains: each heterotetramer of two heavy and two light chains results in two antigen binding sites

• IgM: pentameric (10 heavy and 10 light chains plus joining J chain); initially membrane bound; first antibody released into circulation in response to a new antigen

• IgD: bound to B-cell surface; rarely released into circulation

• IgG: major antibody of immune response; four subclasses (1, 2a, 2b, 3); MW = 140 kD (2 × 50 kD + 2 × 20 kD)

• IgA: monomeric in serum, dimeric (contains joining J chain and secretory fragment) in secretions: milk, saliva, tears

• IgE: most commonly found on surface of mast cells; mediates hypersensitivity reactions

Antibody diversity is generated by genetic rearrangement of the DNA during B-cell maturation; at each splicing, random bases are added by terminal deoxy-transferase (TdT) to generate "non–template directed diversity"

First, heavy chain undergoes D-J joining, then V-DJ joining; VDJ-C splicing (class switching) occurs later at mRNA level; then κ rearranges; if nonproductive, the other κ gene rearranges; if still nonproductive, λ rearranges.

	Chromosome	V	D	J	C
Heavy chain:	8	100–200	>10	6 + 3ψ	5 classes
κ light chain:	2	40–80	—	5	1
λ light chain:	22	>40	—	[6 J-C units]	

On chromosome 8, the heavy chain constant regions are arranged as μ, δ, γ3, γ1, γ2b, γ2a, ε, α

B CELLS

10–20% of circulating lymphocytes

Found in superficial cortex of lymph nodes and white pulp of spleen

• CD10: pre-B cells: common acute lymphoblastic leukemia antigen (CALLA)

• CD19 (Leu12): pre-B to mature B cells; not on plasma cells

• CD20 (Leu16, L26): pre-B (after CD19) to mature B; not on plasma cells

• IgM: surface receptor

[handwritten: 4 binds MHC 2 / 8 bind MHC 1]

T CELLS

Arise in bone marrow, mature in thymus; 80–90% of circulating lymphocytes

Paracortical areas of lymph nodes; periarteriolar sheaths of spleen

• CD1 (Leu 6): expressed on immature thymocytes

• CD2 (Leu 5): sheep RBC receptors; all T cells, natural killer (NK) cells

• CD3 (Leu 4): all T cells; associated with the T-cell receptor

• CD4 (Leu 3a): 60% of T cells; helper and delayed-type hypersensitivity reactions; binds MHC class II

• CD8 (Leu 2): 30% of T cells; cytotoxic and "suppressor"; binds MHC I

• CD5 (Leu 1): all T cells (peripheral and thymic)

• CD7 (Leu 9): all T cells

• CD25: IL-2 receptor (activated T, B, and monocytes)

• α/β receptor: 95% T cells; associated with CD3

• γ/δ receptor: 5% T cells; CD4- and CD8-; associated with CD3

T-cell receptor (chromosome 7) undergoes VDJ rearrangement:

	V		D	J	C
α chain	50–100		—	50–100	1
β chain	75–100	β1 unit	1	6	1
		β2 unit	1	7	1
γ chain	8 + 7ψ	γ1 unit	—	1 + 2ψ	1
		γ2 unit	—	1 + 2ψ	1
δ chain	4		2	3	1

The δ chain sequences are located between the V and J sequences of the α chain; therefore, when α rearranges, the δ chain gene is deleted

CD3, associated with the TCR, transduces activating signals

NK CELLS (LARGE GRANULAR LYMPHOCYTES)

Can lyse tumor cells or virus infected cells without prior sensitization; insert pore forming proteins (perforins) into victim, making them leaky

- CD16: all NK cells and granulocytes; low affinity Fc receptor
- CD56 (Leu19) and CD2 positive
- CD3 *negative*

K cells, which mediate antibody-dependent cell-mediated cytotoxicity, are probably a subset of NK cells

MACROPHAGES
Arise from circulating monocytes
Antigen-presenting cells—lots of MHC class II on surface
- CD11b: receptor for C3b; monocytes, granulocytes, NK
- CD13: blood monocytes and granulocytes
- CD33: myeloid stem cells and mature monocytes

CYTOKINES (INTERLEUKINS)
IL-1: made by monocytes, macrophages, endothelium, etc.; activates resting T cells, chemotactic (via endothelial effects), induce fever
IL-2: made by activated T cells; autocrine stimulation of T cells; stimulate B cells, NK cells; activates monocytes
IL-3: made by activated T cells; stimulates stem cells
IL-4: growth and differentiation of B and T cells
IL-5: differentiation of activated B cells to plasma cells
IL-6: maturation of T and B cells, inhibits fibroblast growth
Gamma-interferon: made by sensitized T cells; activates macrophages, induces expression of HLA class II molecules on macrophages and endothelial cells, direct antiviral effects

MAJOR HISTOCOMPATIBILITY COMPLEX
AKA: MHC (Chromosome 6)
Human leukocyte antigen (HLA)
Part of immunoglobulin supergene family
CLASS I
CD8
HLA-A, HLA-B, HLA-C
A,B,C
Heterodimer of 44 kD protein (three Ig domains) with 11.6 kD β_2-microglobulin (chromosome 15; 1 Ig domain)
Present on all nucleated cells and platelets
Involved in restricting the action of CD8+ cytotoxic T cells
Disease associations:
- B27: ankylosing spondylitis, postgonococcal arthritis, acute anterior uveitis, Reiter's syndrome
- A3: hemochromatosis
- BW47: 21-hydroxylase deficiency
- A1, B8: Addison's disease

CLASS II (IMMUNE RESPONSE GENES)
CD4 APC
DR DP DQ
HLA-D region: subregions DP, DQ, DR
Heterodimer of alpha and beta (34 kD and 29 kD) chains, each with two Ig domains
Found on monocytes, macrophages, dendritic cells, B cells, some activated T cells; can be induced on endothelial cells, fibroblasts, and renal tubule cells with gamma-interferon
Mixed lymphocyte reaction: T cells proliferate in response to foreign class II
Involved in restricting the action of CD4+ helper T cells
Disease associations:
- DR2: lupus, multiple sclerosis
- DR3: chronic active hepatitis, Sjögren's syndrome, insulin-dependent diabetes, Grave's disease, lupus
- DR4: rheumatoid arthritis, drug-induced lupus, giant cell arteritis, Takayasu's arteritis
- DR5: Hashimoto's thyroiditis
- DR8: Primary biliary cirrhosis

CLASS III
Components of complement system within the MHC gene region; include C2, C4, and Bf
May also include TNF-α and TNF-β

Hypersensitivity Reactions

TYPE I (ANAPHYLACTIC TYPE)
Reaction within minutes—may be systemic or localized
Systemic form can be fatal within an hour from massive laryngeal edema, pulmonary edema, and hemorrhage
Local form (atopy) often hereditary
Bee sting, cutaneous swelling (hives), hay fever, bronchial asthma, allergic gastroenteritis (food allergy)
Antigen binds to IgE on surface of sensitized mast cells and basophils, crosslinking IgE receptors, resulting in degranulation with release of rapidly acting factors (via rapid increase in cAMP) and subsequent production and release of slow acting factors
Some factors can directly induce degranulation independent of IgE: C3a, C5a, codeine, morphine, melittin (in bee venom), trauma, heat, cold, sunlight
Primary (rapidly acting) factors:
- Histamine: bronchial smooth muscle contraction, increased vascular permeability
- Eosinophil and neutrophil chemotactic factors
- Granule matrix derived factors: heparin, proteases
Secondary (slow-reacting substances of anaphylaxis):
- Leukotrienes C_4, D_4: most potent vasodilators known
- Prostaglandin D_2: bronchospasm and vasodilation
- Leukotriene B_4: chemotactic for neutrophils
- Platelet activating factor

TYPE II (ANTIBODY MEDIATED TYPE)
AKA: cytotoxic type (although not always cytotoxic)
Antibodies directed against normal or modified cell surface or tissue components induce cell lysis
COMPLEMENT DEPENDENT
Two mechanisms:
- Direct lysis by complement activation
- Lysis by opsonization (C3b)—often involves RBCs
Examples: transfusion reactions, erythroblastosis fetalis, autoimmune hemolytic anemia or thrombocytopenia, certain drug reactions
ANTIBODY-DEPENDENT CELL-MEDIATED CYTOTOXICITY
Monocytes, neutrophils, eosinophils, or NK cells recognize cells by Fc portion of IgG bound to cell and kill cell without phagocytosis
Example: Goodpasture's syndrome
ANTI-RECEPTOR ANTIBODIES
Noncytotoxic
Examples: myasthenia gravis from antibody to acetylcholine receptor

TYPE III (IMMUNE COMPLEX MEDIATED)
Antigen (Ag)–antibody (Ab) complexes produce tissue damage by activation of serum mediators (primarily complement)
SYSTEMIC FORM
Acute serum sickness is the prototype (described in 1905)
Antibodies are produced by a large dose of administered antigen (~5 days after administration); Ag–Ab complexes are deposited in the tissues, often inducing localized type I hypersensitivity reactions in glomeruli, joints, skin, heart, serosal surfaces, and small blood vessels, where they can activate complement; an inflammatory

reaction ensues (~10 days) with resulting fever, urticaria, arthralgias, lymphadenopathy, proteinuria

Inflammation in and around vessels causes an acute necrotizing vasculitis with fibrinoid deposition and acute inflammation (innocent bystander destruction)

LOCALIZED FORM (ARTHUS REACTION)

Introduction of antigen to which patient has been sensitized

Localized tissue necrosis resulting from acute immune complex vasculitis, usually in the skin

Lesion develops over 4–10 hr; may ulcerate

Histology shows fibrinoid necrosis of vessels, platelet thromboses, edema, hemorrhage, and numerous neutrophils

TYPE IV (CELL MEDIATED)

Mediated by sensitized T cells

DELAYED-TYPE HYPERSENSITIVITY

Examples: tuberculin reaction: reddening and induration begins 8–12 hr after injection; peaks at 24–72 hr

Histology: perivascular cuffing of mononuclear cells in deep and superficial dermis

Induration is caused by fibrin deposition in interstitium

Reaction mediated by CD4+ T cells: memory T cells release lymphokines to amplify response, specifically macrophage chemotactic and activating factors

T-CELL–MEDIATED CYTOTOXICITY

CD8+ cytotoxic T cells kill cells via pore formation; recognize modified self-MHC class I antigens.

ORGAN TRANSPLANT AND REJECTION

Transplants can be autologous (self), syngeneic (monozygotic twins), allogeneic (same species), or xenogeneic (different species)

Donor lymphocytes, etc. in graft have both class I and class II MHC antigens—responsible for increasing rejection

Immunosuppression: cyclosporin suppresses activation of CD4+ T cells; anti-CD3 is new agent

HYPERACUTE REJECTION

Minutes to hours

Mediated by preformed antibodies

Produces Arthus-type reaction with antigen–antibody mediated fibrinoid vasculitis

ACUTE REJECTION

Weeks to months

- Interstitial: cell mediated, CD4+ and CD8+ T cells
- Vascular: humorally mediated: antibody binds to vessel walls—activation induces vasculitis

SUBACUTE REJECTION

Months

Vasculitides with marked thickening of intima of vessels, proliferation of fibroblasts and myocytes, luminal narrowing

CHRONIC REJECTION

Months to years

Intimal fibrosis, interstitial scarring, tissue atrophy

Graft Versus Host Disease

Occurs when immunologically competent cells are transferred into a recipient with an impaired immune system; transferred cells "outreact" the endogenous lymphoid tissue

Most commonly occurs following nonautologous bone marrow transplant

Greatest damage occurs to the skin, intestine, spleen, and liver

Immunologic Deficiency Syndromes

AGAMMAGLOBULINEMIA OF BRUTON

X-linked; restricted to males

Virtual absence of B cells and immunoglobins from serum (small amounts of IgG may be seen), despite normal number of pre-B cells in marrow; abnormal maturation

Severe recurrent infections seen beginning at about 8 months of age, esp. pyogenic organisms (*Staphylococcus, Haemophilus influenzae*); conjunctivitis, pharyngitis, otitis media, bronchitis, pneumonia, skin infections

Normal handling of most viral and fungal infections (normal cell-mediated immunity), except poliovirus, echovirus, hepatitis, enterovirus

High incidence of autoimmune-type diseases

ISOLATED IGA DEFICIENCY

Very common: 1/600 individuals

Familial or acquired in association with toxoplasmosis, measles, or some other viral infection

Respiratory, GI, and urogenital tract infections

Autoimmune diseases more common, esp. systemic lupus erythematosus (SLE) and rheumatoid arthritis (RA)

Defect in differentiation of IgA B cells; 40% have anti-IgA antibodies

DIGEORGE'S SYNDROME (THYMIC HYPOPLASIA)

Selective T-cell deficiency resulting from failure of development of the 3rd and 4th pharyngeal pouches (thymus, parathyroids, C cells of thyroid)

No cell-mediated response, tetany (from hypocalcemia), congenital defects involving the heart, great vessels; may have abnormal-appearing mouth, ears, facies

Not genetic; intrauterine damage before 8th week

Partial DiGeorge's syndrome exists

Nezelof's syndrome: absent thymus but with normal parathyroids

SEVERE COMBINED IMMUNODEFICIENCY DISEASE (SCID)

Heterogeneous disorder: autosomal recessive and X-linked recessive forms

Both T-cell and B-cell immunity impaired; generally greater loss of T-cell immunity

Abnormal differentiation of stem cells caused by either intrinsic defect or abnormal thymic signals for differentiation

Usually succumb to opportunistic infections in 1st year of life: *Pseudomonas, Candida, Pneumocystis, Cytomegalovirus* (CMV), herpes simplex virus (HSV)

50% of patients with the autosomal recessive form lack adenosine deaminase, accumulating deoxy-ATP, which is toxic to lymphocytes

WISKOTT-ALDRICH SYNDROME

AKA: immunodeficiency with thrombocytopenia and eczema

X-linked recessive; vulnerable to recurrent infections

Always progressive T-cell deficit, sometimes also B-cell deficit

Spleen shows near-complete absence of white pulp

Poor antibody response to polysaccharide antigens

IgM levels in the serum are low; IgA and IgE are elevated
Patients prone to develop malignant lymphoma

ATAXIA-TELANGIECTASIA SYNDROME

Autosomal recessive disorder resulting in predominantly a defect of T-cell maturation

Associated clinically with cerebellar ataxia, telangiectasia, decreased serum alpha-fetoprotein levels, ovarian dysgenesis

IgA, IgE, and IgG levels often low; IgM often high

Defect is abnormal repair of x-ray damage, resulting in chromosomal instability

Patients prone to develop lymphoma, leukemia, gastric carcinoma

COMMON VARIABLE IMMUNODEFICIENCY

Heterogeneous group of disorders characterized by hypogammaglobulinemia (usually all immunoglobins, sometimes just IgG)

Term refers to disorders for which no primary defect or secondary cause can be identified

Three types:
• Predominant intrinsic B-cell defect
• Predominant T-cell disorder with T-helper cell defect *or* T-suppressor cell surplus
• Autoantibodies to T or B cells

Hyperplastic B-cell areas

Patients suffer recurrent bacterial infections and parasitic infections (*Giardia* common); also have a high frequency of autoimmune disorders, sometimes progressing to lymphoid malignancy; also spruelike illness and noncaseating granulomas in the liver

LEUKOCYTE ADHESION DEFICIENCY

Autosomal recessive—chromosome 21

Deficiency in synthesis of the common β-chain of adhesion molecules LFA-1, MAC-1, and CD11/CD18 (binding of leukocytes to ICAM-1 on endothelial cells)

CHRONIC GRANULOMATOUS DISEASE OF CHILDHOOD

Most commonly X-linked; affects males

Neutrophils lack the "respiratory burst" upon phagocytosis

Deficient production of hydrogen peroxide due to deficiency in the H_2O_2–myeloperoxidase system

Patients particularly susceptible to infections by coagulase-positive organisms (such as *S. aureus*)

COMPLEMENT DEFICIENCIES

C2: connective tissue diseases (lupus-like syndromes)
C3: bacterial infections
C5-8: recurrent *Neisseria* infections (gonococcal, meningococcal)

CHEDIAK-HIGASHI SYNDROME

Autosomal recessive—appears to be a microtubule defect

Neutropenia, impaired chemotaxis, impaired lysosomal fusion, impaired degranulation

Also, oculocutaneous albinism

Prone to infections; giant lysosomes by electron microscopy

ACQUIRED IMMUNODEFICIENCY SYNDROME

AKA: AIDS

June 1981: five young male homosexuals in Los Angeles reported to Centers for Disease Control (CDC) as having contracted *Pneumocystis* pneumonia; two died

Etiologic agent identified 1983–1984

EPIDEMIOLOGY

Risk factors:
• Homosexuality
• IV drug abuse
• Blood or blood product recipients
• Heterosexual contact with infected individuals

Transmission:
• Venereal: in U.S., homosexual transmission most common, but heterosexual transmission is increasing at a greater rate; in Africa, heterosexual transmission most common
• Parenteral: 90% efficiency for blood products, more common for hemophiliacs because factor VIII is concentrated from multiple donors; also IV drug users
• Perinatal: transplacentally *in utero,* birth canal, or via breast milk

HUMAN IMMUNODEFICIENCY VIRUS (HIV)

Formerly HTLV-III, but unlike HTLV-I and -II, which are transforming, HIV is cytopathic

Spherical retrovirus (related to lentivirus), with two strands of genomic RNA (10 kb genome, at least eight genes)

Core proteins (*gag*), reverse transcriptase (*pol*), envelope glycoproteins (*env*) are gp120 and gp41, plus *vif* (budding), *tat III, rev, nef,* and *vpr* (infectivity)

gp120 shows a high degree of variability and polymorphisms

Related to simian immunodeficiency virus (SIV) and HIV-2, a virus causing an AIDS-like illness in West Africa; HIV-2 and HIV-I are 40% homologous, HIV-2 and SIV are 70%

Infects cells by high affinity interaction between gp120 and CD4 on T-helper cells and macrophages; virus is then internalized and integrated, but not activated until the cell is stimulated

Virus isolated from white cells can only infect white cells; virus isolated from brain can infect both brain and white cells; may be different strains

Activation results in the death of T cells by unclear mechanism; prior to death, cell appears to lose its ability to respond to antigens

Monocytes and macrophages (also express low levels of CD4) can be infected, are usually not killed, and may serve as the reservoir for "latent" infection; infected monocytes are likely to be the mode of transmission into the CNS

Neuroleukin: neuron growth factor with 30% sequence homology with gp120; receptors on neurons may therefore bind HIV

IMMUNE DYSFUNCTION

Loss of CD4+ T cells results in inversion of the CD4:CD8 ratio (normally 2; can go down to 0.5)

CD4+ cells are source of IL-2, IFN-γ, chemotactic factors

AIDS patients typically have hypergammaglobulinemia (polyclonal B-cell activation—may be secondary to CMV, Epstein-Barr virus (EBV), or gp120 itself)

In spite of increased Ig production, AIDS patients cannot mount proper response to new antigens

NATURAL HISTORY

Anti-HIV antibodies detectable 3–17 wk after exposure
2–8 yr incubation or "latency" period

CD4 counts <200 usually seen in clinical AIDS (normal >700)

When CD4 count drops below 50, increased risk of lymphoma

30–50% develop an acute mononucleosis-like illness

Persistent generalized lymphadenopathy

AIDS-related complex (ARC): long-lasting fever (>3 months), weight loss, diarrhea

Secondary infections/neoplasms: *Pneumocystis, Cryptosporidium* (GI), toxoplasmosis, *Cryptococcus* (CNS), candidiasis, *Mycobacterium avium-intracellulare* (MAI), CMV, HSV, progressive multifocal leukencephalopathy (PML); Burkitt's lymphoma, Kaposi's sarcoma, immunoblastic B-cell lymphoma, primary CNS lymphomas, Hodgkin's disease

Autoimmune Diseases

Immunologic Tolerance

Failure of immune system to respond to an antigen

Tolerance can be natural (develops during fetal life) or acquired (develops under immune suppression)

Desensitization: temporary "tolerance" produced by administering large doses of antigen that use up the remote antibodies and cells

Since cooperation between B and T cells is necessary, only need to produce tolerance in one of them

In general, T cells develop tolerance at a lower antigen dose, and this tolerance lasts longer than B-cell tolerance; high doses of antigen can produce tolerance in both T and B cells

Postulated Mechanisms

CLONAL DELETION

Self-reacting clones are deleted

Because normal individuals have lymphocytes with receptors for self-antigens (DNA, myelin, collagen), it is also postulated that some self-reacting immature B cells are inactivated but they are not actually deleted (clonal anergy)

SUPPRESSION OF AUTOREACTIVE LYMPHOCYTES

Suppressor cells: T cells actively limit immune response

IDIOTYPE–ANTI-IDIOTYPE

Antibodies to self-reacting antibodies limit response

ANTIBODY BLOCKING

Potentially responding cells are blocked by presence of circulating antibody

Mechanisms for Overcoming Tolerance

Emergence of a sequestered antigen

Bypass T-helper cell tolerance

• Modification of the antigen by complexing to drugs or microorganisms—recognized by nontolerant T cells

• Crossreaction between nontolerant T cells to infecting organisms and other "self"-antigens

• Polyclonal B-cell activation: direct, nonspecific activation of B cells; for example, bacterial lipopolysaccharide can induce mice to make antibodies to DNA, RBC antigens, etc.

Idiotype bypass mechanisms

• Anti-idiotype antibodies will look like the antigen—these can stimulate the response

• Microbial antigens (or other portions of antibodies directed against them) can crossreact with self-reactive lymphocytes

Imbalance of suppressor-helper function

• Example: T-suppressor activity decreases with age in some mice

Increased expression of class II MHC on tissues

Summary of Autoantibodies

Disease	Antigen
Lupus	dsDNA, Smith antigen
Sjögren's	SS-B (La), SS-A (Ro)
Scleroderma: Diffuse	Scl-70 (DNA topoisomerase I)
Scleroderma: CREST	Centromere
Polymyositis	tRNA synthetase (esp. histidyl)
Hashimoto's	[T-cell defect]; later: thyroglobulin, thyroid stimulating hormone (TSH) receptor
Graves'	TSH receptor
Myasthenia gravis	Acetylcholine receptor
Primary biliary cirrhosis	Mitochondria
Chronic active hepatitis	Smooth muscle
Pemphigus vulgaris	Adherens junction (suprabasal)
Pemphigus foliaceus	Desmoglian (more superficial)
Bullous pemphigoid	Anti–skin basement membrane
Dermatitis herpetiformis	IgA at dermal-epidermal junction
Goodpasture's syndrome	Anti–glomerular basement membrane (GBM)
Pernicious anemia	Parietal cells; intrinsic factor

SYSTEMIC LUPUS ERYTHEMATOSUS

Multisystem disease of autoimmune origin, acute or insidious in onset, chronic, remitting, involving principally injury to the skin, joints, kidney, and mucous membranes

If include all mild forms, as common as 1:2500 in population; female:male = 9:1

By definition, requires 4 of 11 criteria: malar rash, discoid rash, photosensitivity, oral ulcers, arthritis, serositis, renal disorder, neurologic disorder (seizures, psychosis), hematologic disorder (hemolytic anemia, leukopenia, lymphopenia, thrombocytopenia), immunologic disorder (lupus erethymatosus [LE] cells, anti-DNA, anti-Smith antigen, false-positive Venereal Disease Research Laboratory [VDRL] test), antinuclear antibody

Genetic factors: 50–60% concordance in monozygotic twins, familial patterns, associated with HLA-DR-2 and -DR-3, and with C2 deficiency

Nongenetic factors: drugs and UV light can induce or exacerbate symptoms

Fundamental defect in immune regulation and self-tolerance; B-cell hyperactivity, with resulting increased production of both self- and nonself-antibodies; mechanisms include intrinsic defect in B cells, polyclonal activation of B cells, excessive stimulation of normal B cells by hyperactive T cells, and T-suppressor cell defects

Autoantibodies: DNA, histones, nonhistone RNA binding proteins (Smith antigen, SS-A [Ro], SS-B [La]), nucleolar antigens; *antibodies to dsDNA and Smith antigen are strongly suggestive of SLE*

DNA is not very antigenic; anti-DNA antibodies probably represent cross reaction from antibodies to phospholipids, etc.

Tissue injury mediated predominantly by DNA–anti-DNA immune complexes (type III hypersensitivity) but also anti-RBC antibodies (type II)

LE bodies (hematoxylin bodies) are denatured nuclei following antibody attack; when mixed with phagocytic cells that engulf them, form LE cells; LE cell test positive in >70% of patients

Highly variable clinical course

Pathology

Vasculitis of small arteries and arterioles, most common in skin and muscles, with fibrinoid deposits in vessel walls

Onion skinning of vessels of spleen by perivascular fibrosis

Glomerulonephritis (GN):

Class I: no recognized abnormality: rare

Class II: mesangial lupus GN: 10% patients

Class III: focal proliferative GN: typically segmental

Class IV: diffuse proliferative GN: most serious; 40–50%

Class V: membranous GN: 10%

All types caused by deposition of DNA–anti-DNA complexes

Subendothelial deposits are unusual outside of lupus

Skin: immune complex deposition at dermal–epidermal junction; seen in both clinically involved and uninvolved skin

Joints: nonerosive synovitis

Pericarditis

Heart: Libman-Sacks endocarditis (nonbacterial verrucous endocarditis); vegetations predominantly on flow side of mitral and tricuspid valves but may be on back; diffusely distributed over leaflets; small, may extend onto mural endocardium

CHRONIC DISCOID LUPUS ERYTHEMATOSUS

Skin lesions; systemic manifestations rare

Face and scalp most commonly; LE cell test rarely positive, positive antinuclear antibodies (ANAs) in 35%; anti-dsDNA rare; no Ag–Ab complexes in uninvolved skin

SUBACUTE CUTANEOUS LUPUS ERYTHEMATOSUS

Intermediate between SLE and discoid lupus

Widespread superficial skin involvement, mild systemic

Anti-SS-A antibodies

DRUG-INDUCED LUPUS ERYTHEMATOSUS

Seen with hydralazine, procainamide, isoniazid, and D-penicillamine most commonly

ANAs common, esp. anti-histones

Renal and CNS involvement rare

Associated with HLA-DR4

SJÖGREN'S SYNDROME

Dry eyes and dry mouth resulting from autoimmune destruction of the lacrimal and salivary glands; may see dysphagia, fissuring of mouth, ulceration of cornea; often see parotid gland enlargement

90% of affected patients are women 40–60 yr

May occur as an isolated disorder (sicca syndrome or primary form) or in association with another autoimmune disease (secondary form), the most common being RA, but also SLE, polymyositis, scleroderma, etc.

Histology shows infiltration of glands with predominantly T cells, predominantly CD4+, in a periductal distribution; tubulointerstitial nephritis can also be seen in the kidney

ANAs detected in most patients; most specific are antibodies to the ribonucleoproteins SS-A (Ro) and SS-B (La), especially the latter

Lymph nodes often show pseudolymphomatous enlargement, but there is also a 40-fold increased risk of true lymphoma

Associated with HLA-DR3

SCLERODERMA (PROGRESSIVE SYSTEMIC SCLEROSIS)

Progressive fibrosis of predominantly the skin, but also GI tract, kidney, heart, muscles, lungs; death often from renal failure or cardiac failure

Female:male = 3:1, mean age 40 yr

Often present with Raynaud's phenomenon (episodic vasoconstriction of the arteries and arterioles of the extremities)

Fibroblasts of affected patients synthesize abnormally large amounts of collagen, although the collagen is normal

Etiology involves cytokine activation of fibroblasts and/or damage, and fibrosis of small blood vessels; initiating factor is likely to be some as yet uncharacterized Ab–Ag interaction

Pathology: dermal fibrosis, atrophy of appendages, and thinning of epidermis; fibrous replacement of muscularis of the gut (particularly esophagus); inflammatory synovitis; renal vascular fibrosis; pulmonary alveolar fibrosis

DIFFUSE SCLERODERMA

Widespread skin involvement at onset, with progression to internal viscera

Antibody to DNA topoisomerase I (Scl-70) present in 70%

Anti-centromere antibody seen in 20–30%

CREST SYNDROME

More limited involvement; more benign course; involvement of viscera only much later

Calcinosis, Raynaud's, Esophageal dysmotility, Sclerodactyly, Telangiectasia

Anti-centromere autoantibody seen in 80–90%

"LOCALIZED SCLERODERMA" (E.G., MORPHEA)

Skin involvement only; no visceral involvement

Usually limited in distribution, may be widespread

Probably not related to progressive systemic sclerosis

MIXED CONNECTIVE TISSUE DISEASE

Characterized by simultaneous features suggestive of SLE, polymyositis, and scleroderma

Includes most cases of scleroderma

High titer antibodies to nuclear ribonucleoproteins

Better long-term prognosis than SLE or scleroderma alone; responds well to corticosteroids

May simply be a variant

POLYMYOSITIS-DERMATOMYOSITIS

Chronic inflammatory myopathies of uncertain cause

- Group I: adult polymyositis (no skin involvement)
- Group II: adult dermatomyositis
- Group III: I or II with malignancy
- Group IV: childhood dermatomyositis
- Group V: either polymyositis or dermatomyositis associated with another immune disorder

Autoantibodies against tRNA synthetase (particularly histidyl) are seen in >25%

May be related to cross reaction to Coxsackie B group viruses, particularly in the childhood form

Myositis affects proximal muscles first: pelvic and shoulder girdle, then neck, posterior pharynx, intercostals; this is in contrast to most dystrophies (primarily distal muscles) and myasthenia gravis (ocular muscles)

Skin rash classically is a lilac discoloration of the upper eyelids with periorbital edema, accompanied by a scaly erythematous eruption over the knuckles, elbows, knees

Visceral cancers more common in patients with dermatomyositis, approaching 15–20%, and involving the breast, ovary, lungs, and stomach

AMYLOIDOSIS

Probably a disease resulting from derangement of the immune apparatus

Proteinaceous substance insidiously deposited in tissues throughout the body, encroaching on structures and inducing pressure atrophy

Defect may be an inability to properly digest/degrade

AMYLOID

Not a single compound; chemically, several types; derived from circulating precursor protein

All types have same structure and appearance

Homogenous, amorphous, pink hyaline on H&E; pink to red staining with Congo red, which imparts an apple-green birefringence

Electron microscopy: nonbranching, long, 7.5–10 nm diameter fibers (90% mass), accompanied by P component (10%): doughnut-shaped pentagons with 9 nm external and 4 nm internal diameter composed of 180–220 kD alpha-1 serum glycoprotein—homologous to C-reactive protein

Amyloid fibrils aggregate yielding a cross-β-pleated sheet

Types:
- AL (amyloid light chain): Ig light chain derived (Bence Jones protein), usually λ; when partially cleaved, can accumulate
- AA (amyloid-associated): 8.5 kD protein (76 amino acids) derived from 12 kD serum amyloid–associated protein (SAA) made by the liver
- AF: mutant form of transthyretin (formerly called prealbumin, because it electrophoreses just before albumin but has no relation to it; involved in transport of thyroxin and retinol) seen in familial amyloid polyneuropathies and senile cardiac amyloidosis
- Hormones: calcitonin, proinsulin, etc.
- Others

IMMUNOCYTE DYSCRASIA–ASSOCIATED (PRIMARY) AMYLOIDOSIS

AL type; systemic in distribution

Most common form in U.S.

Occurs in 5–15% of patients with multiple myeloma; also can be seen in Waldenström's macroglobulinemia, heavy chain disease, solitary plasmacytoma, follicular lymphomas

Most patients have no underlying overt B-cell neoplasm; these cases are referred to as *primary amyloidosis*

Most common sites: heart, GI tract, peripheral nerves, skin, tongue

REACTIVE SYSTEMIC (SECONDARY) AMYLOIDOSIS

AA type; systemic in distribution

Occurs secondary to underlying chronic inflammatory condition such as tuberculosis (TB), bronchiectasis, chronic osteomyelitis, rheumatoid arthritis (14–26%), inflammatory bowel disease (IBD), heroin users; also seen with renal cell cancer and Hodgkin's disease

Most common sites: kidneys, liver, spleen, lymph nodes, adrenals, thyroid

Better prognosis than immunocyte-associated amyloidosis

ENDOCRINE AMYLOID

Derived by enzymatic conversion of polypeptide hormones

Medullary carcinoma of thyroid, islet tumors of pancreas, pheochromocytoma, undifferentiated carcinoma of lung

HEMODIALYSIS-ASSOCIATED AMYLOIDOSIS

Deposition of β_2-microglobulin in synovium, joints, and tendon sheaths; seen in patients on hemodialysis; cannot be filtered through dialysis membranes

HEREDOFAMILIAL AMYLOIDOSIS

- Familial Mediterranean fever: attacks of fever with inflammation of serosal surfaces; AA protein
- Familial amyloidotic polyneuropathies: autosomal dominant; AF protein (mutated transthyretin)

LOCALIZED AMYLOIDOSIS

Tumor-like nodule

Lung, larynx, skin, urinary bladder, tongue, periorbital

At least some are AL protein

AMYLOID OF AGING

- Senile cardiac amyloidosis: usually asymptomatic but can lead to heart failure; usually transthyretin (not mutated)
- Senile cerebral amyloidosis: deposition of A4 (beta-amyloid) in "senile plaques" of Alzheimer's disease

Pathology

Kidney: most common cause of death; enlarged, waxy, firm; involves primarily glomeruli but also peritubular interstitium, arteries, arterioles

Spleen: begin perifollicularly; two patterns of deposition
- Sago spleen: splenic follicles—granular on gross exam
- Lardaceous: walls of sinuses, fusing

Liver: first in space of Disse, then hepatic parenchyma

Heart: interstitial deposits with pressure atrophy of myocytes

2

INFECTIOUS AGENTS

VIRUSES

General Features of Viral Diseases
Can cause a wide variety of symptoms and diseases
Same virus can cause different diseases, depending upon the route of infection, and can cause disease of differing severity in different individuals
Similar clinical and pathological presentations can be caused by different viruses
The presence of a virus does not necessarily mean that it is responsible for the observed disease

DNA Viruses

Nonenveloped

PARVOVIRUS
18–26 nm, defective (adeno-associated), icosahedral capsid, ssDNA
Adenosatellovirus

PAPOVAVIRUS
45-55nm, icosahedral capsid, circular dsDNA
PAPILLOMAVIRUS
Human papilloma virus: many types, producing verruca vulgaris, condyloma acuminata, laryngeal papillomas
POLYOMAVIRUS
Polyoma virus
SV-40
Progressive multifocal leukoencephalopathy virus (JC virus)
BK virus: often isolated from urine samples, but not yet linked to any specific human clinical syndrome

ADENOVIRUS
70–90 nm, icosahedral capsid, dsDNA
MASTADENOVIRUS
Adenovirus: conjunctivitis, pharyngitis, pneumonia; infected cells have enlarged nuclei and show two types of inclusions: clumped eosinophilic bodies with surrounding halo, or "smudge cell": large, ovoid nucleus filled with granular amphophilic to deeply basophilic mass and an indistinct nuclear membrane

Enveloped

HEPADNAVIRUS
42 nm, icosahedral capsule (28 nm), dsDNA
HEPATITIS B

HERPESVIRUS
120–200 nm, icosahedral capsid (100 nm), dsDNA
ALPHAHERPESVIRUS
Herpes simplex I: predominantly oropharyngeal infections
Herpes simplex II: predominantly urogenital infections
Varicella-zoster virus: Chickenpox and shingles
BETAHERPESVIRUS
Cytomegalovirus (salivary gland virus); cytomegalic inclusion disease, when acquired perinatally, can (10%) develop into a full-blown illness resembling erythroblastosis fetalis, involving salivary glands, kidneys, liver, lungs, gut, pancreas, thyroid, adrenals, and brain; CNS involvement can be fatal; get both large nuclear and smaller cytoplasmic inclusions
GAMMAHERPESVIRUS
Epstein-Barr virus: Infectious mononucleosis: virus infects B cells and incorporates into its genome; expression of viral antigens on surface of B cells induces a marked expansion of T cells, with many T-killer cells; these T cells are responsible for the atypical circulating cells and lymphadenopathy and splenomegaly (spleen may get so enlarged as to rupture)

POXVIRUS
250–400 nm, complex structure (brick-shaped), dsDNA
ORTHOPOXVIRUS
Variola (small pox)
Vaccinia
Cowpox
Molluscum contagiosum
Paravaccinia (milker's nodules)
Contagious pustular dermatitis (orf)

RNA Viruses

Nonenveloped
PICORNAVIRUS
24–30 nm, icosahedral capsid, ssRNA
ENTEROVIRUS
Poliovirus   Polio, paralysis

Coxsackie A virus	Meningitis, acute respiratory infections
Coxsackie B virus	Myocarditis of newborn, pericarditis
Echovirus	Usually local infections only
Enterovirus	

RHINOVIRUS
Many strains: major cause of the "common cold"
Generally remain confined to the upper respiratory tract

APHTHOVIRUS
Foot and mouth disease virus

HEPATITIS A

REOVIRUS
60–80 nm, icosahedral capsid, dsRNA

REOVIRUS
ORBIVIRUS
Colorado tick fever virus

ROTAVIRUS
Epidemic acute gastroenteritis: can be visualized by negatively stained stool ultrafiltrates; oral-fecal transmission; children and elderly most susceptible; peak incidence in winter months; mixed inflammation, shortening of villi, crypt hyperplasia

Enveloped

TOGAVIRUS
40–70 nm, icosahedral capsid (30 nm), ssRNA

ALPHAVIRUS (GROUP A ARBOVIRUS)
Eastern equine encephalitis virus: 70% mortality; survivors usually have mental defects; meningoencephalitis with acute vasculitis and fibrinoid necrosis
Semliki Forest virus

FLAVIVIRUS (GROUP B ARBOVIRUS)
St. Louis encephalitis virus: 30–40% mortality; lesions most severe in substantia nigra and thalamus
Dengue virus: fever, rash, muscle and joint pains; can cause severe hemorrhagic disease
Yellow fever virus: vicerotrophic for liver; midzonal necrosis
Hepatitis C virus (see liver outline)

RUBIVIRUS
Rubella virus (German measles): short, benign course, but when transmitted from mother to fetus can cause severe congenital malformations, predominantly cardiac

BUNYAVIRUS
90–120 nm, helical capsid (9 nm), ssRNA
California encephalitis virus
Crimean hemorrhagic fever
Hantavirus: causes marked noncardiogenic pulmonary edema; has recently caused several deaths in southwestern U.S.; natural reservoir: deer mouse

RETROVIRUS
80–140 nm, icosahedral capsid (70 nm), ssRNA

CISTERNAVIRUS A
ONCOVIRUS B
Mouse mammary tumor virus

ONCOVIRUS C
Rous sarcoma virus
Murine sarcoma virus
Human T-lymphocyte virus I and II (HTLV)

ONCOVIRUS D
LENTIVIRUS E
Visna virus
Human immunodeficiency virus (HIV)

SPUMAVIRUS F

CORONAVIRUS
80–160 nm, helical capsid (10–20 nm), ssRNA
Common cold syndrome

ARENAVIRUS
50–300 nm, complex capsid, ssRNA
Lymphocytic choriomeningitis virus
South American hemorrhagic fever virus

ORTHOMYXOVIRUS
80–120 nm, helical capsid (9–15 nm), ssRNA
Influenza: generally remains confined to respiratory tract; evades host defenses by antigenic shift/drift

PARAMYXOVIRUS
125–250 nm, helical capsid (18 nm), ssRNA
Viruses enter body through respiratory tract; may produce local symptoms or pass through without local reaction to cause systemic disease

PARAMYXOVIRUS
Parainfluenza virus: most common cause of croup in children
Mumps virus: Contagious childhood disease (peak incidence 5–15 yr), characterized by swelling of parotid glands (bilateral in 70%) and occasionally other salivary glands; may involve pancreas, gonads (20%, usually unilateral), CNS; in adults, tissue destruction may be more marked; salivary gland infiltrated by histiocytes, lymphocytes, plasma cells, which compress acini and ducts, occasionally with focal necrosis; similar pathology also seen in testes, where swelling can induce more necrosis

MORBILLIVIRUS
Measles virus: measles (rubeola); acute febrile illness with spotty lesions inside the mouth (Koplik's spots—blister and ulcerate; diagnostic), conjunctivitis, lymphoreticular hyperplasia, blotchy erythematous rash; largely eliminated, but increasing in U.S.; lymphoid tissue shows multinucleated giant cells with eosinophilic nuclear inclusions (Warthin-Finkeldey cells); measles virus can also cause subacute sclerosing panencephalitis in children and young adults

PNEUMOVIRUS
Respiratory syncytial virus (RSV): croup or pneumonia; can also cause otitis media, meningitis, myelitis, myocarditis

RHABDOVIRUS
Bullet shaped (130–240 × 70–80 nm), helical capsid (15 nm), ssRNA

LYSSAVIRUS
Rabies virus: primarily a disease of animals; transmitted to humans via bite from rabid animal; replicates locally and travels to brain via peripheral nerves; initial symptoms include malaise, fatigue, headache; this is followed by neurologic symptoms, including disorientation, hallucinations, seizures, coma, death; cytoplasmic inclusions in neurons (especially Purkinje cells), called Negri bodies, are pathognomonic

VESICULOVIRUS
Vesicular stomatitis virus (VSV)

Unclassified

Hepatitis delta virus: 36 nm particle with an envelope ("viroid"); defective virus that requires coinfection with hepatitis B virus; produces a fulminant hepatitis
"Slow viruses": unclassified, unidentified infectious agents

Other Terms

ARBOVIRUSES (ARTHROPOD-BORNE VIRUSES)
Sometimes used to refer collectively to the alphavirus and flavivirus genera of the togavirus family

Sometimes also includes bunyavirus, reovirus, arenavirus, and rhabdovirus families

PSEUDOMYXOVIRUS
Refers collectively to the Morbillivirus and Pneumovirus genera of the paramyxovirus family

BACTERIA

Gram-Positive Cocci

STAPHYLOCOCCUS
Non–spore-forming gram-positive cocci, usually unencapsulated, in clusters
- *S. aureus* (coagulase positive)
- *S. epidermidis* (coagulase negative)
- *S. saprophyticus* (coagulase negative)

S. aureus generally produces most severe disease and when causes sepsis, often fatal; however, even *S. epidermidis* can be fatal in immunocompromised patient

Normal inhabitant of nasopharynx and skin

Infective only following large dose inoculation

Most often form suppurative lesions with walled-off abscesses or spreading cellulitis

Regional lymphadenitis, usually mild

S. aureus sepsis is a medical emergency—often fatal

SKIN INFECTIONS
Furuncles (boil): focal superficial suppurative inflammation of skin beginning in a single hair follicle

Carbuncles: deeper subcutaneous suppuration spreading laterally, generally involving skin of upper back or neck

Impetigo: see *Streptococcus*

Surgical wound infection: sutures and foreign bodies favor persistent infections; will not heal unless pus is drained

PNEUMONIA
Generally destructive bronchopneumonia, which may rupture into pleura (empyema)

ENDOCARDITIS
Left or right sided

Most frequent destructive vegetative endocarditis

TOXIN-RELATED DISEASES
Staphylococcal food poisoning: caused by toxin in contaminated food; acute, self-limited; onset 1–6 hr after consumption

Toxic shock syndrome: sporadic, related to infected tampons; intractable shock, sometimes fatal

Scalded skin syndrome: caused by exfoliation toxin; subepidermal blistering and exfoliation with minimal inflammation; seen in children

STREPTOCOCCUS
Gram-positive cocci (slightly oval) in pairs and/or chains
- Beta-hemolytic (complete hemolysis on blood agar plates)
  - *S. pyogenes:* group A; local and systemic invasion, poststreptococcal disorders
  - *S. agalactiae:* group B; can cause perinatal infections
  - *S. faecalis* (AKA: enterococcus): group D; urinary tract infections (UTI), cardiovascular infections, meningitis
- Alpha-hemolytic (partial hemolysis on blood agar plates)
  - *S. viridans:* group H, K, others: endocarditis
  - *S. pneumoniae* (AKA: pneumococcus)

Two disease patterns: suppurative inflammation and post-streptococcal hypersensitivity disease (rheumatic fever, glomerulonephritis, erythema nodosum)

Asplenic patients particularly susceptible

SCARLET FEVER
Acute streptococcal pharyngitis accompanied by rash caused by erythrogenic toxin

3–15 yr of age

Raspberry or strawberry tongue

Notoriously associated with post-streptococcal sequelae

IMPETIGO
Superficial skin infection, usually occurring in children

Can be caused by *Streptococcus* or *Staphylococcus*

Streptococcus often produces lymphangitic spread (red streaks)

BRONCHOPNEUMONIA
S. pneumoniae (diplococcus)

Causes most cases of lobar pneumonia

Polysaccharide capsule responsible for virulence

Same organism can also cause a bacterial meningitis

Gram-Positive Bacilli

BACILLUS
Large gram-positive rods, square ended, in chains; spore forming; aerobic
- *B. anthracis:* major pathogen (anthrax)
- *B. subtilis:* pathogenic only in immunocompromised patients
- *B. cereus:* food poisoning

ANTHRAX
Organism itself produces minimal inflammation; hemorrhage, inflammation, and edema caused by exotoxin

Predominantly a disease of sheep

In humans, forms a malignant pustule at entry site, which blisters; necrosis, edema, inflammation

If becomes systemic (sepsis), usually fatal

CLOSTRIDIUM
Gram-positive motile rods, anaerobic, spore forming, widely distributed in soil

Invade only under conditions of low oxygen tension, previous tissue damage, or poor phagocytosis

Disease usually caused by a specific exotoxin that can be fatal, even in the absence of tissue invasion—antitoxin only effective if given while toxin still circulating, before it binds to its target cells

Toxin liberation often requires growth without interference from competing flora

CLOSTRIDIUM TETANI
Tetanospasmin: neurotoxin that disseminates through the blood stream, binds to peripheral nerve endings, ascends to cell body in CNS, all without causing any harm; when it passes into the presynaptic terminals of inhibitory spinal interneurons, it produces loss of sympathetic inhibition

Increased muscle tone, tachycardia, hypertension: muscles of face first, then trunk, producing tonic contractions

Minimal morphologic changes

Mortality today ~20%

CLOSTRIDIUM BOTULINUM

Spores can resist boiling for many hours

Food poisoning caused by ingestion of preformed, heat labile toxin that is resistant to gastric acidity—readily absorbed into blood; attaches to synaptic vesicles of cholinergic nerves and blocks release of acetylcholine

Descending paralysis beginning with cranial nerves (ptosis, dysphagia, dysphonia, dry mouth, paralytic ileus, etc.)

15% mortality

CLOSTRIDIUM PERFRINGENS

Invasive infection

- Necrotizing cellulitis: foul odor, thin serosanguineous exudate, sloughing of skin
- Myonecrosis (gas gangrene): produces gas bubbles in tissues (can cause crepitus) and extensive necrosis of muscle; toxins induce active hemolysis: hematocrit can drop rapidly, even to 0!

CLOSTRIDIUM DIFFICILE

Pseudomembranous colitis, with inflammatory exudate spewing out from crypts

Seen particularly with clindamycin, lincomycin, and cephalosporins; treated with vancomycin

CORYNEBACTERIUM

Gram-positive rods, nonmotile, non–spore forming, club-shaped ends, often arranged in smears as "Chinese characters"

CORYNEBACTERIUM DIPHTHERIAE

Acute communicable disease, usually of children 2–15 yr old

Induces formation of an inflammatory "pseudomembrane" in the respiratory tree overlying an ulcerated necrotic surface

Exotoxin (encoded by a lysogenic phage) is heat labile, 62 kD, and can be lethal in a dose of only 0.1 μg/kg; fragment B required for transport into cell; fragment A is enzymatically active: ADP-ribosylates elongation factor-2, causing necrosis; the toxin can have far-reaching effect, esp. myocardial fiber necrosis and polyneuritis with degeneration of the myelin sheaths

Gram-Negative Cocci

NEISSERIA

Gram-negative, nonmotile diplococci, small (0.8 μm), strict aerobes

NEISSERIA MENINGITIDIS

Gram-negative diplococcus

Colonizes upper respiratory tract, can invade

Two thirds of all invasive infections produce meningitis

Characteristically produces cluster infections

NEISSERIA GONORRHOEAE

Causes common gonorrheal urethritis ("clap")

Easily transmitted sexually or by other contact

Retrograde spread to internal genitalia where a chronic purulent inflammation is produced

If untreated, can spread into peritoneum in females (perihepatitis: Fitz-Hugh-Curtis syndrome) or systemically (septic arthritis) in either sex, but this is rare

Most common cause of pelvic inflammatory disease

In smears, often identified *within* phagocytes

Organisms under constant programmed genetic variation

Gram-Negative Coccobacilli

HAEMOPHILUS

Encapsulated coccobacillary (pleomorphic) gram-negative

HAEMOPHILUS INFLUENZAE

Currently primary pathogen for children under 1 yr

Meningitis, upper respiratory infection, epiglottitis, pneumonia, endocarditis

Meningitis peaks at 1 yr (2 months to 7 yr), usually sporadic, rapidly progressive, not infrequently fatal

Lesions are rich in neutrophils and fibrin, giving a plastic quality that resolves slowly and may scar

Acute epiglottitis is a pediatric emergency

HAEMOPHILUS DUCREYI

Causes chancroid (soft chancre), a sexually transmitted disease

BORDETELLA

Small, pleomorphic gram-negative coccobacillus

BORDETELLA PERTUSSIS

Causes whooping cough: highly communicable, usually self-limited childhood disease with violent coughing paroxysms

Organism does not invade but produces exotoxin

Extensive coughing spells can lead to subcutaneous emphysema or hypoxia-induced convulsions

BRUCELLA

Gram-Negative Bacilli

The family Enterobacteriaceae, all facultative anaerobes or aerobes, includes the following genera: *Enterobacter, Escherichia, Klebsiella, Proteus, Salmonella, Serratia, Shigella*

All are found in the GI tract

ESCHERICHIA

ESCHERICHIA COLI

Forms mass culture in human gut lumen, perhaps preventing colonization by more harmful bacteria

Most common cause of uncomplicated UTIs; infections arising secondary to stone or obstruction are more likely caused by *Proteus, Pseudomonas,* or *Enterobacter*

Also common: acute appendicitis, cholecystitis, diverticulitis

When it causes gram-negative bacteremia, endotoxin-induced disseminated intravascular coagulation (DIC) and/or shock ensues: 50% fatal

Enteroinvasive form produces a Shigella-like picture

Toxigenic form produces a watery diarrhea similar to that of cholera; causes one third of cases of "Montezuma's revenge" in travelers not immune to the organism; no mucosal injury

Most versatile source and recipient for gene exchanges

KLEBSIELLA, ENTEROBACTER, AND SERRATIA

KLEBSIELLA PNEUMONIAE AND ENTEROBACTER AEROGENES
Closely related organisms with similar disease spectrums
Severe pneumonia, UTI—not enterotoxic
Pneumonia is often lobar

SALMONELLA
Gram-negative coliform organisms with flagella
Common cause of food- and water-borne enteric infections
Numerous serotypes and species
Lack enterotoxins but invade mucosal cells, inducing brush border degeneration, ulceration; can live in macrophages and neutrophils for a while

SALMONELLA TYPHI
Causes typhoid fever
Penetrates into blood stream—bacteremia results in lymphoid proliferation, especially of Peyer's patches, which can subsequently ulcerate (form oval ulcers elongated in direction of stool flow, vs. TB, which produces circular or transverse ulcers)
Neutropenia in peripheral blood, hemophagocytosis in lymph nodes (LNs), spleen, and liver
Culture of organism from blood in 1st week is diagnostic

"FOOD POISONING"
Mildest expression of *Salmonella* disease spectrum
Short incubation period, superficial lesions limited to colon, with mixed inflammatory infiltrate

SALMONELLA TYPHIMURIUM
Generally causes disease intermediate between food poisoning and typhoid fever

SHIGELLA
Gram-negative coliform facultative anaerobes
Infectious only for humans; infectious even in small numbers
Cause bacillary dysentery: invade colonic mucosa, multiply in lamina propria and mesenteric LNs; unlike salmonella, do not cause bacteremia
Endotoxin release causes mucosal necrosis and a fibrino-purulent exudate, forming a gray-yellow pseudomembrane—ulcerations usually remain superficial

PSEUDOMONAS

PSEUDOMONAS AERUGINOSA
Low virulence in noncompromised hosts; readily phagocytosed
Common secondary invader (when normal host barriers circumvented by other means)
Number one source of sepsis in burn units
Exotoxin A ADP ribosylates EF-2 (like diphtheria toxin)
Histology: necrotizing vasculitis with thrombosis, hemorrhage, large masses of proliferating organisms

CAMPYLOBACTER

CAMPYLOBACTER JEJUNI
Responsible for 5–10% of hospital acquired dysentery
Inflammation can involve entire gut from jejunum to anus, with superficial erosions, crypt abscesses, villus atrophy

CAMPYLOBACTER (now *HELICOBACTER*) *PYLORI*
Causes an antritis

VIBRIO
Comma-shaped gram negative

VIBRIO CHOLERAE
Does not invade
Heat labile enterotoxin, ADP-ribosylates a G-protein regulator of adenylate cyclase, generating excess cAMP, marked mucosal secretion, and a watery diarrhea
Lymphoid hyperplasia often seen—may be due to other organisms

YERSINIA
Gram-negative bacillus; safety pin appearance with methylene blue stain

YERSINIA ENTEROCOLITICA
Major cause of enteritis in pediatric population
Upper and lower GI tract involvement, with ulceration and spread to LNs
Lymph nodes and intestinal mucosa show "granulomas" with stellate microabscesses rimmed by histiocytes—can mimic cat scratch granulomas

YERSINIA PESTIS
Causes bubonic, pneumonic, and septicemic plagues—total hemorrhagic necrosis of infected tissues
Bubonic form limited to skin and LNs; most common; now mortality <20%; pneumonic and septicemic forms worse

Spirochetes

BORRELIA
Tick-borne, loosely wound spirochetes measuring up to 30 μm
Stain well with Wright-Giemsa stain

BORRELIA RECURRENTIS
Relapsing fever caused by bouts of bacteremia with symptom-free intervals of about 1 wk duration
Recurrences caused by programmed antigenic variation

BORRELIA BURGDORFERI
Lyme disease
Spreading, migrating erythema at inoculation site with sharp margins and central blanching
Untreated, may progress to arthralgias, myocardial involvement, or CNS involvement

TREPONEMA
10–13 μm corkscrew-shaped spirochete
Produces minimal tissue damage, no known toxins
Lesions linked to host immune response
Low virulence, long latencies, but very high infectivity
Two types of host antibody response:
• Nonspecific antibodies; detected by STS, VDRL tests; can be falsely positive in mononucleosis, leprosy, autoimmune diseases, viral hepatitis, heroine users
• Specific antibodies—detected by fluorescent treponemal antibody (FTA)

TREPONEMA PALLIDUM
Causative agent of syphilis (AKA lues)
Sexually transmitted; also maternal-fetal transmission
Three stages of disease, all marked histologically by plasmacytosis and proliferative (obliterative) endarteritis
• Primary: chancre at site of inoculation
• Secondary: generalized, flat, red-brown elevations (condylomata lata); contain numerous spirochetes
• Tertiary: may occur years or decades later; only seen in about one third of untreated cases

• Medial necrosis of aortic base and valve ring
• Neurosyphilis
• Syphilitic gumma, most common in liver

Congenital syphilis characteristically shows interstitial keratitis, Hutchinson's teeth (screwdriver-shaped incisors), and 8th nerve deafness

TREPONEMA PERTENUE AND TREPONEMA CARATEUM

Cause yaws and pinta, respectively

Others

MYCOBACTERIUM

Slow dividers, facultative intracellular invaders
Modest infectivity, but marked persistence in tissues
Acid-fast (Ziehl-Neelsen) staining due to waxy cell wall components
Strict aerobes—do not grow in areas of low oxygen tension
Grow slowly in culture (doubling time 48 hr)

ATYPICAL MYCOBACTERIA

Mycobacterium avium-intracellulare most common in U.S.
Infection acquired from environment, not person to person
Seen in immunocompromised patients, but also in chronic obstructive pulmonary disease

MYCOBACTERIUM LEPRAE

Cause of leprosy; AKA: Hansen's disease
Obligate intracellular organism
Low communicability
Two forms of disease:
• TT (polar tuberculoid form): vigorous T-cell response with local activation of macrophages and granuloma formation
• LL (polar lepromatous form): deficient T-cell immunity, poor host response, macrophages stuffed with bacteria, bacteremia, seed cooler areas of body: skin, peripheral nerves, eyes, upper airways, testes, hands, feet

MYCOBACTERIUM TUBERCULOSIS

AKA: Koch bacillus
Infection used to be seen mostly in children and young adults; now more common in 50–60 yr olds
Two species: one predominantly infects humans (transmitted by inhalation); second is a bovine strain (now much less common but would cause GI infections from infected milk)
Hallmark lesion is caseating granuloma (soft tubercle), although may have a cellular center (hard tubercle)
Ghon focus: 1–1.5 cm gray-white inflammatory consolidation seen at the periphery of the upper part of lower lobe or lower part of upper lobe (greatest volume of air flow) that becomes granulomatous and then centrally necrotic by the 2nd week: primary infection focus, usually clinically silent
Ghon complex: combination of primary lung lesion and ipsilateral LN involvement
Rarely, primary focus will rapidly enlarge, erode into bronchi, giving rise to satellite lesions—may seed blood stream, resulting in miliary dissemination or meningitis
Secondary TB arises from reactivation of old primary lesions; presents as apical or posterior segment lesions (tuberculoma), may be bilateral; can scar down, create progressive pulmonary TB, lead to tuberculous empyema, intestinal TB (if aspirated material is swallowed), or miliary seeding
Isolated distant organ involvement also seen (cervical LN, meninges, kidneys, adrenals, bones, fallopian tubes, epididymis)

Secondary TB usually accompanied by fever, night sweats, weakness, fatigability, loss of appetite

ACTINOMYCETES

Closely related to mycobacteria, with some similarity to fungi
Long, filamentous, gram-positive; do not stain on H&E

NOCARDIA

Infect chronically ill, immunosuppressed
Form necrotizing walled-off abscesses (predominantly in lung); no granulomata
Stain with acid-fast stain (unlike *Actinomyces*)

ACTINOMYCES

Chronic suppurative infection of neck, lung, or abdomen
Grossly visible yellow colonies: "sulfur granules"
Can infect normal hosts—invade only when tissue is devitalized by trauma (strict anaerobe)
Cervicofacial, thoracic, and abdominal actinomycosis

FUNGI

CANDIDA

AKA: moniliasis; most common fungal infection
Nonbranching boxcar-like chains of tubular cells (pseudohyphae) and small 2–4 μm yeast forms
Infect oral cavity, GI tract, and vagina of normal individuals
Bacterial growth inhibits; when bacteria killed, *Candida* can proliferate and become invasive
Thrush: Candidal infection of oral cavity
Vaginal: more common during pregnancy and in oral contraceptive users
Invasive, systemic: renal (numerous microabscesses in both cortex and medulla), cardiac valves, lungs, meningitis

ASPERGILLUS

Second most common infective fungus, esp. in hospitals
45° angle branching septate hyphae; 5–10 μm
Three types of infection:
• Allergic: inhalation of large numbers of spores, producing a hypersensitivity reaction in bronchi or alveoli
• Colonizing: growth of organisms in pulmonary cavity, forming a mass (aspergilloma) without invasion
• Invasive: opportunistic infection involving primarily lung but also heart valves, brain, kidneys: targetoid lesions with necrotizing center and hemorrhagic border; propensity for invasion of vessel walls (like mucormycosis)

MUCORMYCOSIS (PHYCOMYCETES)

Broad (6–50 μm), irregular, empty-looking, nonseptate hyphae with wide-angle branching; ribbon-like
Opportunistic infections
Tendency to invade blood vessel walls (arterial)
Rhinocerebral, via nasal sinuses, seen in diabetics
Lung and GI involvement seen in advanced malignancy, leukemia, lymphoma, immunosuppression

HISTOPLASMA CAPSULATUM

Tiny 2–5 μm yeast forms with occasional unequal budding

Dust inhalation from soil contaminated with bird/bat droppings

Lesions and disease patterns are very similar to those of TB

Histologically, collections of macrophages filled with yeast

BLASTOMYCES

Large 25 μm yeast forms; thick, refractile, double-contoured capsule, with broad-based budding

Male : female = 9 : 1; limited to North America

Chronic focal suppurative or granulomatous lesions in lungs and skin (in skin, striking pseudoepitheliomatous hyperplasia)

CRYPTOCOCCUS NEOFORMANS

5–10 μm yeast with wide capsular halo and narrow-based unequal budding; no hyphal forms in tissue

May infect healthy individuals, but usually opportunistic in patients with Hodgkin's, leukemia, lymphoma, AIDS

Capsule stains bright red with mucicarmine

Most frequent manifestation is meningitis or encephalitis

Small cysts filled with organisms and their mucinous secretions, creating the "soap bubble" lesion

COCCIDIOIDES IMMITIS

20–60 μm spheres with endospores and capsule (spherule)

Infections seen in southwest U.S.: "valley fever"

Primary pulmonary lesion similar to TB—suppurative or granulomatous

60% of infections asymptomatic

Results in delayed hypersensitivity to coccidioidin antigen

PROTOZOA

ENTAMOEBA HISTOLYTICA

15–40 μm trophozoite with small nucleus, foamy cytoplasm

Often ingests red cells; very motile on wet preps

Infects cecum and ascending colon; sometimes whole colon

Can cause mild to very bloody diarrhea

Invades lamina propria from deep in crypts; does not go past muscularis mucosa; spreads out, undermining site of invasion (flask-shaped lesion); as spreads, cuts into blood supply of overlying mucosa, causing liquefactive necrosis with minimal inflammatory response

In ~40% of cases, enters blood vessels and travels to liver, where can form a unilocular cyst, often large, often hemorrhagic (chocolate-colored anchovy paste; *not* malodorous)

Lung and brain abscesses can also be formed

NAEGLERIA FOWLERI

Free-living ameboflagellate; large nucleus

Enters arachnoid space through the cribriform plate while swimming in infected waters: causes meningoencephalitis

Organism has large nucleus; easily mistaken for human cell

GIARDIA LAMBLIA

World's most prevalent gut protozoan

Trophozoites (sickle-shaped) live in brush border of duodenum and give rise to infective cysts

Mucosa: normal to moderately inflamed with blunting of villi

Can cause mild indigestion to copious, watery diarrhea, with flatulence, cramps, malodorous stools

CRYPTOSPORIDIUM

Mild diarrhea in children to severe malabsorption in AIDS

Live in intestine adherent to brush border and surrounded by host cell membrane (intracellular)

Nuclei of infected cells become enlarged and hyperchromatic

Intraepithelial lymphocytes common

MICROSPORIDIUM

Small protozoa that infect GI tract, causing an intractable diarrhea in 60% of AIDS patients

ENTEROTOZOON BIENNEUSI (DISCOVERED IN 1985)

Single organisms: infect only enterocytes

Treated with metronidazole

SEPTATA INTESTINALIS (DISCOVERED IN 1993)

Infects all cells (enterocytes, fibroblasts, neutrophils, macrophages, etc.)

Multiple organisms found as clusters in all stages of maturation, but separated by "septa" of cytoplasm

Treated with albendazol

TRICHOMONAS VAGINALIS

Most frequent venereal parasitic infection

15–18 μm long, turnip-shaped flagellate

Lives in postpubertal vaginas and male urethra (prepubertal vagina has wrong bacterial flora)

Only small fraction of patients are symptomatic (itching, burning, esp. during micturition)

May be asymptomatic, even when present in large numbers

PNEUMOCYSTIS CARINII

4–6 μm cysts

Ubiquitous opportunistic parasite; essentially all children have acquired antibodies to it by age 2

In protein-malnourished children and immunosuppressed adults, can cause an interstitial pneumonia

Foamy alveolar exudate with proliferating parasites

PLASMODIA

Four species; all cause different types of malaria

Life cycle split between human and mosquito

When infected into skin by bite of a carrier female mosquito, sporozoites travel to liver, enter hepatocytes, grow, and transform to merozoites, which reenter the blood and RBCs and grow to become trophozoites; some undergo sexual division into gametes, which can then again be picked up by mosquitoes and transform into sporozoites

Infected individuals show relapsing high fever with chills, rigor, headache, body ache, delirium; then sweating, fever, and lassitude

Parasites can be found in the blood, and brown-black malarial pigment (hemozoin) can be found in histiocytes in the spleen and in Kupffer cells in the liver

Sickle-cell hemoglobin (HbS) carriers limit parasitemia by forcing parasite to leave the red cell as its heme starts sickling

PLASMODIUM VIVAX, PLASMODIUM OVALE
Benign tertian malaria: fever spikes 48 hr apart; rarely fatal
P. vivax can only infect RBCs with the Duffy blood group factor

PLASMODIUM MALARIAE
Benign quartan malaria: fever spikes 72 hr apart; long latency periods

PLASMODIUM FALCIPARUM
Malignant tertian malaria: fever spikes at 48 hr intervals, progressive damage to RBCs, high parasitemias; can spread to CNS, which accounts for most of the fatalities

BABESIA MICROTI
Babesiosis: acute, sometimes prolonged illness with headache, fever, chills, myalgia, fatigue
Commonly seen on eastern U.S. seaboard, especially Nantucket and Martha's Vineyard
Transmitted by tick

TRYPANOSOMA
TRYPANOSOMA RHODESIENSE, TRYPANOSOMA GAMBIENSE
Acute febrile attack with purpura and DIC, then chronic episodic fever with lymphadenopathy and splenomegaly, then progressive brain dysfunction, "sleeping sickness," cachexia, and death
Transmitted by insect (tsetse flies); live in blood stream
Genetically programmed antigenic variation

TRYPANOSOMA CRUZI
Causes Chagas' disease; AKA: American trypanosomiasis
Intracellular parasite
Acute, myocarditis; chronic, progressive cardiac failure
In the heart, occasional cells stuffed with organisms; inflammation far out of proportion to number of organisms

LEISHMANIA
Tiny <3 μm intracellular parasite; on smears, two basophilic dots (nucleus and kinetoplast)
Limited cutaneous infection or generalized visceral infection

TOXOPLASMA GONDII
3×6 μm tachyzoites
Definitive hosts are domestic cats; when shed in feces, oocysts are highly infective by any route
In normal adults, produces a limited lymphadenopathy, often cervical, with follicular hyperplasia, monocytoid B cells, and epithelioid histiocytes
Fetal, neonatal, or immunocompromised infections rapidly lead to CNS involvement, progressive encephalitis, death

HELMINTHS

Effective infections rely upon longevity of individual worms rather than large reproduction rates; most helminths must cycle through the environment for reproduction

Individual worm burdens in humans tend to be stable and long-lasting; individuals harboring worms are generally more resistant to superinfection by the same worm
Only a small percentage of "infections" result in disease
Disease can be caused by:
• Competition with host for essential nutrients
• Mechanical obstruction
• Blood digestion
• Inflammation and malabsorptive changes in the gut
• Host hypersensitivity

Nematodes (Roundworms)

ASCARIS LUMBRICOIDES
Largest (up to 35 cm) and most common intestinal roundworm
Fecal-oral transmission
In most infected individuals, remains commensally in gut, not causing disease; eventually dies and is passed
Infections most common in children
Disease caused by hypersensitivity, GI obstruction, perforation of appendix or bile duct with peritonitis

TRICHURIS
AKA: whipworm
Small intestine, up to 5 cm long with attenuated anterior end
Rarely causes disease, and then only with massive infections and only mild disease

ENTEROBIUS VERMICULARIS
AKA: pinworm
Tiny, up to 1.3 cm long, prominent lateral ridges
Causes enterobiasis; AKA: oxyuriasis
Female worms migrate to anus at night to lay eggs; causes intense pruritus, insomnia, and irritability in children
Not infrequently found incidentally in appendix

NECATOR AMERICANUS, ANCYLOSTOMA DUODENALE
AKA: hookworms
1 cm long
Sharp mouth plates penetrate into duodenal or jejunal mucosa; worms feed on blood, most of which is excreted into the intestinal lumen (each worm uses 43 μl blood/day)
Heavy infections needed to produce iron deficiency anemia
Eggs hatch in gut, deposited in feces, enter skin of human feet, travel to lungs, coughed up, swallowed, reenter gut

STRONGYLOIDES STERCORALIS
Very small (1 mm long), intestinal luminal dweller
Burrow into mucosal crypts; can damage absorptive surface of gut, leading to chronic enteritis
Only intestinal nematode that can reproduce within host
Larvae can invade and migrate to lung, liver, CNS

DRACUNCULUS MEDINENSIS
AKA: guinea worm
Long (120 cm), thin worm that enters by drinking larva-infested water; mature worms migrate to skin

Blistering, ulcerating skin lesions (often outer malleolus of foot); occasionally can see head of worm in fresh lesion
Worm used to be removed by winding it up on a stick; this is the probable origin of the caduceus

TRICHINELLA SPIRALIS

Trichinosis acquired by eating improperly cooked contaminated meat (pork, bear, wild game); larvae released into stomach by digestion of cyst wall, attach to duodenal mucosa, mature to adult worms, produce numerous new larvae that invade blood stream and spread to skeletal muscles and convert muscle cell to a nurse cell, encyst, and in time may die and calcify
Most common muscles: diaphragm, eye muscles, laryngeal muscles, deltoid, gastrocnemius, intercostals

FILARIA

Long stringlike nematodes whose fertilized females release tiny microfilariae into the lymph, blood, and skin
Can survive for many years, producing microfilariae
Mosquito borne
WUCHERERIA BANCROFTI
10 cm long; invade lymphatics, producing lymphedema of scrotum, penis, vulva, leg, breast, or arm
ONCHOCERCA VOLVULUS
Largest of human filariae (50 cm)
Transmitted by black flies
Lives in skin; discharges microfilariae into subcutaneous tissue
In addition to skin lesions, can get blindness from millions of microfilariae accumulating in eye chambers

Cestodes (Flatworms)

AKA: tapeworms, platyhelminths
Can achieve lengths of 3–6 meters
Scolex is head region: generates thousands of proglottids that articulate with each other and make up bulk of worm
Two types of infections: adult worm attached to intestinal wall or invasion by larval forms into various organs

TAENIA

Ingestion of undercooked meat; larvae excyst and mature into adults, attach to bowel wall by scolex, can grow to great lengths
Can obstruct GI tract or lead to B_{12} deficiency
Diagnose by finding proglottids or eggs in stool
To cure, must remove scolex; a vermifuge can be used
CYSTICERCOSIS
Usually *Taenia solium*
Acquired by consumption of eggs; invade through gut and disseminate to brain, muscles, skin, heart
Can block spinal fluid reabsorption
Ovoid, white to opalescent
Often calcify or degenerate
Minimal inflammation when alive, extensive when die

ECHINOCOCCUS GRANULOSUS

Main host is dog
Human ingestion of eggs leads to hatching in duodenum and invasive embryos, which usually go to liver (66%) but also to lung (5–15%) or bones, brain, etc.

In target site, lodge within capillaries, incite an inflammatory reaction, and if survive encyst; this "hydatid cyst" grows in size over years and can reach 10 cm or more
Cysts unilocular (*E. multilocularis* causes multilocular cysts)

Trematodes (Flukes)

SCHISTOSOMA

6 species, including *S. mansoni, S. japonicum, S. haematobium*
Infective form burrows through skin of feet into blood stream; pauses in lung at 4–14 days until reaches liver; matures in intrahepatic portal radicals; eventually descends to mesenteric or pelvic venules, where mates and lays eggs
Hypersensitivity granulomas in liver can lead to fibrosis
Generally minimal host tissue reactions to adults until die
Eggs produce significant inflammation; often calcify
Predisposes to squamous cell carcinoma of the bladder

FASCIOLA HEPATICA

Liver fluke
Worms migrate through liver (predominantly subcapsular); settle in gallbladder or bile ducts; can cause obstruction

FASCIOLOPSIS BUSKI

Large intestinal fluke (7 cm), principally small bowel
Attaches to mucosa, hemorrhagic inflammation, can lead to abscesses and mucosal destruction

PARAGONIMUS WESTERMANI

Lung fluke; small, 1.2 cm long
Causes cystic inflammatory lesions, usually in lung
Source: uncooked crayfish or crabs

OTHER INFECTIOUS AGENTS

CHLAMYDIA

Obligate intracellular parasites with both RNA and DNA
Live within phagocytic vacuoles in cells; prevent fusion of lysosomes
Synthesize own nucleic acids, but not own ATP
Do not dictate host cell synthesis of new products
Inclusions can be identified with fluorescent antibodies
Giemsa stain can demonstrate either large "initial" (1 μm) bodies or smaller (0.2–0.3 μm) "elementary" bodies
Two species: *C. psittaci* and *C. trachomatis,* the latter with numerous serotypes
ORNITHOSIS (PSITTACOSIS)
Caused by inhalation of contaminated bird excrement
Infection can be asymptomatic, flu-like, serious, or fatal
Fatality has ranged from 5% to 40%
URETHRITIS
Asymptomatic in women
Often recognized by persistence following treatment for gonorrhea

TRACHOMA

Chronic suppurative eye disease

Mostly seen in dry, sandy regions

One of the leading global causes of blindness

LYMPHOGRANULOMA VENEREUM (LGV)

Venereally transmitted disease; marked lymphadenopathy

In males, invariably inguinal nodes; in females, can be deep pelvic or perirectal nodes

Stage I: small epidermal vesicle; granulomas; chlamydial inclusions

Stage II: suppurative granulomatous inflammation with stellate abscesses rimmed by epithelioid histiocytes

Stage III: chronic inflammatory infiltrates and dense fibrosis, plasma cells

RICKETTSIA

Small, gram-negative obligate intracellular bacteria; inhabit ticks, mites, fleas, lice; don't damage arthropod hosts

Infect humans either by arthropod bite or by contact of abraded skin with arthropod excreta

In humans, multiply in small vessel endothelium; enter cell by induced endocytosis, escape into cytoplasm and begin dividing; can fill cell with organisms, may burst

TYPHUS FEVER

Caused by *Rickettsia prowazekii*

Generally, no eschar is formed at site of inoculation

Limited to skin in milder cases, but can cause necrosis of fingertips, nose, ear lobes, scrotum, penis, vulva; internal hemorrhages involve brain, heart, testes, lungs, kidneys

Endothelial proliferation and swelling in capillaries, arterioles, venules; may narrow lumen or thrombose vessels but rarely destroy vessel walls

Cuff of inflammation, mixed leukocytes, surrounding vessels

In the brain, focal microglial proliferations mixed with leukocytes, referred to as "typhoid nodule"

ROCKY MOUNTAIN SPOTTED FEVER

Caused by *Rickettsia rickettsii*

Organisms penetrate deeply into vessels, causing acute necrosis, fibrin extravasation, thrombosis; may mimic necrotizing vasculitis

Generally forms eschar at site of inoculation

Distribution of lesions similar to that for typhus

BACILLARY ANGIOMATOSIS AND PELIOSIS HEPATIS

Caused by *Rochalimaea henselae* or *R. quintana* species, or a related organism

Intracellular parasite that leads to death of infected cells and a degree of vascular proliferation

MYCOPLASMA

AKA: Eaton agents; pleuropneumonia-like organisms (PPLOs)

Resemble L forms of bacteria: tiny, 0.125–0.35 μm polymorphous organisms

Extracellular human parasite

Frequent cause of primary atypical pneumonia

In 40% of cases, elicits Ig production, which agglutinates human group O red cells at 4°C (cold agglutinins)

3

CONGENITAL SYNDROMES

Terminology

Pleiotropism: single gene with multiple effects

Genetic heterogeneity: multiple genotypes, same phenotype

Variable expressivity: same genotype, variable phenotypes

Penetrance: same genotype, same phenotype, but expressed to a varying degree

Malformation: intrinsic developmental abnormality that occurs in <4% of the general population

Variation: structural abnormality that occurs in >4% of the general population

Deformation: structural abnormality due to external mechanical factors (e.g., oligohydramnios)

Disruption: secondary destruction of an originally normal structure

Syndrome: nonsequential group of abnormalities that occur together, not clearly explainable by a single event but thought to be pathogenetically related

Associations: nonrandom concurrence of multiple anomalies

Sequence: varieties of causes producing a pattern of abnormalities

Field defects: pattern of anomalies resulting from disturbance of development of a single region/field

Metacentric: centromere near center

Submetacentric: centromere eccentrically placed

Acrocentric: centromere near end

Reciprocal translocation: no genetic material lost

Robertsonian translocation: fusion of long portions of two acrocentric chromosomes; small chromosome formed by two small portions is often lost

Isochromosome: centromere divides in transverse plane, resulting in one chromosome with two p arms and one with two q arms

Inversion: both break sites on same side (paracentric) or opposite sides (pericentric) of centromere

Ring chromosome: loss of telomeres of p and q arm with fusion of resulting sticky ends

Lyonization: inactivation of all but one X (Mary Lyon, 1961)

General

13% newborns have one minor malformation, most in head, neck, or hands

0.75% newborns have two minor malformations; 1/2000 have three

Causes of malformations: 8% single gene disorders, 6% chromosomal, 20% multifactorial, 5% environmental

Cytogenetic Disorders

Abnormalities of the sex chromosomes are more common and much better tolerated than autosomal abnormalities

TRISOMY 21 (DOWN SYNDROME)

Most common chromosomal disorder (1/1000 newborns), most common genetic cause of mental retardation

Incidence increases with maternal age (1/1550 live births in mothers <20 yr, 1/25 in mothers >45 yr)

95% are true trisomy; 4% are translocations (Robertsonian) of 21 to 14, 22, etc.; 1% are mosaics

Involves 21q22 band: this area includes the GART gene (purine biosynthesis)

Clinical features: Mental retardation, flat facies, oblique palpebral fissures, congenital heart disease (40%), dysplastic ears, horizontal palmar creases

Often see papillary muscle calcification and cystic dilatation of Hassall's corpuscles in the thymus

Increased risk for Alzheimer's, infections, acute lymphoblastic leukemia (ALL)

Life expectancy: now ~30 yr

TRISOMY 18 (EDWARDS' SYNDROME)

1/3000−7000 live births

90% true trisomy, 10% mosaic

Marked mental retardation; seizures; micrognathia; hypertonicity; flexion deformities of fingers; *rocker-bottom feet;* cardiac, renal, and intestinal defects; abnormal-shaped head with low-set ears

Usually die in 1st year of life

TRISOMY 13 (PATAU'S SYNDROME)

1/5000 live births

80% true trisomy, 10% translocation, 10% mosaic

Marked mental retardation, microcephaly, arrhinencephaly, microphthalmia, retinal dysplasia, cleft lip, polydactyly, abnormal ears, cardiac dextroposition and defects, hyperconvex nails, club feet, flexed trigger thumbs, GI and GU abnormalities

Usually die in 1st year of life

CHROMOSOME 5p− (CRI DU CHAT SYNDROME)

Deletion of short arm of chromosome 5

Most patients have a distinctive cry—sounds like a kitten

Mental retardation, cardiac defects (ventricular septal defect), microcephaly

May survive to adulthood

Adults develop myelodysplastic syndrome with picture similar to refractory anemia but does not progress to acute myeloblastic leukemia (AML)

XO (TURNER'S SYNDROME)

XO in 57% (most common abnormal phenotype—only 3% of XO survive to birth), rest are partial deletions

Primary cause of primary amenorrhea

Short stature, streak (atrophied) ovaries, webbing of neck, peripheral lymphedema, coarctation of the aorta

XXX (MULTI-X SYNDROME)

1/1200 live female births

XXX normal; mental retardation increases with number of Xs

XXY (KLINEFELTER'S SYNDROME)
82% XXY; occasionally XXXY, etc. or mosaics
1/850 live births—some increase with maternal age
Most common cause of male infertility
Hypogonadism, eunuchoid body habitus, gynecomastia, female distribution of hair; mental retardation is seen increasingly with increasing numbers of X chromosomes

XYY SYNDROME
1/1000 live male births
Phenotypically normal
May be excessively tall, have severe acne
1–2% show antisocial behavior

TRUE HERMAPHRODITISM
Both testicular and ovarian tissue present, either separately or combined (ovatestis)
Very rare; most are 46XX with translocation of part of the Y chromosome to one of the Xs

PSEUDOHERMAPHRODITISM
By definition, a disagreement between gonadal (histology of gonad) and phenotypic sex
Female pseudohermaphrodite: XX with normal internal genitalia but virilized external; often due to increased androgenic steroids, usually from congenital adrenal hyperplasia
Male pseudohermaphrodite: XY with testis, but external genitalia partially to completely female; most common cause is mutation of the androgen receptor (testicular feminization)
Dihydrotestosterone directs development of male external genitalia; in absence, female genitalia develops

Mendelian Disorders

Factors such as penetrance and variable expressivity often complicate strict dominant/recessive designations

MARFAN'S SYNDROME
Autosomal dominant, probably multiple genes involved, at least one localized to 15q21.1
Some cases involve defect in fibrillin, an elastin binding scaffolding protein
70–85% are familial; in sporadic cases, risk increases with increasing paternal age
Skeletal abnormalities: long extremities, lax joints, pectus excavatum or pigeon breast, kyphoscoliosis
Ocular abnormalities: bilateral dislocation of lens (usually upward and outward); very rare except in Marfan's
Cardiovascular abnormalities:
• Cystic medionecrosis of the root of aorta, causing dilatation and aortic incompetence; rupture is cause of death in 40% of patients with this disorder
• Floppy mitral valve with regurgitation
Average age at death 30–40 yr

NEUROFIBROMATOSIS TYPE I (VON RECKLINGHAUSEN'S DISEASE)
AKA: peripheral neurofibromatosis
Autosomal dominant: gene on 17q11.2; 100% penetrance
1/3000 live births; 50% of cases are spontaneous
Multiple plexiform neurofibromas (superficial and deep); superficial lesions often with overlying hyperpigmentation; deep lesions become malignant in 3% of patients
Cutaneous café au lait macules (>6), present in 90% of patients
Lisch nodules (pigmented iris hamartomas) in 95% of patients over 6 yr old

Can also show erosive defects of bone and have a twofold increased risk of developing other tumors (e.g. Wilms', rhabdomyosarcoma, AML, unilateral acoustic neuromas, optic gliomas, meningiomas, pheochromocytomas)

NEUROFIBROMATOSIS TYPE II (ACOUSTIC FORM)
AKA: central neurofibromatosis
Bilateral acoustic neuromas, café au lait spots ± skin tumors; no Lisch nodules
Autosomal dominant: gene on 22q11

TUBEROUS SCLEROSIS
AKA: Bourneville's disease, Pringle's disease
Adenoma sebaceum of face (actually are angiofibromas), seizures, and mental retardation
Autosomal dominant with incomplete penetrance
Also get numerous hamartomas: CNS—periventricular nodules ("tubers"), angiomyolipoma of kidney, subungual fibromas, cardiac rhabdomyomas, pulmonary lymphangioleiomyomatosis
30% fatal by age 5; 75% fatal by age 20, usually from seizures

VON HIPPEL-LINDAU SYNDROME
Autosomal dominant: maps to 3p25
Patients have a variety of benign and malignant neoplasms, including hemangioblastoma of retina, cerebellum, medulla oblongata, and spinal cord; angiomas of the liver or kidney; adenomas of the kidney and epididymis; renal cell carcinoma; pheochromocytoma; cysts of the pancreas, kidney, liver, and epididymis
Over half die of hemangioblastomas of the CNS; renal cell carcinoma is another leading killer

CYSTIC FIBROSIS (MUCOVISCIDOSIS)
Autosomal recessive, variable penetrance; 1/20 whites are carriers; 1/2000 whites are affected
Gene is on chromosome 7q32: encodes "CFTR" gene, a putative chloride transporter (1480 amino acids long)
Most common (95%) mutation is deletion of amino acid Phe508, resulting in defective anion transport, particularly Cl^- and HCO_3^-, with subsequent abnormal water movement
In sweat glands of skin, sweat ducts cannot take up Cl^- back from secretions: sweat high in NaCl
In lungs, decreased Cl^- transport into lumen results in viscous secretions, which plug airways; infections by *Staphylococcus* and *Pseudomonas* common, often fatal (major cause of death)
In pancreas, ducts do not secrete enough bicarbonate, resulting in viscous secretions, plugging of ducts, and eventually destruction of exocrine pancreas
In liver, bile stasis leads to biliary cirrhosis in 5%
Most affected males are sterile

FAMILIAL HYPERCHOLESTEROLEMIA
Normally, liver secretes very low density lipoprotein (VLDL), which transports lipids to fat and muscle, being converted to intermediate density lipoprotein (IDL); IDL is then re-taken up by the liver, either before or after conversion to low density lipoprotein (LDL) in plasma and other sites, via the LDL receptor
Patients have either reduced levels (heterozygous) or absent (homozygous) LDL receptor, resulting in increased circulating LDL levels and increased cholesterol synthesis in the liver (less feedback inhibition)
• Class I: absent receptors (macrophages pick up LDL by non–receptor-mediated mechanism)
• Class II: defective receptor binding
• Class III: defective transport
• Class IV: failure of receptor to aggregate in pits

Brown and Goldstein won the Nobel Prize in 1985 for elucidating these pathways

ALBINISM

Inability to synthesize melanin

Two variants: oculocutaneous albinism (many types, all autosomal recessive) and ocular albinism (rare; limited to eye; usually X-linked recessive)

Divided into tyrosinase positive and negative (more severe)

FRAGILE X SYNDROME

X-linked (Xq27.3) usually recessive, can occur in women

Familial mental retardation, enlarged testes

ALKAPTONURIA (OCHRONOSIS)

Autosomal recessive

Lack of homogentisic oxidase results in block of phenylalanine metabolism: buildup of homogentisic acid causes black discoloration of urine and cartilage of ears, nose, cheeks

Accumulation in cartilage of joints results in severe arthritis

PHENYLKETONURIA (PKU)

Autosomal recessive; characterized by lack of phenylalanine hydroxylase (PAH), leading to hyperphenylalaninemia and mental retardation

PAH normally converts Phe to Tyr

Metabolites of Phe can be found in the urine

First clinical signs appear within 3–4 months: seizures, bizarre behavior

Disease progression controlled by dietary restriction of Phe and supplementation with Tyr

3–10% cases have normal PAH activity but defects in other enzymes

GALACTOSEMIA

Two forms; both autosomal recessive defects in galactose metabolism

In one, absence of galactokinase; results only in cataracts

Major form is lack of galactose-1-phosphate uridyl transferase, leading to accumulation of galactose in blood, then in urine, with aminoaciduria

1/40,000–60,000

Severe mental retardation results if galactose intake not restricted

Histology: also see fatty liver with bile stasis and eventually cirrhosis

LYSOSOMAL STORAGE DISEASES

Collection of disorders, usually autosomal recessive, resulting from deficiency of some enzyme needed for metabolism and leading to accumulation of secondary lysosomes in brain, heart, bones, liver, spleen

Commonly, infants are normal at birth (no products accumulated yet) and develop normally initially, but become symptomatic between 6 months and 2 yr, depending on rate of accumulation

Sphingolipidoses

TAY-SACHS DISEASE (GM₂ GANGLIOSIDOSIS TYPE I)

Become symptomatic at 6 months—CNS deterioration; death by 2–3 yr of age

Most prominent among Ashkenazi Jews (1/30 are carriers)

Deficiency of hexosaminidase A (chromosome 15), resulting in accumulation of GM_2 ganglioside in neurons of CNS and retina (as well as liver, spleen, etc.)

Ballooning and loss of neurons with microglia proliferation

Electron microscopy: whirled inclusions in lysosomes with onion skin layers

Retina shows cherry-red spot at macula

FABRY'S DISEASE

AKA: angiokeratoma corporis diffusum universale

X-linked recessive

Skin lesions consist of slightly elevated red-blue nodules

Deficiency of lysosomal enzyme trihexosylceramide alpha-galactosidase, with systemic accumulation in blood vessel endothelial and smooth muscle cells, ganglion cells, and in reticuloendothelial, myocardial, and connective tissue

GAUCHER'S DISEASE

Lack glucocerebrosidase (chromosome 1q21), resulting in glucocerebroside accumulation in phagocytic cells throughout body: liver, spleen, bone marrow, lymph nodes, thymus, Peyer's patches, and neurons—types II and III

Gaucher cells: enlarged, swollen (up to 100 μm) cells with PAS-positive "crumpled tissue paper" inclusions

Three forms:
- Type I (classic): most common (80%); adult type (noncerebral form); late onset
- Type II: infantile acute cerebral pattern; death at early age from CNS complications
- Type III: intermediate between I and II

KRABBE'S DISEASE (GLOBOID CELL LEUKODYSTROPHY)

Deficiency of galactocerebroside B galactosidase

Early onset of symptoms (rigidity, instability)—fatal by 1 yr

NIEMANN-PICK DISEASE

Most common type (type A) shows lack of sphingomyelinase, resulting in severe infantile-onset neurologic involvement and death by 1–3 yr of age

Sphingomyelin accumulates as foamy macrophages in liver, spleen, bone marrow

Electron microscopy: membranous cytoplasmic bodies resembling lamellated myelin (zebra bodies)

Mucopolysaccharidoses (MPS)

HURLER'S DISEASE (TYPE I MPS)

Lack of iduronidase

Normal development until 20 months, then dementia begins

Usually fatal by 6–10 yr, often due to involvement of cardiac valves, resulting in stenosis or incompetence

Electron microscopy: zebra bodies (secondary lysosomes filled with lamellated inclusions)

Scheie's disease is a milder form

HUNTER'S SYNDROME (TYPE II MPS)

X-linked recessive

Deficiency of L-iduronosulfate sulfatase, which circulates

Transplantation of normal fibroblasts subcutaneously has led to correction of the defect in some individuals

SANFILIPPO'S SYNDROME (TYPE III MPS)
MORQUIO'S SYNDROME (TYPE IV MPS)

Mucolipidoses

Defect in transport of lysosomal enzymes into lysosomes

Four types; type II is also known as I-cell disease

Glycogen Storage Diseases (Glycogenoses)

Group of disorders of glycogen metabolism
- Types 0 and I result in hypoglycemia and accumulation
- Types II–XI result in accumulation of glycogen in liver, spleen, heart, brain

Many of these disorders do not involve lysosomal enzymes, so glycogen storage diseases are often segregated from lysosomal storage diseases

VON GIERKE'S DISEASE (GLYCOGENOSIS I)

Glucose-6-phosphatase deficiency

Predominantly hepatic and renal accumulation

POMPE'S DISEASE (GLYCOGENOSIS II)
Alpha-L4-glucosidase (acid maltase) deficiency (a lysosomal enzyme)

Glycogen accumulates predominantly in skeletal and cardiac muscle, but also in other organs

Accumulation is in *membrane bound vacuoles* (lysosomes), unlike all other glycogenoses, in which it is cytoplasmic

Progressive weakness, hypotonia, macroglossia, cardiomegaly

Death usually by age 2 yr from heart failure

MCARDLE'S SYNDROME (GLYCOGENOSIS V)
Muscle specific phosphorylase deficiency

Accumulation of glycogen in skeletal muscle only

Muscle cramps with exercise; persistent exercise can cause massive rhabdomyolysis

Debilitating, but usually not progressive

Multifactorial Inheritance

Usually multiple genes and environmental factors involved

2–7% risk of recurrence (9% with two affected children)

20–40% concordance between identical twins

EHLERS-DANLOS SYNDROMES
Heterogeneous group (10–12 types) of disorders of collagen synthesis and structure

Affect predominantly skin, ligaments, joints: hyperextensible and hypermobile; skin is stretchable but also fragile and vulnerable to trauma

• Type I: Diaphragmatic hernia
• Type IV: abnormalities of type III collagen, at least three distinct mutations/forms; spontaneous rupture of large blood vessels or intestines
• Type VI: most common, autosomal recessive, reduced lysyl hydroxylase activity, affects only type I and III collagen; ocular fragility with corneal rupture and retinal detachment
• Type VII: abnormal conversion of type I procollagen to collagen; two distinct mutations (autosomal recessive [enzyme] and autosomal dominant [structural gene])
• Type IX: defect in copper metabolism, altering lysyl oxidase activity; X-linked recessive

Others

BECKWITH-WIEDEMANN SYNDROME
Macroglossia, omphalocele, characteristic ear creases, hemihypertrophy and/or visceromegaly; also see adrenal cytomegaly, pancreatic islet hyperplasia (often with associated clinical hypoglycemia), and renal medullary dysplasia

Cancer develops in 5%, usually Wilms' tumor

Association with 11p15 duplication, the site of the EGF-2 gene, an insulin-like growth factor; receptors are present in large numbers in the tongue and adrenal cortex

STURGE-WEBER SYNDROME
AKA: encephalo-trigeminal angiomatosis

Variably described as autosomal dominant or recessive

Must have at least two of following:
• Congenital port wine nevus of face (nevus flammeus) in distribution of trigeminal nerve
• Leptomeningeal angiomatosis (may calcify)
• Seizures

• Mental retardation
• Hemiatrophy/hemiparesis (contralateral to facial nevus)
• Eye or choroidal angiomas
• Abnormal development of vessels of head and neck; malformation occurs at 4–8 wk gestation

FIELD DEFECTS
BILATERAL RENAL AGENESIS (POTTER SYNDROME)
1/3000–10,000; male : female = 3 : 1

Failure of development of early ureteric bud from mesonephric duct

Usually sporadic, but somewhat higher than expected recurrence rate

Absent kidney, renal artery, ureter; if bilateral, may have absent bladder

Oligohydramnios: low-set ears, limb deformities, club feet

ASSOCIATIONS
VATER
Frequently seen in stillborns, especially infants of diabetic mothers

Vascular (75%): ventricular septal defect, atrial septal defect, tetralogy of Fallot, patent ductus arteriosus

Vertebral (60%): hemivertebrae or absent pedicles

Anus (60%): imperforate

Tracheo-esophageal fistula (60%)

Renal (75%): hydronephrosis, agenesis, horseshoe kidney

Radius (45%): hypoplastic radii and/or thumbs

Acquired Neonatal Syndromes

RESPIRATORY DISTRESS SYNDROME
AKA: hyaline membrane disease

Most common in males, preterm, appropriate for gestational age, maternal diabetes, cesarean delivery

OK at birth, but within 30 min breathing becomes difficult, rate increases, oxygen requirement increases

Caused by deficiency of surfactant; production of surfactant by type II pneumocytes increases after 35 wk and is stimulated by corticosteroids and thyroxin, inhibited by insulin

Lungs are very solid with thickened septa, loss of lining cells, and formation of hyaline membranes if infant survives several hours

Overall mortality is 20–30%

Complications:
• Bronchopulmonary dysplasia (BPD): epithelial hyperplasia, squamous metaplasia, peribronchial and interstitial fibrosis caused by mechanical ventilation and oxygen toxicity
• Patent ductus arteriosus (PDA): immaturity, hypoxia, acidosis delay closure; left to right shunt → congestive heart failure
• Intraventricular hemorrhage (IVH): germinal matrix area has fragile vessels, susceptible to increased cerebral blood flow accompanying hypoxia
• Necrotizing enterocolitis (NEC): risk increases in respiratory distress syndrome
• Retrolental fibroplasia (RLF): destruction of the retina by oxygen toxicity

ERYTHROBLASTOSIS FETALIS
Most common cause used to be due to Rh antigen (D antigen); maternal antibodies (IgG) cross the placenta to react with the second Rh+ infant in an Rh− mother; in

general, ABO incompatibility prevents sensitization of the mother by clearing Rh incompatible cells quickly

Now that mothers are treated with anti-D Rh antibody to prevent sensitization, the most common cause is ABO incompatibility, seen almost exclusively in type O mothers; even this is limited because A and B antigens are expressed only in low levels on fetal red cells

Infants develop hemolytic anemia, hyperbilirubinemia, and jaundice; hypoxic damage to heart and liver, hypoalbuminemia, anasarca (hydrops fetalis)

Kernicterus: deposition of unconjugated bilirubin in the basal ganglia, leads to significant dysfunction—pigment fades within 24 hr, even in formalin, so must cut brain immediately in suspected cases

SUDDEN INFANT DEATH SYNDROME (SIDS)
AKA: crib death, cot death

Sudden unexpected death in otherwise healthy baby that remains unexplained even after a complete autopsy and examination of the death scene

0.5–2/1000 in U.S.

90% occur before 6 months, most between 2 and 4 months

Death usually occurs during sleep

Factors associated with SIDS
- Maternal: <20 yr, unmarried, smoker, drug abuse, low socioeconomic status, short intergestational interval
- Infant: premature, low birth weight, male, not first sibling, SIDS in a prior sibling, prone sleeping position, bottle feeding (vs. breast feeding)

May be multiple causes, may be related to sleep apnea

1–2% recurrence risk

RUBELLA SYNDROME
Occurs in mothers who become infected in first 16 wk

Risks for malformations in the 1st, 2nd, and 3rd months are 50%, 20%, and 7%

Major triad: cataracts, heart disease, deafness

Other defects include microphthalmia, microcephaly, mental retardation, hepatomegaly, splenomegaly

4

NEOPLASIA

DETECTION OF TUMORS
1,000,000 (10^6) cells weighs ~1 mg; $1 \times 1 \times 1$ mm
10^9 cells weighs ~1 g; $1 \times 1 \times 1$ cm
10^{12} cells weighs ~1 kg; $10 \times 10 \times 10$ cm, usually fatal

METASTATIC ABILITY
Attachment to matrix components (laminin, fibronectin) is important:
- Cells with increased numbers of laminin receptors have greater metastatic potential; some also secrete laminin, which binds to own receptors and then to basement membrane
- RGD-containing peptides, which block the fibronectin receptor on tumor cells, can inhibit metastasis formation

Tumor cells with higher levels of collagenase IV have increased metastatic potential

Platelet coating of tumor cell aggregates in the blood stream improves survivability and implantability

KARYOTYPE CHANGES IN TUMORS

Acute myeloblastic leukemia (AML)-M1	t(9;22)
AML-M2	t(8;21)
AML-M3	t(15;17)
Chronic myelocytic leukemia (CML), (abl), Philadelphia chromosome	t(9;22)(q34;q11)
Acute lymphocytic leukemia (ALL)	t(9;22), t(1;19), t(4;11)
Chronic lymphocytic leukemia (CLL)	+12
Burkitt's (c-myc)	t(8;14)(q24;q32) [90%]
Follicular small cleaved (bcl-2)	t(14;18)(q32;q21)
Neuroblastoma	del 1p
Ewing's sarcoma and PNET	t(11;22)(q24;q12)
Retinoblastoma	del 13q (band q14)
Medulloblastoma	del 17q
Small cell carcinoma (ca.)	del 3p
Renal cell carcinoma	del 3p
Wilms' tumor	del 11p (band p13)
Colorectal carcinoma	del 17p, t(17;*)
Papillary cystadenocarcinoma, ovary	t(6;14)
Mesothelioma	del of 1p, 3p, or 22q
Meningioma	del 22
Leiomyoma	t(12;14); del 7
Leiomyosarcoma	del 1p
Liposarcoma (myxoid)	t(12;16)(q13;p11)
Liposarcoma (well differentiated)	Ring chromosome 12
Fibrosarcoma (infantile)	+8, +11, +17, +20
Myxoid chondrosarcoma	t(9;22)(q31;q12)
Synovial sarcoma	t(X;18)(p11;q11)
Rhabdomyosarcoma (alveolar)	t(2;13)(q35;q14)
Rhabdomyosarcoma (embryonal)	+2q, +8, +20
Clear cell sarcoma	t(12;22)(q13;q12)
Desmoplastic small round cell tumor	t(11;22)(p13;q12)
Dermatofibrosarcoma protuberans	Ring chromosome 17

PREDISPOSITION TO CANCER

CANCER INCIDENCE
Males: Prostate, lung, colorectal, bladder, lymphoma, leukemia, stomach, pancreas
Females: Breast, colorectal, lung, endometrium, lymphoma, pancreas, cervix, leukemia
Single most important environmental factor is smoking

CANCER DEATHS
Males: lung, colorectal, prostate, pancreas
Females: lung (recently passed breast), breast, colorectal, ovary, uterus, pancreas
Steady decrease in deaths from cervical, gastric, and hepatic carcinoma

CHEMICAL CARCINOGENESIS
Multistep ($\geq$two stage) process: requires initiation and promotion
Initiation is irreversible (permanent change in DNA of target cells) and rapid; results from exposure to a carcinogen; dose is cumulative over lifetime because irreversible
Promotion is reversible, must follow initiation (cannot induce tumors by itself or before exposure to initiator), and probably also directly affects DNA
Some carcinogens (complete) can both initiate and promote; others (incomplete) only initiate
Chemical carcinogens can act either directly (e.g., alkylating or acylating agents: all are highly reactive electrophiles) or indirectly (procarcinogens: need to be modified, usually by P-450 mixed function monooxygenase)
Ames test: uses Salmonella typhimurium deficient in histidine synthesis; expose to potential carcinogen (usually with liver homogenate to activate if necessary) and grow on histidine-free medium; count number of colonies that have acquired a mutation activating the histidine synthetase; this test relies on the fact that essentially all carcinogens are in fact mutagens
There is not perfect correlation between in vitro mutagenicity and in vivo carcinogenicity; many DNA insults can be repaired; key mutations may involve the activation of protooncogenes
Promoters: include phorbol esters, phenols, hormones, drugs; most widely used is 12-O-tetradecanoyl phorbol-13-acetate (TPA); promoters are not electrophilic and do not damage DNA; TPA activates protein kinase C by acting as a diacylglycerol analog

29

Promoter action seems to involve epigenetic alterations in expression of genetic information in cells

CARCINOGENIC CHEMICALS

Alkylating agents: (cyclophosphamide, chlorambucil, busulfan; other anti-cancer drugs); activation independent; weak carcinogens; induce lymphoid neoplasms

Polycyclic aromatic hydrocarbons: (benzo-a-pyrene, benzanthracene; produced by combustion of tobacco and from broiling or smoking animal fats); require activation to dihydrodiol epoxides; most potent carcinogens known; induce a wide variety of neoplasms

Aromatic amines and azo dyes: (food dyes); require activation in liver by P-450; hepatocellular carcinoma, bladder cancer (inactive form reactivated by glucuronidase in the bladder)

Naturally occurring carcinogens: aflatoxin B_1 from *Aspergillus flavus;* potent hepatic carcinogen

Nitrosamines: require activation

Others: asbestos (bronchogenic carcinoma, mesothelioma, GI carcinoma); vinyl chloride (hemangiosarcoma of the liver); chromium and nickel (lung cancer); arsenic (skin cancer)

RADIATION CARCINOGENESIS

ULTRAVIOLET RADIATION

UVA (320–400 nm); UVB (280–320 nm); UVC (200–280 nm)

Causes squamous cell carcinoma (SCC), basal cell carcinoma, melanoma in sun-exposed areas

Mechanism is due to formation of pyrimidine dimers in DNA

Individuals with deficient excision repair pathways (e.g., xeroderma pigmentosum) have increased risk, as do other chromosome instability syndromes

In mice, UV light also activates T-suppressor cells, permitting the emergence of highly antigenic tumors

IONIZING RADIATION

Electromagnetic radiation (x-rays, gamma rays) and particulate radiation (alpha, beta particles; neutrons) cause cancer

Dose, dose rate, radiation quality (linear energy transfer values), and host repair pathways all affect efficiency

Leukemia is most common radiation-induced malignancy (except for CLL, which never follows radiation)

Thyroid cancer following radiation in children (~9%) is 2nd most common

Others include breast, lung, salivary glands; more resistant are skin, bone, GI tract

VIRAL ONCOGENESIS

DNA Viruses

Infection of a permissive cell results in full virus life cycle and cell death, so no transformation can occur

Transformation occurs following integration in nonpermissive cells in which expression of early genes is still possible (not damaged by integration)

Mechanisms of oncogenesis are diverse

T-antigens (three in polyoma virus, two in SV-40); polyoma large T immortalizes cells in culture but does not confer malignant phenotype; subsequent action of middle T (binds to cellular *src*) results in malignancy

HUMAN PAPILLOMA VIRUS (HPV)

2,4,7: benign squamous papillomas of skin (warts)

6,11: anogenital and laryngeal papillomas; verrucous carcinoma (genital)

16,18,33: cervical and oral carcinoma

5,8,14: SCC of skin in patients with epidermodysplasia verruciformis (EV)

EPSTEIN-BARR VIRUS (EBV)

Associated with endemic form of Burkitt's lymphoma

Binds C3 receptor on B cells

Found in 100% of nasopharyngeal carcinoma

HEPATITIS B VIRUS

200-fold increased risk of hepatocellular carcinoma

RNA Viruses

All are retroviruses; have three groups of genes (gag [core-proteins]; env [envelope proteins]; pol [reverse transcriptase]) flanked by two (LTRs) long terminal repeats

ACUTE TRANSFORMING VIRUSES

All except rous sarcoma virus are deficient—need helper

Contain a viral oncogene

Rapid induction of tumors

SLOW TRANSFORMING VIRUSES

All are replication competent; contain no oncogenes

Tumorigenicity requires integration near protooncogene

Protooncogenes activated by increased expression or introduction of a mutation

HUMAN T-CELL LEUKEMIA VIRUS

Only known human RNA tumor virus

Binds to CD4 on T cells

Genome contains *tat* genes in addition to *gag, env, pol tat* genes (3) are tumorigenic; activate IL-2, IL-2R, etc.

• HTLV-I: associated with adult T-cell leukemia

• HTLV-II: implicated in hairy cell leukemia

ONCOGENES

Carcinogenesis is a multistep process; no single oncogene will transform normal cells in culture; need combinations of two or more oncogenes

abl

Chromosome 9q34

Abelson murine leukemia virus

CML: translocation of *abl* at 9q to 22q (Philadelphia chromosome), forming a chimeric protein *abl-bcr* (breakpoint cluster region) with tyrosine kinase activity

bcl-1 (PRAD-1)

Chromosome 11q13

PRAD = parathyroid adenomatosis

Protein has sequence similar to that of cyclins

Intermediate (mantle zone) lymphomas: translocation with Ig heavy chain region on 14q32

bcl-2

Chromosome 18q21

Outer mitochondrial membrane protein (25–26 kD) that blocks programmed cell death when overexpressed

Block of apoptosis occurs late in pathway because many causes of apoptosis can be blocked by *bcl*-2

Follicular lymphomas (translocation with Ig region on 14q)

bcl-6

Chromosome 3q27

706 amino acid protein, 90 kD, six zinc fingers on C terminus (DNA binding); localizes to nucleus

Expressed in high levels in B cells (mature); not present in pre-B or plasma cells

Translocations show strong association with diffuse large cell lymphoma

Appears to be involved in decision of B cell to become memory cell, plasma cell, or undergo apoptosis

erb-A

Chromosome 17

Thyroid hormone receptor
Associated with erythroleukemia

erb-B1
Chromosome 7p11-12
Avian erythroblastosis virus
Epidermal growth factor (EGF) receptor tyrosine kinase
Squamous cell carcinoma (amplification)

erb-B2
See *neu,* later

fes (fps)
Chromosome 15q25-26
Feline sarcoma virus
Plasma membrane bound and cytoplasmic tyrosine kinase
AML (translocation)

c-myc
Chromosome 8q24
Avian myelocytomatosis virus
Nuclear protein that regulates transcription; can accelerate apoptosis as well as stimulate mitogenesis
Burkitts lymphoma (translocation of *myc* to Ig heavy chain gene at 14q32)
Also rearranged in some glioblastomas

neu (erb-b2, her-2)
Chromosome 17q11-12; 185 kD phosphoprotein
Resembles truncated EGF receptor; tyrosine kinase
Appears to function in development and growth; increased expression makes cells more sensitive to growth factors
Breast cancer (amplification)

ras
Chromosome 6q16-22
Murine sarcoma virus
Gene product is a 21 kD, highly conserved GTP-binding protein with GTPase activity
Activation of *ras* usually involves point mutation in the 12th, 61st, or 13th codon
Most common mutation seen in human tumors; mutated in 10–15% of all human tumors, 90% pancreatic, 50% lung, 40% colonic adenocarcinoma; also in bladder carcinoma, leukemia, neuroblastoma
H-*ras* (11p15); H = Harvey
K-*ras* (6p11-12; 12p12); K = Kirsten
N-*ras* (1p11-13)

src (pp60)
src 1; chromosome 20q13; *src* 2; chromosome 1p36
Rous sarcoma virus
Plasma membrane bound tyrosine kinase
Interacts with vinculin; no known human tumor

OTHER TYROSINE KINASES
fgr: (1p36) Gardner-Rasheed feline sarcoma
fms: (5q34) feline sarcoma virus; macrophage colony stimulating factor-1 receptor analog; no human tumor
mos: (8q11-22) Moloney murine sarcoma virus; serine/threonine kinase; cytoplasmic distribution
raf: (3p25) serine/threonine kinase
ret: medullary and papillary carcinomas of the thyroid
ros: avian sarcoma virus; related to growth factor receptors
yes: (18q21) avian sarcoma virus; no human tumor

OTHER NUCLEAR PROTEINS
ets: (21q22) supplements action of *myb*
fos: murine osteosarcoma virus; nuclear transcription factor
jun: AP-1 transcription factor
myb: (6q22-24) colon carcinoma (amplification)
L-*myc:* (1p32) small cell carcinoma of lung (amplification)
N-*myc:* (2p23-24) neuroblastoma (amplification)
rel: reticuloendotheliosis
ski: (1q22-24) carcinomas

OTHERS (MISCELLANEOUS)
erb-A: (17q11-12) thyroid hormone receptor; supplements action of *erb*-B
int-2: (11q13) mouse mammary tumor virus; FGF-like
met: (7q22) osteosarcoma
sis: (22q13) simian sarcoma virus; platelet derived growth factor (PDGF)–like, cytoplasm

TUMOR SUPPRESSOR GENES (ANTI-ONCOGENES)

rb (RETINOBLASTOMA) GENE
Chromosome 13q14
Gene spans 150 kb, transcribes as a 4.7 kb mRNA, which encodes the 105 kD "RB protein" (a nuclear DNA binding protein)
Prototype for Knudson's two-hit model
Patients with autosomal dominant hereditary disease carry one mutation in their genome (first hit)
Mutations result in an increased frequency of retinoblastoma and also childhood osteosarcoma

p53
Chromosome 17p13.1; 393 amino acids
Negative regulator of cell cycle
Normally present in low levels and with short half-life
Loss of function mutants have an increased half-life; levels accumulate to 5–100 × normal
Some p53 mutants actually stimulate cell division and can act in a dominant fashion
Mutations in region from amino acid 130–290
Hot spots for mutations: 175, 248, 273
Mutations seen in cancers of colon, breast, lung, and in leukemias, sarcomas
Progression of follicular lymphoma to diffuse large cell lymphoma may be accompanied by p53 mutation

WT-1
Chromosome 11p13
50 kb gene; 52–54 kD nuclear protein; interacts with p53
In embryo: expressed in kidney, mesothelium, gonadal ridge, spleen, CNS
In adults: expressed in kidney, ovary, testis, uterus
Binds same DNA sequence that is bound by a variety of growth factor receptors
Translocations seen in Wilms' tumor and in desmoplastic small round cell tumor

EWS
Putative tumor suppressor gene
Chromosome 22q12
40 kb gene, 17 exons; 61 kD protein
Expressed ubiquitously in all tissues
Translocations seen in Ewings sarcoma/PNET, soft tissue clear cell sarcoma, desmoplastic small round cell tumors, myxoid liposarcoma, AML

brca-1
Chromosome 17q21
Mutations in this gene seen in 5% of all breast cancers, but in 40% of breast cancers of patients from families with two or more individuals with breast cancer
Large gene; different mutations seen in different patients
The product of the altered gene is absent, supporting a role as a tumor suppressor

OTHERS
APC: (5q21) familial adenomatous polyposis coli; carcinomas of colon, stomach, pancreas
DCC: (18q21) carcinomas of colon, stomach
NF1: (17q11) schwannomas, neurogenic sarcomas
NF2: (22q12) schwannomas (central), meningiomas

PARANEOPLASTIC SYNDROMES

Symptom complexes in cancer-bearing patients not readily explainable by the local or distant effects of the tumor itself

- Hypercalcemia: most common paraneoplastic syndrome; can result from destruction of bone by tumor or from secretion of parathyroid hormone (PTH)-like substances by the tumor: SCC (lung, cervix, ovary), clear cell carcinoma (ovary, kidney), dysgerminoma
- Cushing's syndrome: lung (small cell), pancreatic, neural, thymic carcinoid; ectopic production of adrenocorticotropic hormone (ACTH)-like substance
- Syndrome of inappropriate antidiuretic hormone (ADH): small cell carcinoma (lung), intracranial tumors
- Migratory thrombophlebitis (Trousseau's phenomenon): pancreas, lung
- Carcinoid syndrome
- Neuromyopathic syndromes (myasthenia gravis, cerebellar degeneration): lung, breast carcinoma, thymoma
- Acanthosis nigricans (gray-black patches of verrucous hyperkeratotic skin): stomach, lung, uterus
- Dermatomyositis: lung, breast
- Hypertrophic osteoarthropathy (finger clubbing): lung
- Polycythemia: hepatocellular carcinoma, cerebellar hemangioma
- Anemia: thymus

TUMOR ANTIGENS

No unequivocal human tumor specific antigens
However, there is evidence that immune defenses play a role in combating neoplasms

- Immunodeficient individuals have 200-fold increase incidence of tumors (5% of congenital immunodeficients)
- In experimental animals, tumor resistance can be achieved by immunizing with killed tumor cells
- T-cell sensitization occurs in melanomas, neuroblastomas, Burkitt's lymphoma, leukemia, osteosarcoma
- Treatment of patients with IL-2 (or IL-2 treatment of lymphocytes isolated from excised tumor) that induces proliferation of stimulated T cells can lead to partial or complete regression of metastases in patients with renal cell carcinoma or melanoma

ORGAN SYSTEMS

5

HEAD AND NECK

EMBRYOLOGY

Head and neck structures develop largely from the branchial arches (numbered cranial to caudally)

Four branchial arches are well developed and visible on the external surface of the embryo by the 4th wk; the 5th and 6th branchial arches are small and internal

Branchial arches are separated by clefts called *branchial grooves* on the external surface and *pharyngeal pouches* on the internal surface; all branchial grooves but the 1st are obliterated

Each arch consists of mesodermally derived mesenchyme covered externally by ectoderm and internally by endoderm

Ectodermally derived neural crest cells migrate into the mesenchyme, proliferate, and give rise to many mesenchymal structures (bone, muscle, cartilage) in the head and neck

Each branchial arch is supplied by the appropriately numbered aortic arch and has an associated cranial nerve (5, 7, 9, and 10, respectively)

BRANCHIAL ARCHES

1: Mandibular arch: splits into two prominences
  • Smaller (maxillary) forms maxilla, zygomatic bone, part of temporal bone
  • Larger (mandibular) forms mandible
  Cartilage of first arch (Meckel's) forms malleus and incus
2: Hyoid arch: overgrows 3rd and 4th to form cervical sinus; also forms part of hyoid bone, muscles of facial expression; cartilage of second arch (Reichert's) forms stapes, styloid
3: Part of hyoid bone, stylopharyngeus muscle
4 + 6: Laryngeal cartilage, cricothyroid and pharyngeal muscles

PHARYNGEAL POUCHES

1: Together with 1st branchial groove, forms external meatus, middle and inner ear structures, eustachian tube
2: Palatine tonsils
3: Inferior parathyroids and thymus (descend to below the 4th pouch structures)
4: Superior parathyroids
5: [Rudimentary]

DENTAL LAMINA

Primitive epithelium overlying free margins of jaws; origin of primary and permanent teeth; epithelial rests are responsible for odontogenic cysts and tumors

ANOMALIES OF THE BRANCHIAL STRUCTURES

BRANCHIAL SINUS (LATERAL CERVICAL SINUS)

Failure of obliteration of the 2nd branchial groove
Usually a blind pit
If extents into pharynx, forms a branchial fistula

BRANCHIAL CYST

Remnants of cervical sinus or 2nd branchial groove
Often not symptomatic until early adulthood, when enlarges owing to accumulation of fluid and cellular debris

FIRST ARCH SYNDROME

Treacher Collins syndrome: autosomal dominant; malar hypoplasia, defects of lower eyelid, deformed external ear
Pierre Robin syndrome: mandibular hypoplasia, cleft palate, eye and ear defects

CONGENTIAL THYMIC APLASIA (DiGEORGE SYNDROME)

Failure of differentiation of the 3rd and 4th pouches
No thymus and no parathyroids

EAR

Inflammatory

EXTERNAL EAR

KERATINOUS CYSTS

Some related to branchial cleft
Lined by keratinized squamous epithelium
Periauricular cysts may be of pilar type

CAULIFLOWER EAR

Acquired deformity of auricle secondary to cartilage degeneration induced by trauma
Seen in boxers and wrestlers

CHONDRODERMATITIS NODULARIS CHRONICA HELICIS

AKA: Winkler's disease
Small, painful nodular lesion of the helix (usually upper) occurring in the elderly, with a raised center containing a crust or scale; may be confused with basal cell carcinoma or actinic keratosis
Epithelial hyperplasia with inflammation of the underlying collagen and/or cartilage degeneration
No premalignant connotation; treat with simple excision

RELAPSING POLYCHONDRITIS

Episodic acute inflammatory destruction of the cartilage of the helix (not the tragus)
Can also involve nose, ribs, trachea (latter may be fatal)
May be autoimmune, mediated by antibody to type II collagen
Many cases associated with polymyalgia rheumatica

MALIGNANT EXTERNAL OTITIS

Necrotizing inflammation of external canal, often involving bone, caused by *Pseudomonas*
Occurs in diabetics and immunocompromised patients
If not aggressively debrided, will often lead to meningitis, brain abscess, osteomyelitis of base of skull, and death

GOUT
Deposits of sodium urate crystals (tophus) in helix and anti-helix, which can ulcerate

Urate will dissolve in water—not present in histologic sections

MIDDLE EAR
OTITIS MEDIA
Acute form: caused by *Streptococcus pneumoniae* or *Haemophilus influenzae;* bulging hyperemic tympanic membrane

Chronic form: persistent drainage, tympanic membrane perforation, polypoid granulation tissue

CHOLESTEATOMA
Tumor-like lesion of middle ear or mastoid area, grossly resembling a pearl; usually presents in 20s–30s

Epidermal cystic structure filled with desquamated keratin debris and cholesterol crystals

Probably arises from ingrowth of squamous epithelium into middle ear following chronic otitis media with drum perforation; congenital form arises from squamous rests

INNER EAR
OTOSCLEROSIS
Autosomal dominant, variably penetrant, most common cause of conductive hearing loss in young adults

Bone deposition around stapes causing fixation to oval window

Neoplastic
EXTERNAL EAR
All tumors of skin and skin appendages can occur here

MIDDLE EAR
CHORISTOMA
Salivary gland or glial tissue
PARAGANGLIOMA (CHEMODECTOMA)
Glomus jugulare or glomus tympanicum

Most common neoplasm of middle ear after squamous cell carcinoma
MIDDLE EAR ADENOMA
Gray-white, firm lesion producing conductive hearing loss

Solid, glandular, or trabecular growth pattern with cuboidal or cylindrical cells

Benign, but may be locally aggressive with bone destruction
MENINGIOMA
6% of all meningiomas arise from arachnoid villi of the petrous bone and may invade middle ear

INNER EAR
ACOUSTIC NEUROMA
Benign tumor of Schwann cells of VIIIth cranial nerve

Usually internal auditory canal and cerebellopontine angle regions

ORAL CAVITY

Odontogenesis
Epithelial buds on alveolar ridge grow down into primitive stroma

The mandible grows around the developing teeth

An invagination forms and deepens
- Epithelium: ameloblasts (form enamel of tooth)
- Stroma: odontoblasts (form dentin of tooth)

Inflammatory/Non-neoplastic

NONSPECIFIC INFLAMMATORY LESIONS
GINGIVITIS/PERIODONTITIS
Inflammation of soft tissue around teeth or surrounding alveolar bone, respectively

Acute gingivitis can become necrotizing ("trench mouth"), particularly in setting of poor oral hygiene, smoking, stress
APHTHOUS ULCERS (CANKER SORES)
Single or multiple shallow, fibrin-coated ulcers with mononuclear underlying infiltrate

Etiology unknown

Painful
PYOGENIC GRANULOMA (LOBULAR CAPILLARY HEMANGIOMA)
Inflammatory "tumor" composed of granulation tissue

Most commonly maxillary labial gingiva
PALATAL PAPILLOMATOSIS (INFLAMMATORY PAPILLARY HYPERPLASIA)
Multiple foci of epithelial hyperplasia and pseudoepitheliomatous hyperplasia, usually associated with poorly fitting dentures

Not a premalignant condition
PERIPHERAL GIANT CELL TUMOR (EPULIS)
Unusual inflammatory reaction (not neoplastic), characteristically protruding from the gingiva close to teeth

Predilection for females

Intact or ulcerated overlying mucosa

Numerous multinucleated osteoclast-like foreign body giant cells with scant fibroangiomatous stroma

Well delimited and easily excised

SPECIFIC INFLAMMATORY LESIONS
ORAL CANDIDIASIS
AKA: thrush, moniliasis

Proliferates during extensive antibiotic therapy, immunosuppression, severe debilitation
HERPETIC STOMATITIS
More commonly herpes simplex virus (HSV)-I

Lesions can vary from isolated cold sore to blistering lesions over much of the oral mucosa

Initially intra- and intercellular edema, ballooning degeneration, acantholysis, intraepidermal vesicle

Intranuclear inclusions identifiable

ODONTOGENIC CYSTS
Occur around teeth and are derived from remnants of the dental lamina epithelium

Cysts are lined by hyperplastic squamous to thin squamous or cuboidal epithelium; often histologically similar to epidermal inclusion cysts; named most commonly by location (except odontogenic keratocyst)

Types:
- Odontogenic keratocyst: squamous lined cyst with parakeratosis and palisading basal cells; usually posterior, usually multilocular; can be aggressive or destructive; high recurrence rate (Note: this histology

overrides epidermal inclusion cyst [EIC]-like cyst of any location because of its aggressiveness)
- Radicular (periapical) cyst: most common, usually maxillary molars; occurs at apex of tooth root on account of severe pulp inflammation/death from infection or trauma
- Dentigerous cyst: surrounds the crown of an unerupted permanent tooth; can be destructive or deforming
- Eruption cyst: forms over the site of a future tooth eruption; can prevent tooth from coming in
- Primordial cyst: develops where a tooth never was
- Paradental cyst: laterally associated with the crown; essentially exclusively mandibular
- Lateral peridontal cyst: develops in alveolar bone between teeth
- Calcifying odontogenic cyst (Gorlin cyst): painless enlargement of the mandible; may be a tumor, or may just be frequently associated with odontogenic tumors
- Gingival cyst: whitish nodules in the gingiva of infants; looks most like an EIC

FISSURAL CYSTS

Occur at junction points of developing structures, presumably arising from entrapped epithelial tissue
Lined by stratified squamous epithelium or pseudostratified columnar epithelium
- Nasopalatine cyst: most common; usually 30s–50s; occurs in bone or soft tissues
- Median palatine cyst: occurs in posterior midline of palate
- Nasoalveolar cyst (nasolabial): most commonly soft tissues of upper lip, lateral to midline
- Globulomaxillary cyst: occurs in bone at site where globar process and maxillary process fuse

LEUKOPLAKIA

Clinical term: *white plaque;* premalignant lesion
Sharply demarcated; can occur anywhere in oral mucosa
May be orderly mucosal thickening with epidermal hyperplasia and hyperkeratosis, or disorderly hyperplasia with varying degrees of dysplasia up to carcinoma in situ
Erythroplasia (red plaque) more likely to be dysplastic

Neoplastic

SQUAMOUS CELL CARCINOMA

<5% of all malignancies
>90% of all oral malignancies
More common in men
Sites include gingiva, buccal mucosa, floor of mouth, tongue, lip, palate
May have papillary, basaloid, small cell, or spindle cell (pseudosarcomatous) morphology

Staging

T1	≤2 cm	N1	Single ipsilateral LN
T2	2–4 cm		≤3 cm
T3	>4 cm	N2	Ipsilateral LN 3–6
T4	Invades adjacent		cm or multiple LNs
	structures	N3	LN >6 cm diameter

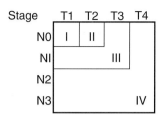

Stage	T1	T2	T3	T4
N0	I	II		
NI			III	
N2				
N3				IV

ODONTOGENIC TUMORS

Epithelial

AMELOBLASTOMA (ADAMANTINOMA)

Most common odontogenic tumor with aggressive potential
Most commonly posterior mandible (80%) in middle 30s
May be associated with dentigerous cyst or impacted (20%) tooth
Almost always at least partially cystic, usually multilocular
Numerous histologic patterns: follicular (most common), acanthomatous, plexiform, unicystic, granular cell, desmoplastic, vascular, basal cell (least common); mixed pattern often seen
Outermost cell layer of tall, columnar, palisading cells with reversed polarity (apically situated nuclei); inner layers of cells form variety of patterns, often with "stellate reticulum cells"
Slow growing; curettage almost always results in recurrence, although may take 10–20 yr; complete excision recommended
Radiation is contraindicated because it too frequently induces malignant transformation
When malignant cytologic features present, often referred to as *ameloblastic carcinoma*

ADENOMATOID ODONTOGENIC TUMOR (ADENOAMELOBLASTOMA)

Anterior maxilla; usually in teens (mean = 18 yr); male : female = 1 : 2
Slow-growing, painless, well-defined (often encapsulated) proliferation of pre-ameloblasts forming rosettes and duct-like tubules
Benign; conservative surgery usually curative

CALCIFYING EPITHELIAL ODONTOGENIC TUMOR (PINDBORG'S TUMOR)

Most commonly mandible; usually 30–40 yr old
Sheets of eosinophilic squamoid cells with nuclear pleomorphism and small cystic areas with amyloid-like material that often calcifies, forming psammoma bodies (Liesegang rings)
Generally less aggressive than ameloblastoma

SQUAMOUS ODONTOGENIC TUMOR

Rare
Anastomosing nests and islands of mature stratified squamous epithelium in bland stroma

Mesenchymal

ODONTOGENIC FIBROMA

Children and young adults, usually mandible
Simple: fibrous connective tissue with plump fibroblasts and nests/strands of odontogenic epithelium
WHO type: very cellular fibrous connective tissue

ODONTOGENIC MYXOMA

20–30 yr old, usually posterior mandible
Slow growing, expansile, can destroy bone

Honeycomb or multilocular, with delicate myxoid stroma containing scattered odontogenic epithelial rests (looks like immature dental pulp)

CEMENTOMA

Includes true cementoma (cementoblastoma), periapical fibrous dysplasia, gigantiform cementoma, and central cementifying fibroma

Mixed

ODONTOMA

Usually maxilla; mean age 15 yr; usually asymptomatic

Multiple benign tumors (complex, compound, ameloblastic), which include "completely differentiated" components, including calcification

Arises from enamel organ

AMELOBLASTIC FIBROMA

Posterior mandible; male ≥ female; mean age 15 yr

Islands of odontogenic epithelium with typical reverse polarity in loose fibrous connective stroma that is often myxoid

AMELOBLASTIC FIBROSARCOMA

Similar to ameloblastic fibroma but with a malignant stromal component; epithelial component remains benign

Usually mandible; mean age 30 yr

NASOPHARYNX AND SINONASAL CAVITIES

Developmental

NASAL GLIAL HETEROTOPIA

AKA: nasal glioma (misnomer, not a tumor)

Firm, solid, polypoid mass composed of neuroglial tissue unconnected to the intracranial contents

Usually present at birth; one third are intranasal, two thirds are extranasal

No malignant potential

NASAL ENCEPHALOCELE

Herniation of brain through a bony defect in the skull

NASAL DERMOID

"Teratomatous" cysts lined by squamous epithelium

Occurs in midline

Inflammatory

RHINITIS

Acute rhinitis, almost always viral

Chronic forms: allergic, nonallergic eosinophilic, and vasomotor

MUCOCELE/MUCOPYOCELE

INFLAMMATORY (ALLERGIC) POLYPS

Unusual before age 20; if occurs in children, most likely indicates cystic fibrosis

Loose edematous stroma with neutrophils, eosinophils, plasma cells, lymphocytes; can become quite large; may erode bone

Stroma frequently contains isolated bizarre cells

WEGENER'S GRANULOMATOSIS

Can produce a necrotizing sinusitis

Necrotizing vasculitis with secondary granulomatous inflammation and epithelial ulceration

Giant cells are also found unassociated with granulomas

SARCOIDOSIS

Neoplastic

SINONASAL PAPILLOMA

Benign but locally aggressive neoplasm occurring in nose and paranasal sinuses, usually of older (40–70 yr) men

Present with epistaxis or mass

Proliferating squamous or columnar epithelium intermixed with mucin-containing cells; mild to moderate atypia

Recur if incompletely excised

FUNGIFORM (TRANSITIONAL-CELL) TYPE (50%)

Exophytic lesions arise from septum

Usually occurs in slightly younger age group

Human papilloma virus (HPV) types 6 and 11 present in high proportion of cases

Rarely become malignant

INVERTED (ENDOPHYTIC) TYPE (47%)

Arise from middle meatus or lateral surface

Also associated with HPV

~13% will progress to malignancy

CYLINDRICAL CELL (ONCOCYTIC SCHNEIDERIAN) TYPE (3%)

Do not appear to be associated with HPV

Sharply defined cell borders, oncocytic cytoplasm, cilia on surface, mucin droplets, and intraepithelial spaces with inflammatory cells

May destroy bone via pressure atrophy

~10% become malignant; does not metastasize

NASOPHARYNGEAL CARCINOMA

Bimodal incidence with peaks at 20 and 65 yr of age; male > female

Epstein-Barr virus (EBV) implicated in pathogenesis of type III and some type II

May be very difficult to detect grossly (most common presentation is unilateral lymph node [LN] metastasis) but may form an ulcerating, fungating growth

Insidiously malignant lesions

Vesicular nuclei with single, large eosinophilic nucleolus

Keratin positive, often EMA (epithelial membrane antigen) positive, may be carcinoembryonic antigen(CEA) positive

KERATINIZING (EPIDERMOID; TYPE I) (25%)

Clear-cut keratinization

Older age group; no association with EBV; less common

5 yr survival 20%; *not* radiosensitive

NONKERATINIZING (TYPE II) (10–15%)

Polygonal cells with well-defined cell margins; resembles transitional cell carcinoma

5 yr survival 35%; variable responsiveness to radiotherapy

UNDIFFERENTIATED (LYMPHOEPITHELIOMA; TYPE III) (60–65%)

Common in males from southern China (Kwantung Province)

Strongest correlation with EBV: polymerase chain reaction (PCR) can demonstrate the viral genome in the tumor cells

Abundant *benign* lymphocytic infiltrate in stroma

Indistinct cell borders

Two patterns:

• Reyaud's: well-defined epithelial rests surrounded by fibrous tissue and lymphoid cells

• Schmincke: epithelial and lymphoid cells diffusely intermingle

SINONASAL CARCINOMA
Rather rare, with a surprising left-sided predominance
Often detected late when has already destroyed bone
Most are squamous cell type, but other types include transitional (cyclindric), verrucous, adenocarcinoma, and undifferentiated carcinoma

ESTHESIONEUROBLASTOMA
AKA: olfactory neuroblastoma
Median age 50 yr, but wide range (3–79 yr)
Reddish-gray, highly vascular polypoid mass
Small round cells of neural crest origin, with round nuclei and indistinct cell borders, with or without Homer-Wright rosettes; may also have larger cells growing in solid nests
Cytologic features not predicative of clinical behavior
Highly malignant
Translocation of 11 to 22 seen commonly (same as Ewing's)
Very sensitive to radiation

ANGIOFIBROMA
Present with nasal obstruction and epistaxis
Almost exclusively in adolescent males; androgen dependent
Non-encapsulated intricate mixture of blood vessels (with thin walls, no elastic laminae, minimal if any smooth muscle) and fibrous stroma (dense to edematous, often with stellate plump nuclei, can have giant cells)
Electron microscopy: tight RNA–protein complexes, forming dense, round granules in the nuclei of fibroblasts
Benign, but may bleed extensively during surgery

POLYMORPHIC RETICULOSIS
Variant of peripheral T-cell lymphoma
Clinical term: *lethal midline granulomas,* a syndrome with ulcerating mucosal lesions of the upper respiratory tract, unresponsive to antibiotic therapy
Extensive tissue necrosis, cartilage destruction, vascular thrombosis, large atypical cells in lymphoid aggregates, many of which mark as T cells
Frequently lethal on account of bacterial infection or hemorrhage

OTHERS
ISOLATED "EXTRAMEDULLARY" PLASMACYTOMA
Often polypoid growths into nasal sinuses or nose
Overlying mucosa usually intact
Very radiosensitive (x-ray therapy often chosen over surgery)
SMALL CELL CARCINOMA
MALIGNANT MELANOMA
LOBULAR CAPILLARY HEMANGIOMA
HEMANGIOPERICYTOMA
~10% of all hemangiopericytomas occur in the sinuses
SOLITARY FIBROUS TUMOR OF THE NASOPHARYNX
FIBROUS HISTIOCYTOMA
EMBRYONAL RHABDOMYOSARCOMA
GIANT CELL TUMOR
ANEURYSMAL BONE CYST
MENINGIOMA
Usually transitional cell or menigothelial pattern
MYXOMA

LARYNX

NON-NEOPLASTIC LESIONS
ACUTE EPIGLOTTITIS
Due to infection with *Haemophilus influenzae* type B
Cherry red, markedly edematous epiglottis—can cause complete airway obstruction
NONSPECIFIC "GRANULOMAS"
Usually unilateral vocal cord lesions composed of cellular granulation tissue, often with overlying ulceration
True granulomas are not seen
Believed to be caused by trauma
CONTACT ULCERS OF LARYNX
Pyogenic granuloma-like lesions occurring on the posterior aspect of the vocal cords with overlying epithelial ulceration or hyperplasia
Present with hoarseness, dysphagia, pain, sore throat
Caused by vocal cord abuse: shouting, intubation, gastric regurgitation, persistent coughing
LARYNGEAL NODULE
AKA: singer's nodule, amyloid tumor, "vocal cord polyp"
Non-inflammatory reaction of vocal cord to injury
Usually at junction of anterior one third and posterior two thirds of cord
Stromal edema with fibroblast proliferation, then dilated vessels and stromal hyalinization
Occasionally the term *polyp* is used to refer to a single lesion and *nodules* when bilateral
Telangiectatic, fibrous, hyaline, and edematous–myxoid types

PAPILLOMAS
JUVENILE LARYNGEAL PAPILLOMA
Multiple tumors on true cords, which may spread to the false cords, epiglottis, even tracheobronchial tree; often recur
Related to HPV-6 and 11
Papillary or acanthotic growth of well-differentiated squamous cells with mild atypia and some mitoses overlying fibrovascular core
Repeated treatment may lead to destruction of the cords
ADULT LARYNGEAL PAPILLOMA
Male predominance; usually solitary
More inflammation
Dysplasia more significant; probably precursor to carcinoma
Does not spread or recur
VERRUCA VULGARIS

LARYNGEAL CARCINOMA
2.2% of all cancers in men, 0.4% in women; 96% are male
Most patients in 40s or older; mean age 55 yr
Epidemiologically linked to tobacco and/or alcohol use
Histologically, >95% are squamous cell carcinomas, which are either well, moderately, or poorly differentiated
GLOTTIC (60–65%)
Arise from true vocal cords, almost always anterior one third
Remain localized for long period because surrounded by cartilage; few lymphatics
LN metastases unheard of for T1 lesions, rare even in T2 lesions
May be effectively treated with radiation
SUPRAGLOTTIC (30–35%)
False cord, epiglottis, arytenoid, aryepiglottic fold
Very rarely invades downward to the glottis; amenable to horizontal supraglottic partial laryngectomy

LN metastases in about 40%; 20–35% of clinically negative nodes will be positive

TRANSGLOTTIC (<5%)
Tumor involves laryngeal ventricle
Highest incidence of LN involvement (52%)

SUBGLOTTIC (<5%)
Exclusively subglottic (rare) or true cord lesion, extending more than 1 cm subglottically
Most aggressive site: cervical LN metastases in 15–20%, paratracheal nodes positive in 50%
Frequent extension to trachea and esophagus

Staging

T1   Confined to site of origin; normal cord mobility
T2   Involves adjacent site; normal cord mobility
T3   Confined to larynx with cord fixation
T4   Extension beyond larynx
N1   Single ipsilateral LN ≤3 cm
N2   Single ipsilateral LN 3–6 cm or multiple LNs
N3   LN >6 cm diameter

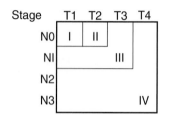

PROGNOSIS

5 yr survivals	I	II	III	IV
Glottic	90%	85%	60%	20%
Supraglottic	85%	75%	40%	15%
Transglottic		50%		
Subglottic		40%		

SPECIAL HISTOLOGIC TYPES
Verrucous: 1–3%, most are glottic, pushing margin, better prognosis
Basaloid: most commonly supraglottic; very aggressive with poor prognosis
Spindle cell (sarcomatoid): most commonly glottic; polypoid mass; stromal component may be truly malignant; epithelial component most commonly metastasizes
Transitional
Small cell

OTHER LARYNGEAL TUMORS
Salivary gland–like tumors
Paraganglioma
Chondrosarcoma
Rhabdomyoma
Synovial sarcoma
Lymphoma
Granular cell tumor

6

SALIVARY GLANDS

NORMAL ANATOMY

Major salivary glands:
- Parotid: largest, main duct (Stensen's) enters oral cavity opposite 2nd maxillary molar
- Submaxillary: 1/4 size of parotid, main duct (Wharton's) empties into floor of mouth
- Sublingual: 1/12 size of parotid; empties into floor of mouth

Minor salivary glands: oropharynx, gingiva, floor of mouth, cheek, hard and soft palates, tonsillar areas, tongue

Terminal portion (intercalated ducts and acini = ducto-acinar unit), esp. reserve cells of intercalated ducts, probable source of most neoplasms

Xerostomia: dry mouth on account of decreased salivary flow

ABNORMAL LOCATION/GROWTH

Heterotopia: within lymph nodes in and near parotid, neck (often associated with cysts or sinuses)

Choristoma: nodule (usually gingival) of disorganized seromucinous salivary tissue plus sebaceous glands

Adenomatoid hyperplasia: localized nodule of hyperplastic glands, usually in hard palate

INFLAMMATORY AND RELATED DISORDERS

SIALOLITHIASIS

Calculi can form in major ducts, sometimes multicentric

Most common in submaxillary gland (higher calcium content, largest duct)

Initially swelling and distention of ducts, then acini

Eventually, destruction of acini, chronic inflammation, induration

CHRONIC SIALADENITIS

May be caused by obstruction of small ducts

In older females, related to rheumatoid arthritis; autoimmune (?)

Granulomatous sialadenitis can result from TB, fungus, sarcoidosis, or secondary to duct obstruction/rupture

NECROTIZING SIALOMETAPLASIA

Self-limited, benign inflammation; lobular necrosis; central acini undergo squamous metaplasia

Most common in palate

CYSTS

Benign lymphoepithelial cysts: epithelial lined with prominent lymphoid infiltrate in walls with germinal centers

Most common sites: lower lip, cheeks, tip of tongue

May be acquired (e.g., HIV), retention, or developmental

Also seen with warthin's tumor, mucoepidermoid carcinoma, benign mixed tumor, sebaceous lymphadenoma

MIKULICZ'S DISEASE (BENIGN LYMPHOEPITHELIAL LESION)

Most common cause of Mikulicz's syndrome, the diffuse, enlargement of bilateral salivary and lacrimal glands

One manifestation of Sjögren's syndrome (also keratoconjunctivitis, rheumatoid arthritis, hypergammaglobulinemia, xerostomia)
- Lymphoid infiltration (often with germinal centers—mixed B and T cell)
- Epimyoepithelial islands: collapsed acini with basal epithelial cells, modified myoepithelial cells, hyaline material (basement membrane), and lymphocytes

May progress to lymphoma, usually large cell, B-cell immunoblastic

Also small cleaved cell lymphomas

OTHERS

Keratinous cysts, amyloidosis, nodular fasciitis, cystic fibrosis

NEOPLASMS

General

Tumors 12× more common in the parotid than submaxillary

Only ~20% parotid tumors are malignant vs. ~40% for submaxillary gland and ~45% for palate; sublingual gland has highest incidence of malignancy

Tumors of submaxillary gland have worse prognosis than the same tumor in the parotid

Pain, facial nerve paralysis, rapid growth suggest malignancy

Benign or low-grade malignancy of superficial parotid can be treated with superficial parotidectomy, sparing facial nerve

Recurrence following excision, short survival

Radiation postoperatively may decrease local recurrence

Staging

T1	≤2 cm	N0	None
T2	2–4 cm	N1	Single ipsilateral LN ≤3 cm
T3	4–6 cm	N2	Single LN 3–6 cm or multiple LNs
T4	a. >6 cm	N3	Any LN >6 cm
	b. Any size with local extension		

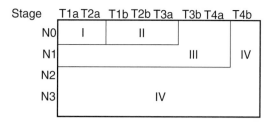

Stage	T1a T2a	T1b T2b T3a	T3b T4a	T4b
N0	I	II		
N1			III	IV
N2				
N3		IV		

PLEOMORPHIC ADENOMA

AKA: benign mixed tumor (BMT)

Despite its name, the entire tumor is of epithelial origin

Most common neoplasm of salivary glands (60–80%)

75% of all parotid neoplasms, <50% of all palatal neoplasms

Parotid : submaxillary : sublingual = 10 : 1 : <<1

75% in superficial lobe of parotid, 25% deep

Most frequently seen in women in 30s; presents as painless, persistent swelling

Gross: rubbery, well-circumscribed, bosselated mass with small extensions; cartilage may be present

Wide variety of histologic appearances, including glandular, spindled, pseudovascular patterns, focal squamous metaplasia

May be focally very cellular, or be predominantly stroma

Stroma can be myxoid or hyalinized; usually some cartilage

Mesenchymal elements derived from myoepithelial cells

Two types of mucin (both actually epithelial in origin):
• Epithelial type: neutral glycoprotein
• Stromal type: highly sulfated glycosaminoglycans

Epithelium is keratin, epithelial membrane antigen, carcinoembryonic antigen (CEA), lysozyme positive

Myoepithelium: keratin, actin, myosin, S-100 positive

Focal areas of penetration of surrounding tissue can result in a high recurrence rate, multifocally, if not widely excised

Recurrences may occur over 50 yr later—may be intractable

MALIGNANT MIXED TUMOR

MALIGNANT TRANSFORMATION OF PLEOMORPHIC ADENOMA

Occurs in 5–10% of benign mixed tumors

Clinical indications: sudden increase in size, pain, paralysis

Sometimes, only hyalinized scar may indicate former benign mixed tumor

Malignancy is limited to the epithelial component: can be any pattern; terminal duct type has best prognosis

If malignancy confined to the benign mixed tumor, excision usually curative; with extension >8 mm beyond capsule, often die of tumor

Metastases to regional LNs, lungs, bone, abdominal organs

TRUE MALIGNANT MIXED TUMOR

AKA: carcinosarcoma; carcinoma ex pleomorphic adenoma

Both epithelial and "stromal" elements are malignant; both metastasize

Aggressive, often rapidly lethal

MONOMORPHIC ADENOMA

Includes benign tumors that are not pleomorphic adenomas

Simple excision usually curative; malignant forms are rare

WARTHIN'S TUMOR

AKA: adenolymphoma, papillary cystadenoma lymphomatosum

More common in men, usually ~60 yr old; often multicentric, bilateral in 10–15%; accounts for 70% of bilateral tumors

Almost exclusive to the parotid

Often cystic with papillary growth of two layers of oncocytic epithelial cells associated with numerous inflammatory cells with germinal centers (predominantly B cells)

May undergo hemorrhagic infarction with necrosis

Epithelial cells, granular, loaded with mitochondria

No myoepithelial cell component

May arise in ectopic salivary gland tissue in LNs

OXYPHILIC ADENOMA

AKA: oncocytoma, mitochondrioma

Solid, well-circumscribed mass; tan

Exclusively composed of oxyphilic cells; granular cytoplasm

Electron microscopy: cytoplasm packed with mitochondria with partitions (dividing?)

Clear cell change can result from cystic dilatation of the mitochondria

BASAL CELL ADENOMA

Some pathologists use the term *monomorphic adenoma* only for this entity because it is the most monomorphic

~2% of all salivary gland tumors; 75% occur in parotid

Mean age 58 yr

Grossly encapsulated, often cystic, generally smaller than benign mixed tumors; most common in parotid

Uniform, monotonous cells with palisading at the periphery of the epithelial nests

Growth patterns: tubular, trabecular, canalicular, solid, dermal eccrine; may be confused with adenoid cystic

Abundant basal lamina material around and within epithelial nests

Canalicular pattern much more common in upper lip

SEBACEOUS ADENOMA

When prominent lymphoid stroma: sebaceous lymphadenoma

Malignant counterparts exist

SIALADENOMA PAPILLIFERUM

Papillary lesion of oral cavity, usually hard palate

Exophytic mass of well-differentiated squamous epithelium covering glandular component with cleftlike cystic spaces lined by cuboidal or columnar epithelium; cells may be oncocytic

INVERTED DUCTAL PAPILLOMA

Small submucosal mass in oral cavity

Well-differentiated, predominantly squamous epithelium associated with microcysts, occasional mucous cells, columnar lining

MYOEPITHELIOMA

Tumor composed "exclusively" of myoepithelial cells: S-100+, SMA+, keratin+

Some pathologists consider this a monomorphic adenoma, some a variant of benign mixed tumor

Three major morphological types exist:
• Spindle cell type: stroma-like, scanty collagen, microcystic formations, myxoid change (most common)
• Hyaline (plasmacytoid) cell type: eccentric nuclei, pleomorphic, no mitoses; diffuse (vs. granular) eosinophilic cytoplasm, polygonal cell margins sharply outlined

- Clear cell type (AKA: glycogen-rich adenoma, tubular carcinoma, epithelial-myoepithelioma): tubules of clear cells with hyaline stroma; glycogen, but no fat or mucin; multinodular growth pattern, partial capsule

Spindle cell and clear cell types occur usually in parotid; hyaline type most common in palate

Hyaline cell type usually benign, clear cell type often malignant: 37% recur locally, 17% LN metastases, 9% die

MUCOEPIDERMOID CARCINOMA

Most common malignant tumor of parotid; most common malignant salivary gland tumor in children

Can range from very indolent to overtly malignant

Four cell types: mucinous, squamous, intermediate, clear

- Low grade: well-circumscribed, cystic areas, predominantly well-differentiated mucinous cells
- High grade: ≥20% of the tumor is more solid, infiltrative; predominantly squamous, intermediate, and clear cells; marked nuclear atypia is generally *not* seen

Mucin or keratin may escape, causing inflammatory reaction

Prognosis: 5 yr survival: 98% for low grade, 60% for high

Recurrences/metastases usually occur within 5 yr, or never

ADENOID CYSTIC CARCINOMA

AKA: cylindroma

3rd most common malignancy in parotid, 1st in minor salivary glands

Grossly: solid, infiltrative

Hyperchromatic angulated nuclei, clear cytoplasm

Three histologic patterns: cribriform, tubular, solid; usually mixed with all three present; classify by most predominant pattern

Pseudocysts with hyaline-like PAS+ material often seen in cribriform areas

Marked propensity for perineural invasion; spread along nerves accounts for high recurrence rate

Mesenchymal areas and squamous metaplasia consistently absent (unlike pleomorphic adenoma)

Immunohistochemically, cells in ducts react like intercalated duct cells (positive for keratin, CEA, S-100), cells in pseudocysts react like myoepithelial cells (positive for S-100, actin, ± keratin); amorphous material positive for laminin and type IV collagen

Slow growing but highly malignant, with late recurrences (good 5 yr survival, but much worse at 15 yr)

15 yr survival based on pattern: 5% for solid, 26% for cribriform, 39% for tubular

Prognosis better when in palate than when in parotid; worst in submaxillary gland

Metastases most commonly to lung (often silent); LN metastases rare

ACINIC CELL CARCINOMA

1–3% of all salivary gland tumors; most in parotid

Male predominance; peak incidence in the 3rd decade

Grossly: encapsulated, solid, friable, gray-white, ≤3 cm

Histologic patterns: solid ("classic"), microcystic (most common), papillary cystic, and follicular (least common); prognosis is independent of histologic pattern

Frequently have a granular, basophilic cells with numerous zymogen granules

Other cell types include: intercalated duct type, clear, vacuolated, nonspecific glandular

When clear cells (glycogen containing) predominate: hypernephroid

May see peripheral lymphoid infiltrate, central psammoma bodies

Survival: 89% 5 yr, 56% 20 yr; completeness of excision most important factor

ADENOCARCINOMA

TERMINAL DUCT CARCINOMA

AKA: lobular carcinoma, polymorphous low-grade adenocarcinoma

Usually restricted to minor salivary glands/oral cavity

Palate most common location (2nd most common type)

Uniform cell type (plump, columnar) with variable patterns: tubular, cribriform, papillary, solid, fascicular, Indian-file

Background can be mucinous or fibrous

Low-grade malignancy: 12% recur, 10% LN metastases, no distant metastases

SALIVARY DUCT CARCINOMA

Elderly males, usually parotid, sometimes submaxillary

Micro: resembles ductal carcinoma of breast: comedo, solid, papillary, or not otherwise specified (NOS)

Highly aggressive: 70% mortality

PAPILLARY ADENOCARCINOMA (PAPILLARY CYSTADENOCARCINOMA)

Less than 3% of all parotid tumors

May become large—hemorrhage and necrosis common

Well-defined papillary structures microscopically, mucinous component, often nuclear atypicality

Low grade vs. high grade based on stromal invasion

ADENOCARCINOMA, NOS

Two thirds occur in major salivary glands

Usually asymptomatic

Designate as low grade or high grade based on cytologic atypia

SEBACEOUS CARCINOMA

Rare; most common in parotid

Pleomorphic, atypical cells arranged in sheets and nests

Often present as painful mass with facial nerve paralysis

OTHER NEOPLASMS

MALIGNANT LYMPHOMA

Prototypical location for mucosal associated lymphoid tissue (MALT) lymphomas

Usually follicular center cell lymphomas, with slow evolution and good long-term prognosis

Those arising in Mikulicz's disease usually immunoblastic with more rapid clinical course

CAPILLARY HEMANGIOMA (BENIGN HEMANGIOENDOTHELIOMA)

Most common salivary gland tumor in infants and children

Permeate through glandular elements, often with mitoses

Do not become malignant; often spontaneously regress

NEURILEMOMA

PILOMATRIXOMA

EMBRYOMA

Highly cellular epithelial parotid tumor of infancy with blastomatous appearance; rare

GIANT CELL TUMORS

EPIDERMOID CARCINOMA

Usually represent metastases to intraparotid lymph nodes

SMALL CELL (ANAPLASTIC) CARCINOMA
Scanty cytoplasm, small cells, solid pattern, many mitoses
Neuroendocrine features found in some

LYMPHOEPITHELIOMA-LIKE CARCINOMA
More frequent among Eskimos and Chinese

Similar to Mikulicz's disease at low power, but epithelial
islands are malignant cytologically
As with lymphoepithelioma (nasopharyngeal carcinoma),
may be EBV related
Overall outcome not too bad

7

LUNG AND PLEURA

NORMAL ANATOMY
Average adult weight 350–435 g
Right is trilobed; left is bilobed, the left "middle" lobe being assumed by the lingula
Bifurcation of trachea at level of 4th and 5th ribs: right main-stem bronchus more vertical and more direct: receives most aspirated material
Trachea and major bronchi have C-shaped cartilage rings; cannot be totally occluded by bronchoconstriction
Bronchi have discontinuous plates of cartilage and submucosal glands
First-order bronchi = lobar bronchi
Second-order bronchi (segmental bronchi) are numbered in order from proximal to distal: 10 on right, 9 on left:

Left upper lobe (LUL): B1–B4	Right upper lobe (RUL): B1–B3
Lingula: B5	Right middle lobe (RML): B4–B5
Left lower lobe (LLL): B6, B8–B10	Right lower lobe (RLL): B6–B10

Bronchioles: no cartilage or submucosal glands; Clara cells secrete nonmucinous lining protein
Acinus: terminal bronchiole plus supplied respiratory bronchioles, alveolar ducts and alveolar sacs
Lobule: 3–5 terminal bronchioles and supplied acini
Pores of Kohn interconnect alveoli
Canals of Lambert: direct accessory bronchioloalveolar connections
Double arterial system: pulmonary and bronchial; single venous system: pulmonary
Pseudostratified ciliated columnar epithelium from larynx to bronchioles (except vocal cords: squamous)
Type I pneumocytes cover 95% alveolar surface
Type II pneumocytes contain lamellar bodies of surfactant
Inhaled particles over 10 μm in size tend to impact on nasal or pharyngeal walls; 3–10 μm impact in large airways; 1–5 μm impact in terminal airways and alveoli; <1 μm tend to remain suspended and are exhaled
Pulmonary defense mechanisms: nasal clearance, mucociliary ladder, alveolar macrophages

Congenital Malformations

TRACHEOBRONCHIAL MALFORMATIONS
LARYNGEAL WEB
Incomplete recanalization of the larynx during the 10th wk
Membranous web forms at the level of the vocal cords, partially obstructing the airways
TRACHEOESOPHAGEAL FISTULA (TEF)
Incomplete division of foregut into respiratory and digestive portions

Five types:
- Focal esophageal atresia: proximal esophagus ends as blind pouch (dilated); distal arises from trachea just above bifurcation; 85% of all TEFs
- Both esophageal segments blind pouches (8%)
- Both trachea and esophagus complete, but connected at level of bifurcation (4%)
- Focal esophageal atresia: proximal esophagus connects to trachea at level of bifurcation; distal arises as blind pouch
- Focal esophageal atresia: both proximal and distal esophageal segments communicate with the trachea

TRACHEAL STENOSIS/ATRESIA
Rare
Usually associated with some tracheoesophageal fistula

PULMONARY SEQUESTRATION
Partial or complete separation of a portion of a lobe from the "surrounding" lung; sequestered segment has no connection to the main bronchial tree
Blood supply from aorta, not from pulmonary arteries
20% of patients have a histology of congenital cystic adenomatoid malformation
INTRALOBAR SEQUESTRATION
Enclosed within pleura of "normal" lung
Usually lower lobe; 60% on the left
More likely to be symptomatic: recurrent infections or bronchiectasis
Usually large systemic arterial supply: 25% arise below diaphragm; may have shunts to pulmonary vessels; subclassified as type I, II, or III for extensive, slight, absent overlap between circulations
Venous drainage is into pulmonary veins
Chronic inflammation, fibrosis, obliteration of vessels
May be congenital or acquired after multiple pneumonias
EXTRALOBAR SEQUESTRATION
Separated from pleural covering of lung; may be found anywhere in thorax or mediastinum; 90% occur on left
Associated with polyhydramnios and edema
Systemic arterial supply, usually small
Venous drainage is into azygous veins

BRONCHOGENIC CYSTS
May occur anywhere in lung; usually single, occasionally multiple; range from microscopic to >5 cm
Usually found adjacent to bronchi or bronchioles
Lined by bronchial-type epithelium; connective tissue may contain cartilage or mucous glands
Cavities usually filled with mucinous secretions or air; when infected, may lead to progressive metaplasia of lining or total necrosis of wall, leading to lung abscess
May rupture into bronchi or pleural cavity

CONGENITAL LOBAR/LOBULAR EMPHYSEMA

Presents in very young children as sudden progressive respiratory distress

Affects upper lobes or RML most commonly

Massive overdistention of airways without tissue destruction

CONGENITAL CYSTIC ADENOMATOID MALFORMATION

AKA: cystic adenomatoid transformation

Seen in neonates with respiratory distress, but occasionally in older children

Solitary lesions, usually lower lobe

Various-sized intercommunicating cysts with an adenomatoid cuboidal pseudostratified epithelium and smooth muscle proliferation; no cartilage

Classification: based on size of cysts and "level of origin" based on histologic appearance (e.g., bronchial to alveolar):

- Type 0 (<5%): main bronchus–like structures
- Type I (65%): large cyst or cysts (~10 cm), often surrounded by smaller cysts; bronchial-like
- Type II (25%): medium-sized (<2.5 cm) cysts surrounded by "normal" lung; bronchiolar-like
- Type III (<10%): large number of small (<1.5 cm) cysts; terminal bronchiolar-like
- Type IV (<5%): flattened epithelium; alveolar-like

Other associated anomalies, pulmonary and extrapulmonary, seen in 50% of patients with type II histology, 12% of patients with type I histology, but no patients with type III

CYSTIC FIBROSIS

AKA: mucoviscidosis

Autosomal recessive; 1/20 whites are carriers

Variable penetrance

Gene is on chromosome 7 (7q22-7q31): encodes CFTR gene, a putative chloride transporter

Results in defective anion transport, particularly Cl^- and HCO_3^-, with subsequent abnormal water movement

In sweat glands of skin, sweat ducts cannot take up Cl^- back from secretions: sweat high in NaCl

In lungs, decreased Cl^- transport into lumen results in viscous secretions, which plug airways; Infections by *Staphylococcus* and *Pseudomonas* common, often fatal (major cause of death)

Pneumonias/Inflammation

LOBAR PNEUMONIA

95% caused by pneumococci, most commonly types 1, 3, 7, 2

Other agents: *Klebsiella, Staphylococcus, Streptococcus, Haemophilus influenza*

Widespread fibrinosuppurative consolidation

Four stages:

- Congestion: (~24 hr) vascular engorgement, intraalveolar fluid, numerous bacteria, few neutrophils
- Red hepatization: Extravasated RBCs, fibrin, increasing numbers of neutrophils
- Gray hepatization: much more fibrin and neutrophils, disintegrating RBCs
- Resolution

BRONCHOPNEUMONIA

Patchy consolidation of lung with foci of acute suppurative inflammation that are poorly defined grossly

Can be extensive, merging to involve an entire lobe

ASPIRATION

Usually right lower lobe, then RUL, then LLL

Can see significant destruction (out of proportion to inflammation), foreign body giant cells

INFECTIOUS

Most commonly basal

Staphylococcus, Streptococcus, Pneumococcus, Haemophilus influenza, Pseudomonas

COMPLICATIONS

Abscess: may be secondarily colonized by mucormycosis or *Aspergillus*

Empyema

Organization

LIPOID PNEUMONIA

AKA: golden pneumonia

Well circumscribed, firm

Lipid accumulation within foamy macrophages

Inflammation, proliferating pneumocytes, ± reactive endarteritis

ENDOGENOUS (OBSTRUCTIVE)

Most commonly from obstruction by tumor, lymph node (LN), abscess

Lipid derived from degenerating type II pneumocytes

Cholesterol clefts, giant cells

EXOGENOUS

Aspiration of lipid materials

Right lung more commonly than left

Multinucleated giant cells

INFECTIOUS GRANULOMATOUS INFLAMMATION

Can assume a variety of patterns and mimic any of the noninfectious granulomatous disorders

Vasculitis of infection more likely to show mural infiltrate of lymphocytes and plasma cells; few neutrophils

HISTOPLASMOSIS

Histoplasma capsulatum: oval-shaped, 1–5 μm, occasional buds

Necrotizing granulomas with cores composed of multiple concentric lamellae, frequently calcified, surrounded by palisading histiocytes and active inflammation, surrounded by zone of acellular collagen

Organisms identified by silver stain in necrotic cores

COCCIDIOIDOMYCOSIS

Coccidioides immitis: numerous small (2–5 μm) endospores within thick-walled spherule (30–60 μm)

Necrotizing granuloma often with prominent eosinophilic infiltrate in surrounding tissue with organisms distributed throughout necrotic and viable zones

CRYPTOCOCCOSIS

Cryptococcus neoformans; soil, pigeon droppings; 2–15 μm

Intracellular collections in histiocytes impart bubbly look

Bright red staining of capsule with mucicarmine

Varying dimensions

Usually necrotizing granulomas; some non-necrotizing

BLASTOMYCOSIS

Blastomyces dermatitidis; 8–15 μm; round

Initially acute inflammation followed by granulomas with centers containing necrotic neutrophils

Numerous round, refractile organisms; stain strongly with mucicarmine

MYCOBACTERIUM TUBERCULOSIS
AKA: Koch bacillus

Infection used to be seen mostly in children and young adults; now more common in 50–60 yr olds

Two species: one predominantly infects humans (transmitted by inhalation) and the second is a bovine strain, which is now much less common but causes GI infections from infected milk

Histology: hallmark lesion is caseating granuloma (soft tubercle), although may have a cellular center (hard tubercle)

Ghon focus: 1–1.5 cm gray-white inflammatory consolidation seen at the periphery of the upper part of lower lobe or lower part of upper lobe (greatest volume of air flow) that becomes granulomatous and then centrally necrotic by the 2nd week—primary infection focus, usually clinically silent

Ghon complex: combination of primary lung lesion and ipsilateral LN involvement

Rarely, primary focus will rapidly enlarge, erode into bronchi, giving rise to satellite lesions—may seed blood stream, resulting in miliary dissemination or meningitis

Secondary TB arises usually from reactivation of old primary lesions; present as apical or posterior segment lesions (tuberculomas), may be bilateral; can either scar down, create progressive pulmonary TB, leading to tuberculous empyema, intestinal TB (if aspirated material is swallowed), or miliary seeding

Isolated distant organ involvement is also seen: cervical lymph node, meninges, kidneys, adrenals, bones, fallopian tubes, epididymis

Secondary TB usually accompanied by fever, night sweats, weakness, fatigability, loss of appetite

DIROFILARIASIS
Dirofilaria immitis: canine heartworm

Most patients asymptomatic

Well-circumscribed coin lesion radiographically

Central "infarct" with surrounding granulomatous inflammation

Organisms within lumen of necrotic artery: ~200 μm diameter with thick, multilayered cuticle with transverse striations

Organisms may calcify with time

ADDITIONAL SPECIFIC INFECTIOUS AGENTS
PNEUMOCYSTIS CARINII
Immunocompromised host

Foamy or honeycombed intraalveolar exudate with an interstitial lymphoplasmacytic infiltrate

Cysts identifiable by silver stain: 5 μm in diameter with single or paired intracystic bodies (1–2 μm); some cysts may be folded or collapsed

CYTOMEGALOVIRUS (CMV)
Immunocompromised host

May be multifocal, miliary, or diffuse

Predominantly mononuclear inflammation with edema and alveolar epithelial hyperplasia

Foci of hemorrhagic necrosis can be seen

Viral inclusions usually found: both nuclear and cytoplasmic

ADENOVIRUS
Bronchocentric; transmural bronchiolitis with marked destructive inflammation; bronchiolitis obliterans

Smudge cells

ASPERGILLUS
Second most common infective fungus, especially in hospitals

45° angle branching septate hyphae

Three types of infection:
- Allergic bronchopulmonary aspergillosis: inhalation of large numbers of spores, producing a hypersensitivity reaction in bronchi or alveoli (see later under Asthma)
- Colonizing (secondary): growth of organisms in pulmonary cavity forming a mass (aspergilloma) without invasion
- Invasive (primary): opportunistic infection involving primarily lung but also heart valves, brain, kidneys: targetoid lesions with necrotizing center and hemorrhagic border; angioinvasive hyphal forms

DIFFUSE ALVEOLAR DAMAGE (DAD)
Severe acute injury from toxic insult: viruses (influenza), mycoplasma, inhalants (>70% oxygen, smoke, noxious gases), drugs (chemotherapeutic, heroin), ingestants (kerosene, paraquat), shock, sepsis, radiation (10% patients receiving chest radiation), acute pancreatitis, heat, burns, uremia, systemic lupus erythematosus, high altitude, molar pregnancy

Etiology cannot be determined histologically

Abrupt onset of severe arterial hypoxia that is not responsive to O_2 therapy

Combination of endothelial and epithelial injury—bilateral and diffuse
- Exudative stage:
  First week following injury
  Initially, edema (interstitial, intraalveolar), hemorrhage
  Fibrin deposition and thrombi in small vessels/capillaries
  Hyaline membrane formation (3–7 days)
  Sloughing of alveolar cells, denudation of basement membrane
  X-ray often normal
- Proliferative stage:
  Begins in 2nd week
  Increasing interstitial inflammation
  Fibroblast proliferation and interstitial fibrosis
  Organization and phagocytosis of hyaline membranes
  Proliferation of type II alveolar lining cells—hobnail
  Bronchiolar damage with atypical squamous metaplasia
  X-ray shows diffuse bilateral infiltrates

Mortality 10–90%, depending on etiology; fibrosis is a bad prognostic sign, but not necessarily irreversible

ADULT RESPIRATORY DISTRESS SYNDROME (ARDS)
AKA: hyaline membrane disease

Clinically: acute onset of dyspnea following known (by definition) inciting agent

Severe hypoxemia and decreasing lung compliance

50% mortality with rapid course (days to weeks)

ACUTE INTERSTITIAL PNEUMONIA (AIP)
AKA: Hamman-Rich syndrome, accelerated interstitial pneumonia

Rapidly progressive interstitial pneumonia for which an identifiable initial insult cannot be found (relatively rare)

Most often young adults (mean age 28 yr)

May follow flulike illness

Distinguish from usual interstitial pneumonia (UIP)/idiopathic pulmonary fibrosis (IPF) by diffuse fibroblast proliferation with relatively little collagen deposition, temporally synchronized

No effective therapy, bad prognosis, 40–50% die within 2 months

BRONCHIOLITIS OBLITERANS— ORGANIZING PNEUMONIA (BOOP)

AKA: cryptogenic organizing pneumonia

Air space filling process combining bronchiolitis obliterans (inflammation of terminal bronchioles) and extension into alveolar ducts and spaces

Pattern of injury seen in many conditions

Etiology: often unknown, but also infections, inhalant, drugs, collagen vascular disease, chronic aspiration

Acute onset of cough, dyspnea, fever, malaise; multiple patchy air space opacities, often bilateral; restrictive picture

Distinctive type of fibrosis: lightly staining, oval to serpiginous, extending along air spaces, with elongated fibroblasts in a myxoid, pale-staining matrix rich in mucopolysaccharides, with lymphocytes, macrophages, plasma cells, neutrophils

Plugs or polyps may occlude distal bronchioles

Foamy macrophages (obstructive lipid pneumonia)

Excellent prognosis: complete recovery usually in a few weeks

OBLITERATIVE BRONCHIOLITIS

Similar to BOOP, but disease restricted to bronchioles (i.e., pure bronchiolitis obliterans)

Air flow obstruction, distended lung fields without infiltrates, poor prognosis

Includes most cases occurring in bone marrow or heart/lung transplant patients, and those with rheumatoid arthritis

USUAL INTERSTITIAL PNEUMONIA (UIP)

When no specific etiology (such as asbestosis, drug injury, radiation) can be identified, referred to as idiopathic pulmonary fibrosis (IPF), idiopathic (or diffuse) interstitial fibrosis, sclerosing alveolitis

Most common of the idiopathic interstitial pneumonias

Insidious onset of dyspnea, initially during exercise, later even at rest (40–70 yr age; male > female) with chronic, progressive 4–5 yr downhill course to death

X-ray shows bilateral infiltrates, more dense at base, but only minimal if any effusion; with progression, get fibrosis and shrinkage of lungs

Pathogenesis may be related to activation of macrophages and "innocent bystander" destruction of pulmonary tissue

Interstitial inflammation and fibrosis that *varies significantly from field to field* in both cellularity and degree of fibrosis, even with focal areas of honeycombed lung

Lymphocytes (predominantly B), plasma cells, germinal centers, alveolar desquamation, cuboidalization of alveolar lining cells, narrowed air spaces, cystic changes

Foci of fibroblasts in loose stroma represent active lesions

Secondary pulmonary hypertensive changes and *smooth muscle hyperplasia*

Tight intraalveolar aggregates of macrophages

Steroid therapy widely used; less than 20% respond

Cyclophosphamide therapy may be beneficial

DESQUAMATIVE INTERSTITIAL PNEUMONIA (DIP)

Some consider this an early form of UIP/IPF

Occurs at mean age of 42 yr (90% cigarette smokers), 30% mortality with 12 yr mean survival; better prognosis than UIP; more responsive to steroid therapy

Numerous large mononuclear cells in air spaces; most are actually macrophages vs. desquamated cells

Macrophages loosely aggregated, evenly dispersed, do not distend lumens

Loss of type I pneumocytes with type II cells lining air spaces

Blue bodies: laminated PAS+ iron-containing bodies within or surrounded by macrophages

Mild thickening of alveolar septa, less fibrosis than UIP

Temporal uniformity vs. heterogeneity of UIP

Differential diagnosis. DIP-like reactions seen in eosinophilic granuloma, asbestosis, around malignant tumors, respiratory bronchiolitis, collagen diseases, pulmonary alveolar proteinosis

RESPIRATORY BRONCHIOLITIS

Similar to DIP but tends to be patchy, not diffuse, with macrophages predominantly in respiratory bronchioles and alveolar ducts; macrophages distend spaces

Macrophages have finely granular yellow-brown pigment

Almost always smoking history

Predominantly lower lobes

Self-limited; corticosteroid therapy unnecessary

May exist independently or as component of interstitial lung disease in continuum with DIP

MISCELLANEOUS INTERSTITIAL PNEUMONIAS

CHRONIC INTERSTITIAL PNEUMONIA (CIP)

Temporally homogeneous lesions; don't fit others

Cellular interstitial inflammation, many plasma cells, variable amounts of fibrosis (inactive)

Associated with many underlying diseases: collagen vascular diseases, drug toxicity, hypersensitivity pneumonitis, severe pulmonary hypertension, mycoplasma

LYMPHOID INTERSTITIAL PNEUMONIA (LIP)

Mixed cellular infiltrate of lymphocytes, plasma cells, epithelioid histiocytes, germinal centers, granulomas

Variable clinical and radiographic picture

Probably early lymphoproliferative lesion of bronchial associated lymphoid tissue

GIANT CELL INTERSTITIAL PNEUMONIA (GIP)

Isolated multinucleated giant cells in alveoli and interstitium of lung otherwise showing changes of UIP

Associated with heavy metals; rare

GRANULOMATOUS INTERSTITIAL PNEUMONIA

Prominent epithelioid histiocytes as well as lymphocytes and plasma cells; may have loosely formed granulomas (vs. sarcoid, which has well-formed granulomas)

Many represent hypersensitivity pneumonia

More responsive to steroids and better prognosis than UIP

END-STAGE FIBROSIS (HONEYCOMB LUNG)

Common endpoint for multiple causes and patterns

Restructuring of distal air spaces, obliteration of small airways leading to macroscopic "emphysematous" cysts separated by areas of scarring (interstitial fibrosis)

Enlarged air spaces lined by plump cuboidal or ciliated columnar cells (ingrowth of bronchial epithelium) with areas of squamous metaplasia

Patients are at increased risk for developing peripheral carcinomas

PROGRESSIVE MASSIVE FIBROSIS (PMF)

May complicate silicosis, asbestosis, coal workers pneumoconiosis, mixed dust fibrosis, etc.

Large amorphous mass of fibrous tissue obliterating and contracting the parenchyma, usually upper lobes

Central cavitation may be necrobiosis or sign of TB

Clinically, patient is dyspneic, eventually even at rest

Poorly localized chest pain is common

May lead to right ventricular hypertrophy

Caplan's syndrome: development of rheumatoid nodules in setting of progressive massive fibrosis (PMF): small, firm tan nodules with central necrosis

HYPERSENSITIVITY PNEUMONIA

AKA: extrinsic allergic alveolitis

Immunologic reaction to inhaled agents (fungus, mold, animal proteins); combination of type III (immune complex) and type IV (cell-mediated) reactions

- Acute: (large exposure): severe dyspnea, cough, fever—self-limited; resolves in 12–18 hr (continued exposure can lead to permanent damage)
- Chronic: prolonged exposure to small doses; insidious onset of dyspnea and dry cough

Patchy chronic interstitial pneumonia, accentuated around bronchioles, temporally synchronized, with uninvolved lung in between

Lymphocytes predominate (most are CD8+ T cells), with plasma cells, histiocytes, rare eosinophils/neutrophils, minimal fibrosis without vasculitis—many will show loosely formed non-necrotizing granulomas

BOOP-like changes can be seen in two thirds

Steroids may help; best therapy is elimination of inciting agent

FARMER'S LUNG
MAPLE BARK STRIPPER'S DISEASE

Ovoid, thick-walled brown spores (*Cryptostroma corticale*) in histiocytes or granulomas

PIGEON BREEDER'S DISEASE

Small aggregates of foamy macrophages in interstitium and alveoli

BYSSINOSIS

Textile workers; inhalation of cotton fibers

ACTINOMYCETES

EOSINOPHILIC PNEUMONIAS

X-ray: patchy bilateral infiltrates, usually more prominent in periphery

Filling of alveoli with eosinophils and large mononuclear cells or giant cells, necrosis of infiltrate, palisading histiocytes

Interstitial infiltrate of eosinophils, plasma cells, lymphocytes

Mild non-necrotizing vasculitis; bronchiolitis obliterans

- Simple (Löffler's syndrome): mild, self-limited, resolves in 1 month, peripheral eosinophilia
- Tropical: high fever, cough, wheezing, eosinophilia—usually caused by microfilaria within pulmonary capillaries
- Chronic: variable clinical presentation; usually chronic asthma; eosinophilia, elevated IgE
- Allergic bronchopulmonary aspergillosis: (see later under asthma)
- Bronchocentric granulomatosis (see later)

Differential diagnosis. Churg-Strauss syndrome (polyarteritis nodosa associated with asthma), *Aspergillus*-related diseases

DRUG-INDUCED LUNG DISEASE

Alkylating Agents

BUSULFAN

Used for chronic myelogenous leukemia (CML); 1st agent shown to cause lung disease

Pulmonary toxicity occurs in 4% of patients receiving busulfan

Latent periods 1 month to 12 yr (mean 3.5 yr)

Poor prognosis; most die within 6 months

Organizing diffuse alveolar damage with bronchiolar and alveolar epithelial atypia: cytomegaly, nuclear pleomorphism, prominent nucleoli

Chronic interstitial pneumonia, pulmonary ossification, and pulmonary alveolar proteinosis have also been reported

CYCLOPHOSPHAMIDE

Unpredictable latent period

Organizing diffuse alveolar damage most common; less epithelial atypia than seen with busulfan

Have also seen chronic interstitial pneumonia, BOOP

CHLORAMBUCIL

Chronic interstitial pneumonia

Nitrosoureas

CARMUSTINE (BCNU)

Used to treat primary brain neoplasms

Direct relationship between cumulative dose and toxicity

20–30% overall incidence of toxicity; 50% for larger doses

Acute and organizing DAD most common lesion; less commonly CIP, venoocclusive disease, pleural disease

Antibiotics

BLEOMYCIN

3–5% incidence; higher for: higher doses, elderly, prior irradiation, recent previous use of bleomycin

DAD most common, predominantly lower lobes, with alveolar hemorrhage, pleural fibrosis, eosinophilic pneumonia

BOOP, pulmonary venous occlusive disease (PVOD) can be seen

Prognosis poor: rapidly progressive to death within 3 months

MITOMYCIN

8% patients; 50% overall mortality; full recovery possible

DAD with fibrinous pleuritis; BOOP, pulmonary edema, hemorrhage

Antimetabolites

METHOTREXATE

5–10% incidence; most recover completely, < 10% die

Peripheral eosinophilia, diffuse pulmonary infiltrates

CIP with nodular interstitial infiltrates of lymphocytes, plasma cells, histiocytes, occasional giant cells

Hypersensitivity pneumonitis, BOOP, DAD can be seen

Antimicrobials

NITROFURANTOIN

Commonly used; therefore, causes most lung disease

Acute reaction in 90%: peripheral eosinophilia, pulmonary edema, DAD

Insidious onset in 10%: UIP, DIP, eosinophilic pneumonia

SULFONAMIDES

Eosinophilic pneumonia is underlying pathology

AMPHOTERICIN B

Diffuse alveolar hemorrhage when given in combination with leukocyte transfusion

Antiinflammatory Drugs

GOLD

1% patients: some MHC associations

Rheumatoid lung disease, DAD, CIP, BOOP

Others

Antiarrhythmics: amiodarone, tocainide

Antihypertensives: hydrochlorothiazide, propranolol, hexamethonium, hydralazine, captopril

Tocolytics: ritodrine, terbutaline, albuterol, $MgSO_4$

Anticonvulsants: phenytoin, carbamazepine
Psychotherapeutics: haloperidol, chlordiazepoxide, amitriptyline, imipramine
Opioids: morphine, methadone, codeine, heroin

Pneumoconioses

Non-neoplastic reaction of the lungs to inhaled mineral or organic dust, excluding asthma, bronchitis, and emphysema
Extent of disease determined by amount of material retained in lungs and by the size, shape, and solubility of material
Particle sizes:
>5 μm   Generally impact high in airway; cleared
<1 μm   Generally remain suspended; exhaled
1–5 μm   Reach terminal small airways; stay there
In general, concomitant cigarette smoking worsens disease
In general, pneumoconioses do *not* predispose to development of carcinoma (exception: asbestosis)

SILICOSIS
Silica: silicon dioxide, e.g., quartz
ACUTE SILICOSIS (ACCELERATED SILICOSIS)
Heavy exposure over 1–3 yr
Looks like pulmonary alveolar proteinosis with variable amounts of interstitial fibrosis
CHRONIC SILICOSIS
After 20–40 yr exposure to dust containing up to 30% quartz (mining, sand blasting, metal grinding, tunneling, ceramics)
Onset and progression can be years after exposure
Proliferation of hyalinized nodules, usually peripheral, usually upper lobes, with variable amounts of black pigment (concomitant exposure to coal dust), well delimited, concentric lamellated hyaline, with rare giant cells or granulomas; necrosis rare
Nodules slowly but progressively expand; can obliterate small airways
Doubly refractile, round particles may be seen (1–2 μm)
Complications:
• Conglomerate nodules
• TB (10–30× relative risk)
• Progressive massive fibrosis
• Caplan's syndrome

ASBESTOSIS
Elongated fibrous particles in two groups:
• Serpentine group (90%), e.g., chrysotile: long, flexible, curled, very thin; generally do not make it to small airways
• Amphibole group (10%), e.g., amosite, crocidolite: brittle, straight, fracture; fragments carried into airways
Causes interstitial fibrosis similar to UIP, beginning as peribronchiolar fibrosis, preferentially lower lobes, with pleural fibrosis/calcification, parietal pleural plaques
Occurs 15–20 yr after exposure; generally requires >10 yr of exposure; insidious onset
Progression can lead to honeycombed lung or PMF
Increased risk of bronchogenic carcinoma: risk relative to unexposed is 5× (relative risk for smokers, 11×; relative risk for smokers exposed to asbestos, 55×)

Increases risk for mesothelioma (both pleural and peritoneal); still more rare than bronchogenic carcinoma; smoking is not a factor

COAL WORKERS PNEUMOCONIOSIS (CWP)
SIMPLE CWP
Occurs after years of exposure to coal dust
Dust macule: interstitial dust-filled macrophages surrounding dilated respiratory bronchioles and in the interlobular septa, usually upper portions of lobes, with minimal fibrosis
Coal nodule: discrete, palpable <1 cm lesion with central hyalinized collagen and pigment-laden macrophages
Minimal functional deficits
2–8% will progress to complicated CWP
COMPLICATED CWP
Progressive massive fibrosis with large black masses and central cavity
Immunologic mechanisms may be involved in pathogenesis

MIXED DUST FIBROSIS
Low proportion of silica; silicotic nodules do not occur
Stellate interstitial fibrous lesion, predominantly in area of the respiratory bronchioles, spreading into surrounding parenchyma irregularly; fibrous zones remain discrete

OTHER PNEUMOCONIOSES
PULMONARY MYCOTOXICOSIS
AKA: organic dust syndrome
Caused by massive inhalation; probably toxic vs. immune
Bronchiolitis with intraalveolar and interstitial neutrophils
SIDEROSIS
AKA: arc-welder's lung, hematite lung
Results from exposure to inert metallic iron or its oxides
Macules and perivascular dust similar to CWP, but with coarse, brown-black particles of iron and gold-brown hemosiderin
BERYLLIOSIS
Acute form produces DAD
Chronic form is a systemic disease (lung, LNs, kidneys, liver, spleen) with a latent period up to 15 yr: interstitial fibrosis with noncaseating subpleural, peribronchiolar, and perivascular granulomas, which may have Schaumann's bodies or asteroid bodies, as in sarcoidosis
OTHERS
Talc, aluminum powder, hard metal pneumoconiosis, alginate powder (dentists), polyvinyl chloride (PVC), fibrous glass

Chronic Obstructive Pulmonary Disease (COPD)

AKA: chronic obstructive airway disease (COAD)
Pulmonary function tests show increased pulmonary resistance, limitation of maximal expiratory flow rates

EMPHYSEMA
Abnormal permanent enlargement of the distal air spaces caused by destruction of the alveolar walls and loss of respiratory tissue
"Obstruction" caused by lack of elastic recoil

Most commonly caused by smoking: produces a combination of emphysema and chronic inflammation (alpha-1-antitrypsin deficiency produces almost pure emphysema)

Most likely pathogenesis involves increased protease or decreased anti-protease activity

Types

CENTROACINAR (CENTRILOBAR) EMPHYSEMA
Affects central (proximal) parts of the acini (respiratory bronchioles) but spares the distal alveoli

More severe in upper lobes, esp. apical segments

Seen in smoking and secondary to coal dust

PANACINAR (PANLOBAR) EMPHYSEMA
Uniform enlargement of all acini in a lobule

May not necessarily involve entire lung; predominantly lower lobes

Alpha-1-antitrypsin deficiency is prototype

PARASEPTAL (DISTAL ACINAR) EMPHYSEMA
Proximal acinus normal, distal part involved

Most prominent adjacent to pleura and along the lobular connective tissue septa

Probably underlies spontaneous pneumothorax in young adults

BULLOUS EMPHYSEMA
Any form of emphysema that produces large subpleural blebs of bullae (>1 cm)

Localized accentuation of one of the previous forms

INTERSTITIAL EMPHYSEMA
Air penetration into the connective tissue stroma of the lung, mediastinum, or subcutaneous tissue

COMPENSATORY "EMPHYSEMA"
Dilatation of alveoli in response to loss of lung substance elsewhere

Actually hyperinflation because no destruction of septal walls

SENILE "EMPHYSEMA"
Change in geometry of lung with larger alveolar ducts and smaller alveoli

No loss of lung tissue; hence, not really emphysema

CHRONIC BRONCHITIS
Clinically defined: persistent cough with sputum production for at least 3 months in at least 2 consecutive yr

Can occur with or without evidence of airway obstruction

10–25% of urban-dwelling adults qualify

Smoking is most important cause

Hypersecretion of mucous with:
• Increased numbers of goblet cells in small airways as well as large airways
• Increased size of submucosal glands in large airways (Reid index: ratio of thickness of mucus glands to thickness of wall between epithelium and cartilage)

Peribronchiolar chronic inflammation

ASTHMA
Increased responsiveness of tracheobronchial tree to various stimuli, leading to paroxysmal airway constriction

Unremitting attacks (*status asthmaticus*) can be fatal

Types: extrinsic (atopic, allergic), most common; intrinsic, (idiosyncratic); now also recognize mixed

Bronchial plugging by thick mucus plugs containing eosinophils, whorls of shed epithelium (Curschmann's spirals), and Charcot-Leyden crystals (eosinophil membrane protein); distal air spaces become overdistended

Thick basement membrane, edema and inflammation in bronchial walls with prominence of eosinophils, hypertrophy of bronchial wall muscle

Therapeutic agents are aimed at increasing cAMP levels, either by increasing production (β_2-agonists, e.g., epinephrine) or decreasing degradation (methylxanthines, e.g., theophylline); cromylyn sodium prevents mast cell degranulation

ALLERGIC BRONCHOPULMONARY ASPERGILLOSIS
Occurs in chronic asthmatics; hypersensitivity to noninvasive *Aspergillus*

Bronchocentric granulomatosis, mucoid impaction of bronchi, eosinophilic pneumonia

Distinctive proximal bronchiectasis (pathognomonic?)

BRONCHIECTASIS
Permanent abnormal dilation of bronchi and bronchioles, usually associated with chronic necrotizing inflammation

Patients have fever, cough, foul-smelling sputum

More common in left lung, more common in lower lobes

Causes:
• Obstruction (tumor, mucus)
• Intralobar sequestration
• Immotile cilia syndrome
• Kartagener's syndrome
• Congenital
• Cystic fibrosis
• Necrotizing pneumonia

Miscellaneous Diseases

PULMONARY ATELECTASIS
Incomplete expansion of lungs or collapse of a previously expanded lung

Reversible disorder

Affected segment is prone to superimposed infections

OBSTRUCTIVE (ABSORPTIVE)
Complete obstruction of an airway: oxygen trapped distal to obstruction is eventually absorbed, leading to collapse of the obstructed segment

If large, mediastinum shifts toward the affected lung

Usually caused by excessive secretions or inflammatory exudate within the smaller bronchi; most commonly seen in asthma, chronic bronchitis, bronchiectasis, aspiration, postoperative patients

COMPRESSIVE
Pleural cavity partially or completely filled by fluid, exudate, tumor, or air

Most commonly seen in patients with cardiac failure

If large, the mediastinum shifts away from the affected lung

CONTRACTION
Localized fibrosis increases the recoil of a focal area

PATCHY
Loss of surfactant (e.g., respiratory distress syndrome)

ALVEOLAR HEMORRHAGE SYNDROMES
Hemoptysis, pulmonary infiltrates, anemia, diffuse intraalveolar hemorrhage, necrotizing interstitial pneumonitis

Generally not used to refer to hemorrhage secondary to necrotizing bronchopneumonia, renal failure, thrombocytopenia, venous congestion

GOODPASTURE'S SYNDROME
AKA: anti–basement membrane disease

Also get renal involvement on account of glomerular destruction

Male : female = 2 : 1

Accumulation of RBCs and hemosiderin in alveoli and alveolar macrophages, some nonspecific thickening of alveoli, *vasculitis usually absent*

Aggressive therapy needed

Prognosis related more to renal disease

IDIOPATHIC PULMONARY HEMOSIDEROSIS

Similar to Goodpasture's syndrome but no renal involvement

Almost exclusively children under 16 yr; male = female

Often improves without therapy, but may be fatal

SARCOIDOSIS

Lungs frequently involved; may be only manifestation

60% cases will be positive on transbronchial biopsy

X-ray: interstitial infiltrates with hilar adenopathy

Non-necrotizing granulomatous inflammation composed of tight clusters of epithelioid histiocytes, occasional giant cells, few lymphocytes; may become hyalinized

Granulomas predominantly in interstitium vs. air spaces, characteristically distributed along lymphatics

Granulomatous vasculitis frequently present

NODULAR SARCOIDOSIS

Large coalesced areas of hyalinized granulomas

Patients may not have hilar adenopathy

NECROTIZING SARCOID GRANULOMATOSIS

First described by Leibow in 1973; rare

May be a form of nodular sarcoidosis, a cross between sarcoid and Wegener's granulomatosis, or a discrete entity

Extensive noncaseating granulomatous inflammation, vasculitis, and foci of parenchymal necrosis

Confluent areas of well-formed granulomas replace large areas of lung and contain irregular zones of necrosis

WEGENER'S GRANULOMATOSIS

CLASSIC FORM

Acute necrotizing granulomas of upper and lower respiratory tract (with giant cells and leukocytes); necrotizing vasculitis in lungs; focal or diffuse necrotizing glomerulonephritis

Peak incidence is in 40s; male > female

Persistent pneumonitis, chronic sinusitis, nasopharyngeal ulcerations, renal disease

If untreated, 80% will die within 1 yr; if treated (immunosuppression, e.g., cyclophosphamide), 90% respond

Serum antineutrophil cytoplasmic antibodies serve as marker for disease activity

Multiple bilateral nodules of liquefactive and coagulative necrosis in lung, creating large geographic lesions with eosinophils, giant cells (not forming well-defined granulomas), leukocytoclastic angiitis (both arteries and veins); only scant numbers of lymphocytes or plasma cells

Fulminant type: predominantly exudative changes

Fibrous scar type: abundant collagen deposition

LIMITED FORM

Confined to lungs; no renal involvement

Histology identical to classic form; more protracted course

EOSINOPHILIC GRANULOMA

AKA: Langerhans cell granulomatosis, histiocytosis X

30% incidental finding; 25% present with pneumothorax

Mean age 30 yr, but large range; most are smokers

Involvement limited to lung in 50%

Patchy, nodular interstitial lesion with bronchiolocentric distribution, most commonly upper lobes, stellate nodules on account of extension along alveolar septa

Histiocytes with variable numbers of eosinophils, plasma cells, lymphocytes

Macrophages often accumulate around lesions (DIP-like)

Electron microscopy: characteristic Birbeck granules

BRONCHOCENTRIC GRANULOMATOSIS

Pathogenesis is immunologic

Granulomatous inflammatory process beginning within bronchiole walls with destruction that may extend slightly into surrounding lung

Histiocytes initially replace bronchiolar mucosa, palisading around lumen, eventually destroying entire wall with necrosis and cell debris and neutrophils surrounded by palisading histiocytes; necrosis often extends to involve cartilage

Maintains peribronchiolar distribution

Mucoid impaction of larger airways, often with fungal hyphae within the mucus, is common

Closely related to chronic eosinophilic pneumonia

Half of patients have asthma, many have allergic bronchopulmonary aspergillosis

COLLAGEN VASCULAR DISEASES

RHEUMATOID ARTHRITIS

Interstitial pneumonia and fibrosis, often indistinguishable from UIP, may have prominent lymphoid aggregates with germinal centers (cellular CIP), BOOP, obliterative bronchiolitis, follicular bronchiolitis

Necrobiotic nodules rare in parenchyma

Vasculitis and/or pulmonary hypertension have been seen

Pleural lesions include nonspecific pleuritis and necrobiotic (rheumatoid) nodules

Better prognosis than UIP

SYSTEMIC LUPUS ERYTHEMATOSUS (SLE)

Pleuritis, pleural effusion, pleural fibrosis

Chronic interstitial pneumonia common, generally without much fibrosis

DAD, intraalveolar hemorrhage, pulmonary hypertension, vasculitis

SCLERODERMA (PROGRESSIVE SYSTEMIC SCLEROSIS)

Interstitial fibrosis, more prominent in lower lobes, varying from UIP-like to honeycombing

PULMONARY ALVEOLAR PROTEINOSIS

AKA: pulmonary alveolar lipoproteinosis

Filling of alveolar spaces with PAS+ proteinaceous material with normal interstitial pulmonary architecture

Associated with immunodeficiencies, underlying malignancies (esp. leukemia and lymphoma), infectious agents, industrial or environmental exposures

Patients present with slowly progressive pulmonary infiltrates, dyspnea, cough, sputum, fever

Treatment: pulmonary lavage

AMYLOIDOSIS

Generally an incidental finding rather than clinically significant

DIFFUSE ALVEOLAR-SEPTAL AMYLOIDOSIS

Most common in primary amyloidosis or multiple myeloma

Deposits in media of vessels and alveolar septa, which may bulge into alveolar spaces

NODULAR PULMONARY AMYLOIDOSIS
Generally not associated with deposits in other organs
Discrete peripheral tumor-like nodules, 1–3 cm, composed of dense, amorphous, eosinophilic material, often with aggregates of plasma cells, lymphocytes, giant cells

TRACHEOBRONCHIAL AMYLOIDOSIS
Rare; deposits confined to bronchial tree

TRANSPLANTATION-RELATED DISORDERS

BONE MARROW TRANSPLANTATION
Pulmonary complications in ~50% of patients
Usually infectious (CMV, bacteria) or interstitial pneumonia, obliterative bronchiolitis, lymphocytic bronchitis

HEART-LUNG TRANSPLANTATION
50% develop obliterative bronchiolitis after mean interval of 10 months; 50% mortality; probably type of chronic rejection
Acute rejection: within 3 months, perivascular mononuclear infiltrate affecting venules and small arteries: small lymphocytes, plasma cells, lymphoblasts

OTHER

LYMPHOMATOID GRANULOMATOSIS
(See Hematolymphoid outline)

PULMONARY ALVEOLAR MICROLITHIASIS
Rare
Laminated calcospherites in the lung in the absence of any known abnormality of calcium metabolism

PULMONARY HYALINIZING GRANULOMA
Slowly enlarging nodules of thick collagen bundles with lymphocytes and plasma cells
Perivascular inflammation and mild vasculitis may be seen

SCLEROSING MEDIASTINITIS
Destructive and infiltrative proliferation of connective tissue in the mediastinum
May be exaggerated hypersensitivity reaction to infection in mediastinal lymph nodes

MESENCHYMAL CYSTIC HAMARTOMA
Multifocal, bilateral, small (<1 cm) cysts lined by metaplastic respiratory epithelium resting on a cellular cambium layer of mesenchymal cells

Pulmonary Vascular Disorders

PULMONARY CONGESTION AND EDEMA

HEMODYNAMIC
Increased hydrostatic pressure, as seen in congestive heart failure, causes increased interstitial fluid
Fluid accumulates only after lymphatic drainage has increased by about 10-fold
Edema is initially interstitial but later becomes alveolar
Alveolar fluid accumulation more prominent in the lower lobes
Alveolar microhemorrhages and hemosiderin-laden macrophages are common ("heart failure cells")

MICROVASCULAR INJURY
Alveolocapillary membrane injury by inflammation, infection, toxins, shock
When diffuse, can lead to adult respiratory distress syndrome

PULMONARY EMBOLISM/INFARCTION
Occlusions of pulmonary arteries by blood clot—almost always embolic in origin
In 95% cases, thrombi from deep veins of the leg
Large emboli (e.g., saddle embolus) often cause sudden death; if not, clinical picture may resemble myocardial infarction
If patient survives, clot may retract and eventually become totally lysed, leaving only small membranous webs
(Note: see also outline on Vessels)

INFARCTIONS
When bronchial artery circulation is intact, embolization does not lead to infarction; thus, only ~10% emboli → infarction
Infarction occurs when bronchial circulation is inadequate; therefore, seen in elderly patients
Infarction most commonly lower lobe (75%), with a wedge-shaped pleural-based lesion, hemorrhagic at first, but then becomes pale as red cells lyse and fibrous replacement begins (at the margins)

PULMONARY HYPERTENSION
Normally, pulmonary arterial pressures are only 1/8 of systemic levels
Atherosclerotic changes in pulmonary arteries generally indicative of pulmonary hypertension (except can see mild atherosclerosis in elderly patients)

Grading
Grades I–III are considered potentially reversible
Grades IV–VI are considered usually irreversible

GRADE I
Medial muscular hypertrophy involving small arteries (media thickness exceeds 7% of external diameter of artery)
Extension of smooth muscle into small vessels in lung periphery

GRADE II
Muscle hypertrophy plus intimal cell proliferation in small muscular arteries
Proliferating cells are not endothelial: smooth muscle or myofibroblast

GRADE III
Concentric lamellar intimal fibrosis of muscular arteries
Eventually, fibrous tissue and reduplicated internal elastic lamina occlude the vascular lumen
Larger elastic arteries show atherosclerosis

GRADE IV
Widespread dilatation of the small pulmonary arteries and arterioles
Plexiform lesions: aneurysmal expansion of the vessel wall of small muscular arteries usually just distal to their origin from a larger vessel: proliferation of tiny vascular channels lined by myofibroblasts resembling endothelial cells

GRADE V
Grade IV changes plus vein-like branches of hypertrophied muscular arteries with minimal media
Angiomatoid lesions: exaggerated form of vein-like branching in which a conglomeration of thin-walled vessels is found adjacent to a muscular artery
Hemosiderin-laden macrophages throughout the lung

GRADE VI
Fibrinoid necrosis and necrotizing vasculitis with neutrophils and eosinophils

Causes

PRIMARY CARDIAC DISEASE—INCREASED FLOW
Atrial septal defect, ventricular septal defect, patent ductus arteriosus

PULMONARY VENOUS CONGESTION
(See earlier)

PRIMARY PULMONARY PARENCHYMAL DISEASE
Increased pulmonary vascular resistance secondary to COPD, interstitial lung disease, recurrent emboli

PULMONARY VENO-OCCLUSIVE DISEASE
Obstruction of small pulmonary veins by concentric or eccentric intimal fibrosis
May overlook (interpret as interstitial fibrosis) unless do elastic stain to outline vessel walls
Can get medial hypertrophy in arteries
>50% of patients are ≤16 yr old
Etiology unknown—venous thrombosis?

PRIMARY PULMONARY HYPERTENSION
May be related to chronic vascular hyper-reactivity, chronic vasoconstriction, and resultant hypertension, intimal and medial hypertrophy

LYMPHANGIOMYOMATOSIS
AKA: lymphangioleiomyomatosis
Haphazard proliferation of smooth muscle cells throughout the interstitium of the lung involving walls of vessels, lymphatics, bronchioles, and septa
Extrapulmonary involvement (lymphatics, lymph nodes in thorax and/or abdomen) may be seen
Occurs exclusively in women in reproductive years
Associated with tuberous sclerosis; may be a limited form
Differential diagnosis: end-stage UIP, which can show smooth muscle proliferation

LUNG—TUMORS

INFLAMMATORY "PSEUDOTUMORS"
Almost always asymptomatic incidental findings on chest x-ray; small, solitary
Some of these entities may be or may progress to true neoplasms

PLASMA CELL GRANULOMA
AKA: fibroxanthoma, histiocytoma
More common in children and young adults
Usually peripheral
Mature plasma cells and lymphocytes in a framework of fibrosis and granulation tissue
Mast cells and foamy histiocytes usually present

SCLEROSING HEMANGIOMA
Usually adult females; usually peripheral, lower lung fields
Well circumscribed but not encapsulated
Compact growth of polygonal cells lining sclerotic cores of papillary projections
Epithelial membrane antigen, keratin positive
No evidence for vascular etiology; probably type II pneumocytes

PSEUDOLYMPHOMA
Similar to LIP but isolated masses vs. diffuse infiltrate
Represents residuum of healing inflammatory lesion
Nodular mass that replaces a portion of the pulmonary parenchyma; scarring most prominent in the center, with densely packed collagen, fibroblasts, and lymphocytes but no necrosis
May have germinal centers

Distinction from lymphoma: no hilar LN involvement, numerous germinal centers, mixed inflammatory cell population; lymphoma more monomorphous and has a lymphangitic distribution

Bronchogenic Carcinoma

General
Increasing in frequency over past 50 yr
More common in males, but difference is decreasing
90% of patients over 40 yr; multiple tumors in 5%
60% incurable at time of detection
Some detected incidentally as coin lesion on chest x-ray; 35–50% of coin lesions turn out to be carcinoma
Indisputable association with smoking, which increases relative risk by factor of 20 (increased risk for all types); also thought to be related to pulmonary fibrosis
Patients may present with extrapulmonary symptoms: clubbing of fingers (hypertrophic pulmonary osteoarthropathy), cortical cerebellar degeneration, encephalomyelitis
Many lung tumors are associated with ectopic secretion of hormones:
• Small cell: adrenocorticotropic hormone (ACTH), serotonin, antidiuretic hormone (ADH), human chorionic gonadotropin (HCG)
• Carcinoids: ACTH, serotonin, HCG
• Squamous cell: parathyroid hormone (PTH)
Bronchogenic carcinomas all presumably arise from bronchial epithelium; therefore, it is not uncommon for the tumors to have mixed or varied histological patterns

Staging
Spread is by direct extension proximally and distally along bronchi; may seed pleura or mediastinum
Lymphatic spread first to hilar nodes, then mediastinal, lower cervical, and less commonly, axillary and subdiaphragmatic
Metastases to liver, other areas in lung, adrenal, bone, kidney, CNS—brain metastases most common for adenocarcinoma

T1　≤3 cm; no invasion proximal to lobar bronchus
T2　>3 cm or pleural invasion or <2 cm from carina
T3　Direct extension (parietal pleura, diaphragm, . . .)
N1　Peribronchial or ipsilateral hilar nodes
N2　Ipsilateral mediastinal LNs
N3　Contralateral LNs or more distant LNs
M1　Distant metastases

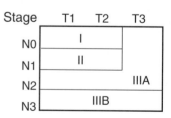

Stage I and II are operable, III is not

Prognosis
60% of patients go to surgery; 60% of these are resectable

Radiation helps, but limited by the fact that 50% have metastases at time of diagnosis

TNM stage best prognostic indicator

Poor prognostic signs: age <40 yr; female sex; vascular invasion, chest wall invasion, presence of a scar, aneuploid

Good prognostic sign: strong inflammatory response

SQUAMOUS CELL CARCINOMA (35–50%)

AKA: epidermoid carcinoma

>80% occur in males; most closely associated with smoking

Most are central (segmental bronchi) and present as hilar or perihilar masses

"Early carcinomas" can be polypoid, nodular, or superficially infiltrating

Generally larger than other lung carcinomas at diagnosis; grows more rapidly but tends to metastasize later

50% show signs of bronchial obstruction

Marked tendency to undergo central necrosis and cavitation

Squamous metaplasia or carcinoma *in situ* common in adjacent bronchial mucosa

Hypercalcemia caused by PTH-related protein is common

Calcification is extremely uncommon

High MW keratin staining is positive

Most curable of the lung cancers; 5 yr survival: 90% for "early lesions," 40% for well differentiated, 20% for moderately, 7% for poorly

ADENOCARCINOMA (15–35%)

50% of all tumors in females—increasing in prevalence (male = female)

Most commonly peripheral; often involve pleura

Usually poorly circumscribed gray-yellowish lesions

Many are associated with a "scar," but it is not always clear if the scar preceded the tumor or vice versa; most tumor-associated scars contain predominantly type III collagen, which is characteristic of a newly formed scar rather than established fibrosis, suggesting the scar follows the carcinoma

Traditionally areas will exhibit gland formation, papillae, and/or secretion of mucin

Wide range of histologic patterns, merging with bronchioloalveolar carcinoma on one end and with undifferentiated large cell carcinoma on the other end; major cell types are bronchial surface cells (without mucus production), goblet cell, bronchial gland cell, Clara cell, type II alveolar cell, and mixed cell types

Low MW keratin, EMA, CEA positive; may be vimentin positive

50% positive for surfactant apoprotein—can be used to distinguish primary from metastatic carcinoma

K-*ras* mutationally activated in some adenocarcinomas

Blood vessel invasion present at resection in >80%; resectability rate ~70% (twice other bronchogenic carcinomas)

5 yr survival 25%, independent of degree of differentiation or histologic type

Most important prognostic factors are metastases (LN or distant) and pleural involvement

Rarely, peripheral adenocarcinoma may spread massively into pleural space, coating both pleural layers, simulating mesothelioma

BRONCHIOLOALVEOLAR CARCINOMA

This term sometimes used to describe a pattern of adenocarcinoma; if restrict term to very well-differentiated single lesions with no alveolar wall scaring and no other carcinoma pattern, accompanied by a slightly better prognosis (50–75% 5 yr survival if resectable solitary lesion)

If multiple lesions present, long-term survival still very poor

Well-differentiated cells lining respiratory spaces without stromal invasion

Can grow as a single peripheral nodule, multiple nodules, or a diffuse pulmonic-like infiltrate; tumor cells tend to grow along spaces: alveolar, perineural, sinusoidal in LNs; generally does *not* form solid mass or invade structures

Three major histologic types:

• Clara cell type (38%)

• Type II pneumocytes (33%): mucin negative; slightly better prognosis

• Mucinous type (29%): more commonly multiple; therefore, worst prognosis

Intranuclear inclusions can be present

Psammoma bodies are present in 13%

SMALL CELL CARCINOMA (10–20%)

80% male, >85% smokers; typically central; may be small

Growth patterns: subepithelial, nodular, mixed, or peripheral

Histology: streaming, ribbons, rosettes, tubules, ductules

Hyperchromatic nuclei with finely dispersed chromatin (salt and pepper) with no obvious nucleoli and a thin nuclear membrane

Usually keratin positive; may also be positive for neural markers: neurofilaments, Leu7, neuron-specific enolase

Electron microscopy: scattered dense-core secretory granules

Tumor may derive from neuroendocrine cells of bronchi

Many of these tumors have a deletion of chromosome 3p

myc gene amplification may correlate with prognosis

Dismal prognosis: <2% 5 yr survival; chemotherapy helps in short term

CYTOLOGIC TYPES

Oat cell (lymphocyte-like): 42%; frequently see crush artifact; Azzopardi effect: basophilic deposits of chromatin surrounding blood vessels in areas of necrosis

Fusiform: (29%); somewhat larger cell size

Polygonal: (29%); medium-sized cells with abundant cytoplasm; often confused with other lung carcinomas

Alternative histologic classification: Oat cell, intermediate cell type (combines fusiform and polygonal), and combined

UNDIFFERENTIATED LARGE CELL CARCINOMA

10–15% of all lung tumors

Pleomorphic tumors without definite evidence of squamous or glandular differentiation (often diagnosis of exclusion)

Probably poorly differentiated variants of other tumor types

Ultrastructural and immunohistochemical features suggest a closer relationship to adenocarcinomas

Some associated with marked peripheral eosinophilia

GIANT CELL CARCINOMA

~1% of all lung tumors; ~5% of large cell carcinomas

Bizarre, multinucleated giant cells and mononuclear forms growing in a solid fashion simulating sarcoma; nuclei are often so large as to suggest CMV infection

Heavy neutrophilic infiltrations between and within tumor cells

Most are peripheral and extensive at time of diagnosis

In some cases, foci of glandular differentiation can be found
LN metastases in nearly 100%; also tends to metastasize to adrenal glands and GI tract
Very aggressive tumor—incurable

CLEAR CELL CARCINOMA
Term should be restricted to cases in which the entire tumor is clear (rare), rather than for other carcinomas which show focal clear cell change
Malignant, mitotically active cells
Keratin, EMA, and LeuM1 positive (just like renal cell carcinoma); however (unlike RCC) tend to be CEA positive and negative for lipid stains
Be sure to consider renal cell carcinoma and sugar tumor

OTHER CARCINOMAS
ADENOSQUAMOUS CARCINOMA
Unquestionable evidence of squamous and glandular differentiation found in the same neoplasm in roughly equivalent amounts
Less than 10% of lung cancers; most are peripheral

BENIGN CLEAR CELL TUMOR ("SUGAR TUMOR")
Rare tumor of unclear histogenesis
Small, bland nuclei; no mitoses; well-defined cell borders
Clear cytoplasm due to accumulation of glycogen; PAS+

CARCINOSARCOMA
Intermingling of carcinoma (usually squamous cell) with malignant spindle-shaped cells simulating fibrosarcoma or malignant fibrous histiocytoma
Osteoclast-like giant cells may be present
Probably carcinoma with sarcoma-like stroma
Prognosis similar to routine bronchogenic carcinoma

PULMONARY BLASTOMA (EMBRYOMA)
May present in adults or children; usually peripheral
Well-differentiated glands in a cellular stroma composed of undifferentiated spindle cells; resembles fetal lung
Stromal component may differentiate toward skeletal muscle, smooth muscle, cartilage, or bone
May be related to carcinosarcoma

Other Tumors

CARCINOID TUMORS
Formerly known as "bronchial adenoma"
Less than 5% of primary pulmonary neoplasms
Younger age of incidence (usually <40 yr)
No association with smoking or other environmental factors
Generally divided into three major types, but there is much overlap—actually a continuum

CENTRAL CARCINOID
Most common type; usually adults, but most common primary lung neoplasm in children
Usually presents as a slow-growing, solitary, endobronchial, often polypoid, mass with high vascularity (hemoptysis)
Most hormonally silent, but may secrete serotonin, ACTH
Overlying mucosa usually intact; grayish-yellow cut surface
Small, uniform cells with central nuclei growing in compact nests, ribbons, festoons, pseudopapillary, papillary, or solid patterns
Dense-core granules by electron microscopy
Variable reactivity for keratin, serotonin, NSE, chromogranin, synaptophysin, Leu7, neurofilaments; CEA positivity may be associated with more aggressive behavior

Metastases to regional LNs in 5%; rare distant metastases
70–80% 10 yr survival
Oncocytic variant exists—similar behavior

PERIPHERAL CARCINOID
More peripheral in origin, often subpleural
Tends to be multiple
Histology: more spindled, simulating smooth muscle; some pleomorphism; few mitoses
Amyloid and melanin may be found, and calcitonin reactivity may be present
Excellent prognosis, metastases rare
Tumorlet: nodular proliferation of small spindle cells around bronchioles—may be minute carcinoids or reactive process

ATYPICAL CARCINOID
Either central or peripheral carcinoid but with increased mitotic activity, nuclear hyperchromasia, or necrosis
LN metastases in 50–70%

HAMARTOMA
AKA: chondroid hamartoma; chondroid adenoma; chondroma
Benign; occurs in adults; usually solitary
Most commonly just beneath pleura
Usually presents as asymptomatic incidental x-ray finding
Composed of islands of cartilage (may calcify), fat, smooth muscle, and clefts lined by respiratory epithelium
An endobronchial variant exists with more adipose tissue and fewer epithelial cells and less cartilage

PARAGANGLIOMA (CHEMODECTOMA)
May rarely occur in the lung; usually peripheral and benign
May be difficult to distinguish from carcinoid: look for S-100 positive sustentacular cells

VASCULAR TUMORS
KAPOSI'S SARCOMA
CAPILLARY HEMANGIOMA
ANGIOSARCOMA
LYMPHANGIOMYOMATOSIS
INTRAVASCULAR BRONCHIOLOALVEOLAR TUMOR (IV-BAT)
Pulmonary form of epithelioid hemangioendothelioma
Young adults; >80% female
Thin rim of plump, acidophilic cells surrounding an eosinophilic mass of hyalinized stroma, sometimes calcified
Polypoid formations fill alveoli, arteries, veins

SALIVARY GLAND-TYPE TUMORS
ADENOID CYSTIC CARCINOMA
Nodular (polypoid) and diffuse (subepithelial) types
MUCOEPIDERMOID CARCINOMA
Low-grade and high-grade varieties
ACINIC CELL TUMOR

LYMPHOMA
Most are B cell, most are small lymphocytic type

Derived from bronchial mucosal associated lymphoid tissue (MALT)

Differential diagnosis from LIP or pseudolymphoma can be very difficult

METASTASES

PLEURA

NORMAL
Pleura (both visceral and parietal) is lined by mesodermally derived mesothelial cells

Mesothelial cells show apical tight junctions, desmosomes, surface microvilli, and a thick glycocalyx

Immunoreactive for low and high MW keratins

Most pleural pathology is secondary to some underlying pulmonary pathology

PLEURAL EFFUSIONS
SEROUS
Normally ~15 ml

If more, usually bilateral and caused by cardiac failure

Also seen with generalized edema (renal failure, cirrhosis)
SEROFIBRINOUS
Pleuritis: pneumonia, tuberculosis, lung infarcts, lung abscess, bronchiectasis

Rheumatoid arthritis, systemic lupus erythematosus

Radiation
SUPPURATIVE (EMPYEMA)
Bacterial or mycotic seeding of pleural cavity, most commonly by contiguous spread from lung, occasionally by hematogenous spread
HEMORRHAGIC
Most commonly, small amount of blood caused by procedure

When bloody serous effusion unrelated to procedure, most common cause is malignancy

Also consider hemorrhagic diathesis, rickettsial disease
BLOOD (HEMOTHORAX)
Almost always ruptured aorta; almost always fatal
CHYLE (CHYLOTHORAX)
Milky-white material that, when allowed to stand, separates into layers, the upper of which is creamy and fatty

Usually indicates pulmonary lymphatic blockage, most commonly caused by malignancy

PLEURAL PLAQUES
Hyalinized fibrous tissue, usually but not always associated with asbestos exposure

Characteristically parietal or diaphragmatic; may calcify

Tumors
Mesothelial cells undergo hyperplastic response to injury or chronic irritation, which can be almost impossible to distinguish from well-differentiated mesothelioma

p53 expression has been noted to be elevated in 70% of mesotheliomas, but is normal in reactive mesothelium

SOLITARY FIBROUS TUMOR OF PLEURA
AKA: solitary fibrous mesothelioma

Well circumscribed, sometimes encapsulated; usually visceral pleura

Usually asymptomatic

May present with pulmonary osteoarthropathy, which vanishes upon tumor resection

No association with asbestos

Firm, lobulated, sometimes pedunculated, with whirled, cut surface; mean diameter 6 cm

Tangled network of fibroblast-like cells with deposition of abundant reticulin and collagen fibers; often referred to as the *patternless pattern;* cellularity varies from densely cellular to edematous to densely collagenous

Probably *not* mesothelial in origin

Tumor cells are CD34 positive

Usually cured by simple excision; may recur

15–20% behave "aggressively," with repeated recurrences

Aggressive signs include >5 cm, absence of pedicle, high cellularity, and mitoses or necrosis

BENIGN MESOTHELIOMA
AKA: pleural fibroma

Relatively common in peritoneal cavity, more rare in pleural cavity

Soft, friable mass; mottled; gray, pink, and/or yellow

Papillary processes lined by one or several layers of cuboidal mesothelial cells

No atypia, solitary, well circumscribed

MALIGNANT MESOTHELIOMA
At least two thirds are related to asbestos exposure

Chronic asbestos exposure carries a 2–3% risk of mesothelioma; risk is not increased by smoking (note: risk of adenocarcinoma much higher); amphiboles (esp. crocidolite) are most carcinogenic; chrysotile is least carcinogenic

Long latency between exposure and tumor: 25–45 yr

Asbestos bodies more commonly found in lung

Multiple gray or white, ill-defined nodules, diffusely thickening pleura; may grow extensively to fill pleural space and encase lung

Pleural effusion almost always present

Prognosis uniformly bad: 50% 1 yr survival
EPITHELIAL TYPE
Papillae or pseudoacini, or even solid nests of cuboidal, columnar, or flattened cells

May be difficult to distinguish from pulmonary adenocarcinoma
SPINDLE TYPE (SARCOMATOID)
More nodular and less plaquelike

Often with hemorrhage, necrosis, cystic changes

Highly cellular, interweaving bundles of spindle cells

Nuclear atypia, mitotic figures common

When large amounts of collagen: desmoplastic mesothelioma

Worse prognosis than epithelial type; more often becomes diffuse

Associated with hypoglycemia, which resolves upon removal of the tumor
MIXED (BIPHASIC)
Combination of epithelial and spindle types

Can resemble synovial sarcoma
SMALL CELL MESOTHELIOMA
Very rare

Distinguishing from Pulmonary Adenocarcinoma

Mesotheliomas produce hyaluronic acid (intracellular and extracellular), which can be stained with Alcian blue in a hyaluronidase-sensitive manner

Mucicarmine or PAS+ droplets in cells favor adenocarcinoma

Electron microscopy: mesothelial cells have long, slender microvilli

Mesothelial cells are keratin, vimentin, EMA, S-100 positive, and almost always CEA, Leu-M1, Ber-EP4 negative

Adenocarcinoma is consistently keratin, EMA, CEA, Leu-M1, Ber-EP4 positive

HMFG-2 stains only cell membranes of mesothelial cells but shows cytoplasmic staining for adenocarcinoma

8

HEART AND PERICARDIUM

NORMAL ANATOMY
Weight: 300–350 g (male); 250–300 g (female)
Right ventricle (RV): 3–5 mm; left ventricle (LV): 13–15 mm
VALVES
Lines of closure of semilunar valves marked by linear thickening, the centers of which have small fibrous nodules called *corpora arantii*

Small fenestrations may exist on the downstream side of the closure line near the commisural attachments

Papillary muscles for the mitral valve: anterolateral is a single large column; posteromedial divided into three to four pillars

Histology: endothelial lined; thin layer of collagen and elastic tissue on atrial side, thick layer of dense collagen on ventricular side, loose myxoid connective tissue (zona spongiosa) in between

CONDUCTING SYSTEM
Sinoatrial (SA) node: posterior wall of right atrium (RA), adjacent to superior vena cava (SVC)

Atrioventricular (AV) node: junction of median wall of right atrium with the interventricular septum

Bundle of His: interventricular septum

CORONARY ARTERIES
Left anterior descending (LAD): apex, anterior LV, anterior one third of RV, anterior two thirds of septum

Right coronary artery (RCA): lateral and posterior RV, posterior LV, posterior third septum

Left circumflex (LCx): lateral LV; in ~20% population, posterior circulation arises from this vessel ("left dominant")

EMBRYOLOGY
The cardiovascular system is the first to function in the embryo; blood begins to circulate by the end of the 3rd wk

Cardiac development begins on day 18–19 in the "cardiogenic area" of the splanchnic mesenchyme; heart forms as two side-by-side longitudinal cellular strands called *cardiogenic cords*

Cardiogenic cords become canalized to form endocardial heart tubes—later fuse to form a single heart tube

Formation of bulboventricular loop on day 23–24 introduces asymmetry

Arterial system develops from paired aortic arches

Venous system develops from venous end of heart

AORTIC ARCHES
1 Maxillary arteries
2 Stapedial arteries
3 Common carotids/internal carotids
4 Proximal right subclavian -and- aortic arch
5 Nothing—may not even develop
6 Right pulmonary -and- left pulmonary/ductus arteriosus

Note: Left subclavian forms from the 7th intersegmental artery, which migrates up the aorta to the arch

NON-NEOPLASTIC CARDIAC PATHOLOGY

Congenital Malformations
0.6–0.8% of live births
5% associated with chromosomal abnormalities
90% are "multifactorial" (unknown etiology)
2–10× more likely in sibling of an affected individual
However, monozygotic twins show only a 10% concordance of ventricular septal defects (VSDs)
Environmental causes: rubella, thalidomide, ethyl alcohol, smoking
Those producing right-to-left shunts (tetralogy of Fallot, transposition of the great vessels) also known as cyanotic heart disease; paradoxical embolization may occur
Those producing left-to-right shunts (VSD, PDA, atrial septal defect [ASD]) are also known as late cyanotic heart disease; the shunt induces pulmonary hypertension, right ventricular hypertrophy, and eventually reversal of the flow through the shunt (Eisenmenger's syndrome)

VENTRICULAR SEPTAL DEFECT
Most common type: 30%
Frequency has been increasing in U.S.
Small VSDs require no intervention; most close spontaneously
90% lie within or adjacent to the membranous septum

PATENT DUCTUS ARTERIOSUS
10% of congenital cardiac anomalies
Joins pulmonary trunk to aorta just distal to left subclavian artery; functionally closes in first day or two of life
Prostaglandin E maintains ductus open
Closure stimulated by increased oxygen tension
Indomethacin induces closure by inhibiting prostaglandin E synthesis

ATRIAL SEPTAL DEFECT
10% of congenital cardiac anomalies
Three types:
• Ostium primum (5%): low in septum, adjacent to AV valves; common in Down's syndrome
• Ostium secundum (90%): at the site of the foramen ovale
• Sinus venosus (5%): high in septum near SVC

PULMONIC STENOSIS/ATRESIA
7% of congenital cardiac anomalies
With atresia, RV hypoplastic
Stenosis usually caused by fusion of the valve cusps

COARCTATION OF THE AORTA
7% of congenital cardiac anomalies

Male : female = 3 : 1, also common in Turner's syndrome

Accompanied by other defects in 50% cases (PDA, bicuspid aortic valve, aortic stenosis (AS), ASD, VSD, . . .)

Usually occurs just distal (localized, adult type) or occasionally just proximal (diffuse, infantile type) to the ductus arteriosus

If not corrected, 60% die before age 40, often of aortic rupture

AORTIC STENOSIS
6% congenital cardiac anomalies

Most commonly bicuspid valve—predisposes to calcification later in life

Both valvular and subvalvular stenosis exist

TETRALOGY OF FALLOT
6% of congenital cardiac anomalies
- VSD, usually large
- Aorta that over-rides the septum
- Obstruction of RV outflow, usually caused by infundibular narrowing but occasionally pulmonic stenosis
- RV hypertrophy

Most common form of cyanotic heart disease

Can survive, even without surgical correction

Heart often boot-shaped on account of RV hypertrophy

Pulmonic orifice generally does not grow with heart, so right-to-left shunting can increase with age; however, pulmonary changes do not occur (stenosis protects lungs), and RV hypertrophy is limited because RV is decompressed into LV and aorta

TRANSPOSITION OF THE GREAT VESSELS
4% of congenital cardiac anomalies; more common in infants of diabetic mothers

Cyanosis from birth—some interatrial communication is required for survival; 60% have PDA, 30% have VSD

Most commonly, aorta arises from morphologic RV and lies anterior to the pulmonary artery

Surgical correction: Ventricles are inverted relative to the atria, so the RA supplies the LV and thus the pulmonary artery

Often, other abnormalities of the AV canal are present

TRUNCUS ARTERIOSUS
2% of congenital cardiac anomalies

Developmental failure of separation of the aorta and pulmonary artery: single large vessel with infundibular VSD

TRICUSPID ATRESIA
1.5% of congenital cardiac anomalies

Complete absence of tricuspid valve, underdeveloped RV, and an ASD

ANOMALOUS CORONARY ARTERIES
Left main arising from pulmonary trunk: early infarcts

Left main arising from right sinus of Valsalva: associated with sudden death in adults

Cardiomyopathies
Congestive Heart Failure
Common endpoint for many forms of heart disease

Decompensation of cardiac function following failure to maintain sufficient output for metabolic needs

LEFT-SIDED FAILURE
Causes: ischemic heart disease, hypertension, aortic or mitral valve disease, myocardial disease

Manifested most commonly by fluid accumulation in the lungs

Dyspnea, orthopnea, paroxysmal nocturnal dyspnea

RIGHT-SIDED FAILURE
Causes: Left-sided failure, increased pulmonary vascular resistance, myocarditis

Manifested by systemic congestion, esp. in the liver, spleen, subcutaneous tissue

ISCHEMIC HEART DISEASE
Causes of 80% of all cardiac mortality (only slightly less than in 1970)

By far, the most common cause of sudden cardiac death

>90% of cases caused by decreased coronary blood flow secondary to atherosclerosis, thrombosis, vasospasm, arteritis, emboli, increased right atrial pressure

Angina
Chest pain just short of irreversible myocardial damage

STABLE
Caused by fixed stenosis, usually in first 2 cm of major coronary artery; 75% stenosis is sufficient to limit flow requirements during increased demand

ST depressions seen on electrocardiogram (ECG): subendocardial ischemia

UNSTABLE (CRESCENDO)
Increasing frequency of pain, precipitated by decreasing efforts or occurring at rest

"Pre-infarction angina," likely to progress to infarction

Probably represents thrombosis of a branch rather than a main coronary artery, with subsequent dilatation of collateral channels preventing infarction (if progresses slowly enough to allow collateral dilatation)

PRINZMETAL'S (VARIANT)
Caused by coronary artery spasm

ST elevations seen on ECG: transmural ischemia

Myocardial Infarction
Predominantly a disease of the LV

25–80% (depending on study) caused by thrombosis, often over an ulcerated plaque, in a main coronary artery

5% occur before age 40; incidence increases with age

Male : female = 4–5 : 1 before age 50, then ratio decreases with age

Two types:
- Transmural ("q-wave infarct"): most common, near full thickness (>60%), >2.5 cm
- Subendocardial: necrosis limited to inner third to half of wall (systolic compression causes subendocardium to be most sensitive to ischemia)

Loss of contractility occurs with 1–2 min of ischemia, ATP is 50% depleted at 10 min, irreversible injury occurs at 20–40 min

GROSS CHANGES
None in first 6–12 hr, although treatment with triphenyltetrazolium chloride (TTC) can impart a red-brown color on noninfarcted myocardium (caused by presence of dehydrogenases), thereby highlighting infarcted areas, even at 3–6 hr postinfarct

18–24 hr: pallor; red-blue cyanotic hue; then yellow

1 wk: hyperemic rim of vascularized connective tissue

7 wk: scarring complete

HISTOLOGIC CHANGES

Waviness of fibers	1–3 hr
Coagulative necrosis	4–12 hr
Neutrophil infiltration	12–24 hr
Contraction band necrosis (reperfusion)	18–24 hr
Total coagulative necrosis	24–72 hr

COMPLICATIONS
Postinfarct arrhythmia (most common cause of death, in 90% of cases)
Congestive heart failure (60%)
Hypotension/shock (10%)
Myocardial rupture (1–5%, 2–5 days)
Papillary muscle infarction/rupture
Subsequent infarct expansion
Fibrinohemorrhagic pericarditis
Mural thrombosis
Ventricular aneurysm (1–2 days)

Chronic Ischemic Heart Disease
Diffuse myocardial atrophy (brown atrophy)
Patchy perivascular and interstitial fibrosis
Progressive ischemic necrosis

HYPERTENSIVE HEART DISEASE
Second most common heart disease; affects 25% of U.S. population
Result of pressure overload on heart
Myocytes form new myofilaments and organelles; nuclei and cells enlarge; *no* new cells are formed
With time, myocyte irregularities, dropout, and interstitial fibrosis is seen

COR PULMONALE
Refers to RV enlargement caused by diseases of the lung and specifically excluding LV hypertrophy as a cause
Seen with chronic obstructive pulmonary disease (COPD), pulmonary fibrosis of any etiology, pulmonary embolism or vascular sclerosis, kyphoscoliosis or massive obesity restricting chest wall movement, chronic atelectasis
Acute form produces RV dilatation
Chronic form produces RV hypertrophy

DILATED CARDIOMYOPATHY
AKA: congestive cardiomyopathy
Refers to disease of unknown etiology in theory, but some causal relationships are suspected
Heart increased in weight, but walls are of normal or reduced thickness
All four chambers usually dilated
Presents as slowly developing congestive failure, which is 75% fatal within 5 yr

ALCOHOLIC CARDIOMYOPATHY
Alcohol and its metabolites are directly toxic to myocardium
Thiamine deficiency and cobalt toxicity (used to be added to beer) also contribute

PHEOCHROMOCYTOMA
Patients with a pheochromocytoma may have foci of apparent ischemic necrosis in myocardium caused by catecholamine release
Mechanism appears related to vasomotor constriction in the face of an increased heart rate

HEMOCHROMATOSIS
Most commonly produces a dilated cardiomyopathy but may produce a restrictive picture

PERIPARTUM CARDIOMYOPATHY
Seen in month before or 6 months after delivery
Likely to be secondary to some nutritional deficiency

ADRIAMYCIN (DOXORUBICIN)
Vacuolization of myocytes caused by dilation of sarcotubular system is earliest change
"Adria cell": loss of cross striations, homogeneous basophilic staining, loss of myofilaments
Minimal to no inflammation
Occurs more frequently after a lifetime dose above 500 mg/m^2
Changes most pronounced in subendocardial region and are enhanced by radiation

CYCLOPHOSPHAMIDE
Hemorrhagic necrosis, extensive capillary thrombosis, interstitial hemorrhage and fibrin deposition

FAMILIAL CARDIOMYOPATHIES
POSTVIRAL MYOCARDITIS

IDIOPATHIC HYPERTROPHIC CARDIOMYOPATHY
AKA: idiopathic hypertrophic subaortic stenosis (IHSS), asymmetric septal hypertrophy (ASH)
May be restricted to septum (15–30 mm thick), but often not
Some degree of LV outflow tract obstruction is often seen (obstructive hypertrophic cardiomyopathy)
Myofiber hypertrophy, myofiber disarray, and interstitial fibrosis; intramyocardial coronary vessels seen in 50%
Endocardial fibrosis of outflow tract
In half of cases, autosomal dominant inheritance; in some cases, the mutation has been localized to the myosin gene (chromosome 14)
Often presents in young adults, either by asymptomatic murmur on routine physical exam or by sudden death during strenuous exercise (mean age 19 yr)

INFILTRATIVE/RESTRICTIVE CARDIOMYOPATHIES
Any disorder resulting in restriction of ventricular filling

AMYLOIDOSIS
As part of systemic amyloidosis (AA type of amyloid) or isolated as in senile cardiac amyloidosis (AF type of amyloid [transthyretin])

ENDOMYOCARDIAL FIBROSIS
Disease of children and young adults in Africa
Endocardial fibrosis extending from apex into outflow tracts of left and/or right ventricle
Scarring may extend into inner third of myocardium and may involve tricuspid and mitral valves
Varying amounts of inflammation, including eosinophils, often seen at edge of scarring

LÖFFLER'S ENDOCARDITIS
AKA: fibroblastic parietal endocarditis with blood eosinophilia
Similar to endomyocardial fibrosis; may be part of same spectrum
Three stages: acute myocarditis (necrotic), organizing thrombus, endomyocardial fibrosis
Eosinophilic infiltration of other organs often seen
Rapid downhill course to death

ENDOCARDIAL FIBROELASTOSIS
Pearly white thickening of endocardium caused by increase in collagen and elastic fibers on surface; most commonly in LV, occasionally in left atrium (LA), RV, RA

Most often seen in children under 2 yr; etiology unclear; may be a common pathway from several injury types

SARCOIDOSIS
Cardiac involvement in 25% of patients with systemic disease
Often present with arrhythmia or other conduction abnormality

GLYCOGENOSIS AND OTHER GLYCOGEN STORAGE DISEASES

HEMOCHROMATOSIS
Normally there is no stainable iron in the myocardium
Iron deposits are greater in the epicardium

MYOCARDITIS
Need to see both inflammation (usually lymphocytic) and myocyte necrosis
Most commonly results in a dilated cardiomyopathy
Deaths are from acute heart failure or arrhythmias

VIRAL
Accounts for most cases of well-documented myocarditis
Coxsackie A and B, ECHO, polio, influenza A and B, HIV
Cardiac involvement follows primary infection by days to weeks

PROTOZOAL
Chagas' disease (caused by *Trypanosoma cruzi*)
In endemic areas, causes 25% of ALL deaths in 25- to 40-year-old age group

HYPERSENSITIVITY
Primarily perivascular inflammation; can see eosinophils and occasional giant cells
Penicillin, sulfonamides, streptomycin

GIANT CELL MYOCARDITIS (FIEDLER'S)
Rare, idiopathic
Widespread myocardial necrosis with numerous giant cells
Seen in young adults; rapidly fatal

OTHERS
Bacterial, fungal, parasitic, spirochetes (Lyme disease), chlamydial disease
Collagen vascular disease, radiation, heat stroke, etc.
Sarcoidosis, Kawasaki disease

ARRHYTHMOGENIC RIGHT VENTRICLE
AKA: right ventricular cardiomyopathy, Uhl's anomaly, parchment RV
Focal thinning to absence of the RV myocardium caused by replacement of muscle by adipose and fibrous tissue (note: a small amount of fatty replacement is normal)
Often familial; usually affects men
Leads to RV dilatation, arrhythmias, and sudden death

Cardiac Transplantation

Myocardial biopsy most sensitive indicator of rejection
Need at least four pieces of tissue with myocardium to be an adequate sampling
Don't mistake a previous biopsy site as indicative of rejection
Quilty: dense subendocardial lymphocyte infiltrate, seen in 15% of post-transplant biopsies, often composed predominantly of B cells (unlike rejection, which is predominantly T cells)
Comment on whether or not there is myocyte necrosis

GRADING OF REJECTION
0   No rejection
I   Mild rejection
    IA: Patchy, perivascular inflammation
    IB: Diffuse, sparse interstitial infiltrate
II Moderate rejection: Single focus of aggressive infiltrate and/or isolated myocyte dropout
III Moderate rejection
    IIIA: Multifocal aggressive interstitial infiltrates
    IIIB: Diffuse inflammation with necrosis
IV Severe rejection: abundant myocyte death with vasculitis, hemorrhage, neutrophils, necrosis; usually not reversible

Valvular Heart Disease

MITRAL VALVE PROLAPSE
AKA: floppy mitral valve
Very common: 5–7% of U.S. population; male : female = 2 : 3; usually 20s–40s; also associated with Marfan syndrome
Midsystolic click; if valve leaks, also late systolic murmur
Intercordal ballooning (hooding), occasionally elongated chordae tendineae
20–40% have concomitant involvement of tricuspid valve; pulmonic involvement in 10%
Histology: myxoid degeneration of zona fibrosa, thickening of zona spongiosa (normal ratio 1 : 1)
Usually asymptomatic; however, can lead to infective endocarditis, mitral insufficiency (gradual or sudden), arrhythmias, or sudden death (rare)

CALCIFICATION OF MITRAL ANNULUS
Stony, hard beading behind valve leaflets at base, without accompanying inflammation, rarely affecting valve function
Seen in elderly patients, usually women, often in association with ischemic heart disease

CALCIFIC AORTIC STENOSIS
Commonly occurs with a congenital unicuspid valve (symptomatic before 15 yr) or a bicuspid valve (50s–60s); may also occur with a normal valve (70s–80s)
Calcified masses within the valve leaflets that protrude from both sides of the cusps, resulting in immobile leaflets and either stenosis, incompetence, or both
Unknown etiology and pathogenesis; more common in men
In bicuspid valves, begins at free ends and progresses toward base; in tricuspid valves, begins at base
Left ventricle undergoes secondary concentric hypertrophy
Treatment: valve replacement, balloon valvuloplasty

RHEUMATIC HEART DISEASE
Incidence steadily declining; now accounts for <10% of valvular heart disease, although still the most common cause of mitral stenosis and still a major cause of cardiac morbidity in the 15–25 yr age group
Rheumatic fever (RF) occurs 1–5 wk following a *Streptococcus* group A pharyngitis (streptococcal infections elsewhere are not rheumatogenic)
Etiology is immune, either on account of antibodies that crossreact with streptococcal antigens or autoantibodies

triggered by streptococcal antigens; antibodies localize to the sarcolemmal membranes

ACUTE RHEUMATIC FEVER
Acute, recurrent disease, usually in children (5–15 yr old)
Fever, migratory polyarthritis (in adults), carditis, subcutaneous nodules (giant Aschoff's bodies), erythema marginatum of skin (targetoid lesions), Sydenham's chorea
Edema, collagen fragmentation, and fibrinoid change dominate in early phase (2–4 weeks after pharyngitis)
Aschoff's bodies: subendocardial or perivascular foci of fibrinoid necrosis with lymphocytes, later with macrophages, which can become epithelioid (granulomatous); after many years, replaced by fibrous scar
Caterpillar cells: large, multinucleated giant cells with chromatin clumping lengthwise in nucleus, appearing owl-eyed on cross section
MacCallum's plaques: maplike thickening of endocardium over lesions, usually in left atrium
Lesions in pericardium, myocardium, and on valves
Valve lesions not well formed Aschoff's bodies: foci of fibrinoid necrosis along the lines of closure and on chordae tendineae; small vegetations may be present
Despite myocarditis, <1% patient die from ARF

CHRONIC RHEUMATIC HEART DISEASE
Develops in only a small number of patients with acute rheumatic fever (ARF), after 10 or more years, more commonly following recurrent ARF or if the initial ARF is severe or occurs early in childhood
Valve leaflets thickened; fibrous bridging across commissures; calcifications; "fish-mouth" deformity
Chordae tendineae thickened, fused, shortened
Mitral involvement alone in 65–70%, mitral and aortic in 25%; tricuspid only when both mitral and aortic involved; very rarely pulmonic

CARDIAC VALVE VEGETATIONS
INFECTIVE ENDOCARDITIS
Colonization or invasion of the valves by infective organisms, which lead to the formation of bulky, friable vegetations on flow side near free edge; often forms polypoid masses of thrombus laden with bacteria, which hang from edge of valve; may extend to back of valve
Acute and subacute forms, depending on the virulence of the organism; acute form usually bulkier, more often on normal valves, and more often erodes or perforates (can be fatal within days); subacute form, though more indolent, is less responsive to antibiotics and blood cultures often negative
Bacteremia seems to be a prerequisite for development of infective endocarditis but is clearly not sufficient
Cardiac abnormalities creating turbulent flow predispose: septal defects, valvular stenosis/reflux, prosthetic valves
Alcohol abuse, immunosuppression, and colon cancer are also predisposing conditions
~30% of cases occur on "normal" valves
65% caused by *Streptococcus* (*S. viridans, S. bovis, S. fecalis,* etc.); relatively low virulence; principal cause of subacute
20–30% caused by *Staphylococcus aureus:* more virulent, leading cause of acute disease
Others include strep pneumonia, *E. coli, Neisseria gonorrhoeae*

IV drug users: *Staphylococcus aureus, Candida, Aspergillus*

Valve Involvement	Left Sided	Right Sided
Acute	70%	25%
Subacute	90%	5–10%
IV drug use	40%	50%

Pulmonic valve almost never involved
In setting of artificial valve, often involve valve ring
Complications: valvular insufficiency or stenosis, abscess, embolization to lungs, brain, spleen, kidneys, metastatic infections, focal or diffuse glomerulonephritis

NONBACTERIAL THROMBOTIC ENDOCARDITIS (MARANTIC ENDOCARDITIS)
Precipitation of small, sterile masses of fibrin on valve leaflets
Usually single vegetation on line of closure, loosely attached
Commonly involves multiple valves
Can become large; indistinguishable from infective endocarditis but without valvular destruction; may be precursor to it
More common in chronic diseases (e.g., malignant tumors, esp. adenocarcinoma)

ENDOCARDITIS OF SYSTEMIC LUPUS ERYTHEMATOSUS (SLE) (LIBMAN-SACKS DISEASE)
Mitral and tricuspid valvulitis occasionally seen in SLE
Multiple small vegetations of the leaflets, usually on the back side (particularly the posterior mitral leaflet) but may be on flow side; diffusely distributed over leaflets; may extend onto mural endocardium
Edema, fibrinoid change, small deposits of nucleic acid
Rarely of clinical significance

LAMBL'S EXCRESCENCES
Small, heaped-up lesions on flow side of valves
Collections of fibrin at sites of endothelial damage

CARCINOID HEART DISEASE
Involves endocardium and valves of right heart, particularly RV outflow tract (pulmonic valve)
Carcinoid syndrome: episodic flushing of skin, cramps, nausea, vomiting, diarrhea—cardiac involvement in half, pulmonary involvement in one third
Plaquelike fibrous thickening of endocardium and valvular cusps with proliferation of smooth muscle and collagen deposition (there are no carcinoid tumor cells in the lesion)
No destruction of valve leaflet

HURLER'S DISEASE
Lack of iduronidase (mucopolysaccharidosis type I)
Sulfated mucopolysaccharides accumulate intracellularly in macrophages in the aortic and mitral valves, resulting in marked thickening with stenosis or incompetence

PROSTHETIC VALVES—COMPLICATIONS
6–9% per patient year
• Thrombosis and thromboembolism
• Infective endocarditis, most commonly *Staphylococcus*
• Calcifications
• Tears in leaflets/structural breakdown of valve

- Paravalvular leaks
- Occlusion or dysfunction caused by tissue overgrowth

CARDIAC TUMORS

Primary tumors are extremely rare; metastases much more likely (30× more likely)

Most common primary tumors (four) are benign and account for 70% of all primary tumors of the heart

Benign Tumors

MYXOMA
Most common primary cardiac tumor (50%)

Sporadic and familial types

Sporadic, tend to be single, and are more common in women; familial more likely to be multiple (one third), are more likely to occur outside of the left atrium, and present at an earlier age

90% located in atria, with 80% of those on the left; favored site is the fossa ovalis

1–10 cm, sessile or pedunculated

Easily confused grossly and histologically with organizing thrombus, esp. when sessile

May actually be a reactive process or a hamartoma

Myxoma cells: stellate or globular

Numerous small vessels in a myxoid acid mucopolysaccharide matrix, hemosiderin

Uncommon findings: mucin-producing glands, cartilage, EMA/CEA positivity

LIPOMA
Well localized, poorly encapsulated, usually subendocardial or subpericardial, but may be within myocardium

Usually left ventricle, right atrium, or interatrial septum

Like myxoma, may represent hamartomas

PAPILLARY FIBROELASTOMA
AKA: fibroelastic hamartoma, fibroma, papilloma, papillary fibroblastoma

Usually located on valves, particularly ventricular surface of semilunar valves and atrial surface of AV valves

Right-sided lesions more commonly in children, left-sided in adults

Cluster of hairlike projections 2–5 mm in length covering a discrete region of the endocardial surface

Central fibroelastic stroma, myxoid matrix, and overlying hyperplastic endothelium

Probably organized thrombi

RHABDOMYOMA
Most common primary cardiac tumor in children

Frequently discovered in 1st yr of life; often multiple; can cause valvular obstruction

Small, gray-white myocardial masses protruding into ventricular chamber

Mixture of large round and polygonal cells with glycogen-rich vacuoles separated by strands of cytoplasm radiating from cell center—*spider cells*—these cells have myofibers

Probably a hamartoma

50% are associated with tuberous sclerosis

40% mortality by 6 months of age; 60% by 1 yr, 80% by 5 yr

OTHERS
CONGENITAL POLYCYSTIC TUMOR OF THE ATRIOVENTRICULAR NODE

AKA: endodermal heterotopia, "mesothelioma of the AV node"

Ductular structures, cysts, and solid nests of epithelial-like cells with desmosomes and microvilli (keratin and CEA positive)

Because of location, may cause complete heart block

EPITHELIOID HEMANGIOMA

Solid or microcystic aggregates of cells with vesicular nuclei (often with deep grooves) and abundant acidophilic cytoplasm, often with vacuoles

Probably metaplastic process

May be mistaken for metastatic carcinoma

Cells are keratin positive (why?)

PARAGANGLIOMA

AKA: extra-adrenal pheochromocytoma

Left atrium most commonly

SCHWANNOMA

GRANULAR CELL TUMOR

Malignant Tumors

ANGIOSARCOMA
Typically in right atrium—large mass with intracavitary extension; may also infiltrate the myocardium

Appearance similar to angiosarcoma elsewhere, but tends to be more poorly differentiated

OTHERS
Kaposi's sarcoma

Liposarcoma

Rhabdomyosarcoma

Metastatic Tumors

In order of frequency: carcinomas of lung, carcinoma of breast, melanoma, lymphoma, leukemia, renal cell carcinoma, choriocarcinoma

Most often involve the pericardium, but may also be multifocal in the myocardium or produce an intracavitary lesion

PERICARDIUM

FLUID ACCUMULATION IN PERICARDIAL SAC
30–50 ml thin, clear, straw-colored fluid normally present

PERICARDIAL EFFUSIONS

Effusions as large as 500 ml can be seen

Serous: congestive heart failure, hypoproteinemia

Serosanguinous: blunt chest trauma, cardiopulmonary resuscitation (CPR)

Chylous: lymphatic obstruction (benign or malignant)

Cholesterol: rare; myxedema, usually idiopathic

HEMOPERICARDIUM
Rupture of heart or intrapericardial aorta (myocardial infarction [MI], dissecting aneurysm, sharp chest trauma)

TAMPONADE
200–300 ml, accumulated rapidly, can cause cardiac compression and death

PERICARDITIS
An acute inflammation; the term *chronic pericarditis* actually refers to healed pericarditis

FIBRINOUS PERICARDITIS
Most frequent type

Seen following myocardial infarction, rheumatic fever, trauma, uremia, radiation, SLE, severe pneumonias

Clinically, hear a loud pericardial friction rub

Rubbery fibrin mass loosely gluing the parietal and visceral pleura together ("bread and butter")

Histology: entangled mass of threadlike eosinophilic fibers or large amorphous mass

May resolve or become organized to produce an adhesive pericarditis

SEROUS PERICARDITIS
Rheumatic fever, SLE, systemic scleroderma, tumors, uremia, virus, or TB can present this way

Mild inflammation of epicardial and pericardial surfaces: both acute and chronic inflammatory cells

Serous fluid, usually 50–200 ml—exudative: thus, develops slowly and rarely alters cardiac function

SUPPURATIVE (PURULENT) PERICARDITIS
Bacterial, mycotic, or parasitic invasion

Male:female = 3:1, 10–40 yr

Enter pericardial space by direct extension, seeding from blood, lymphatic spread, seeding by instrumentation

Inflammation may extend into surrounding mediastinum

Usually results in organization and thus a constrictive pericarditis with clinical sequelae

HEMORRHAGIC PERICARDITIS
TB or malignant neoplasm (from lung or breast)

Can also be seen following cardiac surgery

CASEOUS PERICARDITIS
Almost always TB

CONSTRICTIVE PERICARDITIS
Usually idiopathic, but may follow suppurative or caseous pericarditis (classically TB) or after cardiac surgery or heavy irradiation

Pericardial space obliterated and transformed into a thick (0.5–1 cm) mass of fibrosis and scar tissue, usually with calcification, encasing heart and causing tremendous restriction

When adhesion and fibrosis extends from parietal pericardium into the mediastinum, referred to as *adhesive mediastinopericarditis*

Increased workload on heart induces hypertrophy and dilatation; however, if tightly adherent to the heart, cardiac hypertrophy and/or dilatation cannot occur

SOLDIER'S PLAQUE
Focal pearly thickened epicardial plaque—indicative of a healed pericarditis

9

BLOOD AND LYMPHATIC VESSELS

NORMAL ANATOMY/HISTOLOGY
Three layers: intima, media, adventitia
Veins and lymphatics have "valves"—endothelial folds

Artery Types
LARGE ELASTIC ARTERIES
AKA: aorta, brachiocephalic, subclavian, early common carotid
Intima initially very thin, but thickens with age as myointimal cells proliferate and matrix accumulates
Media contains a large amount of elastic tissue (responsible for maintaining both blood pressure and blood flow during diastole); poor vascular supply (only outer third penetrated by vasa vasorum)
Adventitia poorly defined; many vasa vasorum
MEDIUM-SIZED MUSCULAR ARTERIES
Media well demarcated by internal and external elastic lamina
Elastic laminae are fenestrated, allowing smooth muscle migration into intima
ARTERIOLES (<2 mm)
Thickness of wall is about equal to the diameter of the lumen
As caliber decreases, lose demarcation of layers
Rich nervous supply—responsible for autonomic control of systemic blood pressure

Cell Types
ENDOTHELIAL CELLS
Thromboresistant
Contain numerous pinocytotic vesicles and Weibel-Palade bodies (rod-shaped cytoplasmic organelles 0.1–0.3 μm in length containing an internal structure of parallel tubules; these bodies contain the factor VIII associated antigen, AKA: von Willebrand factor)
Intercellular junction integrity can be adjusted by vasoactive substances
Can actively contract
SMOOTH MUSCLE CELL
Vasoconstriction and dilatation are major roles
Can migrate, proliferate, and can synthesize collagen, elastin, and proteoglycans
Have receptors for low density lipoprotein (LDL)
Responsible for intimal collagenization in atherosclerosis

EMBRYOLOGY
Vascular system develops in week 3 of fetal life from mesodermal cells of the "blood islands" (peripheral cells of islands form endothelium, central cells give rise to hematopoietic elements)
Initially located in region of yolk sac, eventually spread throughout mesenchyme of fetus
Later, pericytes from the surrounding mesenchyme join the primitive vessels and differentiate into the wall layers

NORMAL HEMOSTASIS
Sequence: vascular injury, brief vasoconstriction, binding of platelets to subendothelial connective tissue, activation of platelets with aggregation (primary hemostasis), activation of plasma coagulation cascade (secondary hemostasis)
Balance between antithrombotic and thrombotic activities
ANTITHROMBOTIC
Endothelial surface is nonthrombogenic
Thrombomodulin (endothelial surface protein) binds thrombin, converting it into a protein C activator, which, with protein S, is a potent anticoagulant
Heparin-like molecules on the endothelium accentuate the effects of antithrombin III
Prostacyclin (PGI$_2$) and ADPase activity inhibit platelet aggregation
Tissue plasminogen activator (tPA) promotes fibrinolytic activity by activating plasmin
Blood flow dilutes activated clotting factors—cleared by liver
THROMBOTIC
Subendothelial connective tissue is very thrombogenic
Thromboplastin (tissue factor) and other elements of clotting cascade—von Willebrand factor, thromboxane A$_2$ (synthesized by platelets), and platelet activating factor—induce platelet aggregation
tPA inhibitor limits fibrinolysis
PLATELETS
Alpha-granules: fibrinogen, fibronectin, platelet-derived growth factor, beta-thromboglobulin
Dense bodies: rich in ADP and ionized calcium; also histamine, serotonin (5-HT), epinephrine

NON-NEOPLASTIC VASCULAR PATHOLOGY

Congenital Anomalies

ARTERIOVENOUS MALFORMATIONS
Abnormal communication between arterial and venous systems (without passing through capillaries)
If large, can lead to right-sided heart failure
May be congenital or acquired (e.g., as a result of penetrating injury, inflammatory necrosis, aneurysmal rupture)

BERRY ANEURYSM
Most common vascular malformation of cerebral vessels

Accounts for 95% of cerebral aneurysms that rupture

Occurs at bifurcation of major arteries:
- 40% anterior communicating and anterior cerebral junction
- 34% bifurcation of middle cerebral in Sylvian fissure
- 20% internal carotid and posterior communicating junction
- 4% bifurcation of basilar into posterior cerebral arteries

Multiple in 20–30% of cases

Although referred to as "congenital," most are not present at birth; develop because of a congenital weakness in wall (muscular discontinuity in media at carina of bifurcation)

Straining at stool, lifting, sexual intercourse are associated with rupture: "Worst headache I've ever had"

Likelihood of rupture increased when diameter >1 cm

Most are sporadic, but increased association with polycystic kidney disease and other cerebral arteriovenous malformations

Rupture is fatal in 25–50%; some of the survivors will re-bleed

FIBROMUSCULAR DYSPLASIA

Pathogenesis unknown: no necrosis, calcification, inflammation, arteriosclerosis

Usually develop by 20–30 yr of age

Involves large- and medium-sized muscular arteries: renal, carotid, axillary, mesenteric

Abnormal arrangement of the cellular and extracellular elements of wall, particularly media, with disorderly proliferation and distortion of the lumen

Six distinct types:
- Intimal fibroplasia (1–2%): indistinguishable from proliferative stage of atherosclerosis, but no lipid
- Medial fibroplasia (60–70%): "string of beads," alternating stenosis (intimal fibrosis and medial thickening) and mural thinning/aneurysms
- Medial hyperplasia (5–15%)
- Perimedial fibroplasia (15–25%): fibrosis of outer half of media, with inner portion normal, with circumferential and uniform thickening of vessel and narrowing of lumen
- Medial dissection (5–15%): medial fibrosis; dissecting aneurysms
- Periarterial fibroplasia (1%): perivascular fibrosis and inflammation

Degenerative Conditions

ARTERIOSCLEROSIS

AKA: "hardening of the arteries"

Three distinctive morphologic variants are recognized

ATHEROSCLEROSIS

Term often used interchangeably with *arteriosclerosis*

Most common type; most common cause of death (myocardial infarcts, cerebral vascular accidents)

Atheroma (fibrofatty plaque): raised focal white to whitish-yellow plaque within the intima; core composed of lipid (mainly cholesterol, also cell debris, crystals, foam cells, calcium); overlying fibrous cap (smooth muscle cells, macrophages, foam cells, collagen, lymphocytes [most of which are T cells])

Most common sites: abdominal aorta, proximal coronary arteries, popliteal arteries, descending thoracic aorta, internal carotids, circle of Willis

Atheromas sparse at first, but can coalesce and become "complicated": calcification, necrosis, ulceration, thrombosis, aneurysmal dilatation, hemorrhage

Fatty streak: *may* be precursor lesion of atheromas: yellow lesions composed of lipid-filled smooth muscle cells and macrophages in lumen; present in aortas of all individuals over 1 yr old; distribution different from atheromas

Risk factors
- Age, male, familial predisposition
- Hyperlipidemia: risk correlates best with LDL levels (LDL contains ~70% circulating cholesterol—transports endogenously synthesized cholesterol), cholesterol >220 mg/dl; most important risk factor in <45 yr old
- Hypertension: >140/90 mmHg; diastolic most important correlate
- Cigarette smoking: >1 pack per day increases risk 70–200%
- Diabetes: twofold increase in myocardial infarctions; 150-fold increase in lower extremity ischemia
- Others: sedentary or stressful lifestyles, obesity, oral contraceptives, high carbohydrate intake

Multiple risk factors are more than additive

Theories of pathogenesis
- Reaction to injury: leak of serum proteins and lipids, platelets, monocytes—ingrowth of smooth muscle cells
- Primary smooth muscle proliferation
- Encrustation of small thrombi

ARTERIOLOSCLEROSIS

Two types, both more severe in patients with hypertension

Hyaline arteriolosclerosis

Homogeneous pink hyaline thickening of walls with loss of underlying structure

Commonly seen in diabetes, especially in the kidneys

May be caused by leakage of plasma components

Hyperplastic arteriolosclerosis

More common in severe hypertension (i.e., malignant)

Concentric thickening of wall and narrowing of lumen caused by smooth muscle proliferation

Fibrinoid and acute necrosis can be seen

Kidney, periadrenal fat, gallbladder, peripancreatic, intestine

MÖNCKEBERG'S ARTERIOSCLEROSIS

AKA: medial calcific sclerosis

Calcifications in media of medium to small arteries with no associated inflammation—may ossify

Most commonly: femoral, tibial, radial, ulnar, genital tract

Rare before 50 yr—completely unrelated to atherosclerosis

CYSTIC MEDIAL NECROSIS

Accumulation of amorphous material in the media, often forming cysts or mucoid pools

Disruption of the structure of the tunica media by the appearance of small clefts filled with a slightly basophilic ground substance

Predisposes to dissections

Etiology unclear; seen in Marfan's syndrome

ANEURYSMS

Localized abnormal dilatation of any vessel

Most commonly caused by atherosclerosis and/or cystic medial necrosis; seen in Marfan's syndrome and Takayasu's arteritis

Classified grossly: berry (small), saccular, fusiform

By far the most common site is the aorta, specifically abdominal; also in common iliacs, ascending aorta, descending thoracic aorta, and popliteal artery

When caused by atherosclerosis, rarely seen before age 50 yr

Usually filled with mural thrombus

Thrombus may become superinfected by bacteria (usually *Salmonella, Staphylococus:* embolization from endocarditis) or fungus (*Aspergillus,* mucormycosis)

Complications include embolism of mural thrombus, rupture

Abdominal aneurysms >6 cm carry a 50% chance for rupture within 10 yr; rupture is fatal more than 50% of time

DISSECTING ANEURYSMS
AKA: dissecting hematoma, aortic dissection; both better terms because usually *not* associated with previous aneurysm

40–60 yr age group, male : female = 2–3 : 1; plus pregnant women

Hypertension is present in 95% of patients

Sudden onset of excruciating pain beginning in the anterior chest and radiating to the back

Untreated, 35% fatal within 15 min, 75% within 1 wk

Intimal tear usually (90%) in ascending aorta

Blood tracks through media and adventitia both distally and proximally; proximal dissections are most lethal

Fatalities usually follow secondary rupture into pericardial sac or pleural cavity

Types	Classification System	
	Old	New
Ascending and descending aorta	I	A
Ascending aorta only	II	A
Descending only, above diaphragm	IIIA	B
Descending only, extending below diaphragm	IIIB	B

SYPHILITIC (LUETIC) ANEURYSMS
Confined to thoracic aorta, usually ascending and transverse

Inflammation and destruction (endarteritis obliterans) of vasa vasorum, leading to medial necrosis, inflammation, and scarring; scar retraction gives wrinkled "tree-bark" intima

Dilatation may involve aortic valve ring, leading to incompetence with thickening and rolling of the valve leaflets

MYCOTIC ANEURYSM
Aneurysm secondary to weakening of wall from infectious vasculitis, most commonly bacterial (*Salmonella*)

VARICOSE VEINS
Dilated, tortuous veins, which lead to valvular incompetence, stasis, congestion, edema, and thrombosis

Most commonly involves the legs, often following pregnancy

Pathogenesis related to prolonged elevated intraluminal pressure

More important sites clinically are esophageal and hemorrhoidal varices following portal hypertension

DISTAL AORTIC THROMBOSIS
AKA: Leriche's syndrome

Insidious onset and gradual progression of pain and fatigability of hips, legs, back; claudication, impotence

Often find absent pulses below umbilicus

Thrombotic occlusion of iliac arteries and distal aorta

Probably complication of atherosclerosis with ulceration

CYSTIC ADVENTITIAL DEGENERATION
Rare, almost always the popliteal artery

Mucinous degeneration in the wall leads to deposition of jelly-like material, which bulges into lumen and can cause obstruction

Probably related to pathogenesis of soft tissue ganglion

PHLEBOTHROMBOSIS/THROMBOPHLEBITIS
Terms are interchangeable because always see inflammation in thrombosed vessels

Three major predisposing factors:
- Alteration in blood flow
- Injury to endothelium
- Hypercoagulability of the blood

Most common sites: calf (rarely embolize), femoral, popliteal, iliac, periprostatic/periuterine veins

Risk factors:
- Prolonged bed rest, postoperative state, immobilization
- Myocardial infarction and cardiac failure
- Pregnancy, postdelivery, oral contraceptives
- Cancer
- Others: tissue damage, antithrombin III deficiency, protein C deficiency, prosthetic valves, atrial fibrillation, nephrotic syndrome, hyperlipidemia, smoking

Phlegmasia alba dolens: AKA milk leg: iliofemoral venous thrombosis occurring in 3rd trimester of pregnancy; combination of venous thrombosis and lymphangitis, leading to lymphedema

Vasculitides

Any inflammation of vessels that is not simply a direct extension from surrounding inflammation

Most are noninfectious immunologically mediated inflammations

Anticardiolipin antibodies present in most forms of vasculitis, probably a marker for vascular damage

TEMPORAL (GIANT CELL) ARTERITIS
AKA: cranial arteritis, Horton's disease

Focal granulomatous inflammation (with or without necrosis) of medium and small arteries of the head and neck (although may be seen elsewhere, such as the aorta or mesenteric artery) with destruction of the internal and external elastic laminae

Most common vasculitis: ~1% of all people >80 yr old; male : female = 1 : 3; associated with HLA-DR4

Headache, scalp tenderness, jaw pain, visual loss; markedly elevated erythrocyte sedimentation rate

Temporal artery biopsy positive in 60% of classic cases

Believed to be autoimmune in origin

Rapidly remits with steroid therapy

POLYMYALGIA RHEUMATICA
Flulike syndrome that accompanies half cases of temporal arteritis (TA)

Visual symptoms in 40%

POLYARTERITIS NODOSA (PAN)
CLASSIC PAN
Disease of young adults, male : female = 2–3 : 1

Nodular lesions of small- or medium-sized muscular arteries, esp. renal (85%), coronary (75%), hepatic (65%), and GI tract (50%) (pulmonary circulation spared) with sharp demarcations (segmental lesions); most commonly at branch points

Often present with fever of unknown cause, hematuria, albuminuria, hypertension, abdominal pain and melena, muscular aches, motor peripheral neuritis

Lesions frequently scattered and of various ages

Frequently leads to aneurysms (esp. in intestinal branches) and to thrombosis with infarction of supplied areas

Acute lesions show segmental fibrinoid necrosis, which may be full thickness, with neutrophils, eosinophils, and lymphocytes

Healing lesions show fibroblastic proliferation; elastin stains show disruption of internal elastic lamina

30% of patients have HepB antigen in serum

Antineutrophil cytoplasmic antibodies correlate with disease severity (usually P-ANCA [myeloperoxidase]; not specific)

CHURG-STRAUSS SYNDROME

AKA: allergic granulomatosis and angiitis

Variant of PAN with involvement of tracheal, pulmonary and splenic vessels (arteries, arterioles, capillaries, and veins)

Intravascular and extravascular necrotizing granulomas with eosinophils

Strong association with bronchial asthma and eosinophilia

WEGENER'S GRANULOMATOSIS

Acute necrotizing granulomas of upper and lower respiratory tract (with giant cells and leukocytes), with an accompanying necrotizing vasculitis of the pulmonary vessels and glomeruli, leading to persistent pneumonitis, chronic sinusitis, nasopharyngeal ulcerations, renal disease

Can be isolated to the lung

Peak incidence is in 40s; male > female

Involves predominantly arteries, but also veins

Serum antineutrophil cytoplasmic antibodies serve as marker for disease activity (usually C-ANCA [lysosomal enzymes])

If untreated, 80% will die within 1 yr; if treated (immunosuppression, e.g., cyclophosphamide), 90% respond

BUERGER'S DISEASE

AKA: thromboangiitis obliterans

Acute and chronic inflammation, often granulomatous, of intermediate and small muscular arteries and veins of extremities, usually the legs, leading to focal stenosing or occluding thrombosis

Begins before age 35 yr in most patients, male > > female

Strong correlation with smoking, including relapses

Neutrophil infiltration of wall, occlusive thrombosis, small microabscesses within the thrombus, Langhans' giant cells

Often leads to gangrene of extremities

KAWASAKI'S DISEASE

AKA: mucocutaneous lymph node syndrome

Acute illness of infants and children with fever, conjunctivitis, lymphadenopathy, skin rash; male : female = 1.5 : 1

70% show coronary artery involvement (1–2% mortality)

Acute necrotizing vasculitis (resembles PAN), which can lead to aneurysm formation

Some patients are ANCA positive

May be retroviral in origin

TAKAYASU'S ARTERITIS

Chronic granulomatous arteritis involving adventitia and media and producing intimal fibrosis and fibrous thickening of the aortic arch with marked focal narrowing of the origins of the arch vessels

Common in Orient, male : female = 1 : 3, 15–45 yr old, often HLA-DR4

Ocular disturbances, weakened pulses in upper extremities ("pulseless disease"), subclavian bruits, hypertension, syncope, hemiplegia

GRANULOMATOUS ANGIITIS OF THE CNS

Dense inflammatory infiltrate with necrosis involving small- and medium-sized arteries of the cerebrum and meninges

Rare; affects individuals >40 yr old

HYPERSENSITIVITY VASCULITIS

AKA: leukocytoclastic vasculitis, microscopic polyarteritis

Acute necrotizing inflammation of small vessels (arterioles, venules, capillaries); male = female

May be confined to skin or also involve mucous membranes, lungs, brain, heart, GI tract, kidneys, muscle

All lesions in a patient tend to be of same age

Drugs (penicillin), microorganisms, heterologous proteins, and tumor antigens have been implicated as triggers

Hypersensitivity vasculitis is the histologic pattern seen with the vasculitis of connective tissue diseases (SLE, rheumatoid arthritis), malignancies (lymphoproliferative), mixed cryoglobulinemia, Henoch-Schönlein purpura, drug reactions, serum sickness, amphetamine use, etc.

INFECTIOUS ARTERITIS

Usually suppurative or granulomatous

Bacterial: usually spread from nearby necrotizing inflammation

Fungal: aspergillosis and mucormycosis are angioinvasive, and thus very prone to produce vasculitis and thrombosis

Other Non-Neoplastic Lesions

RAYNAUD'S DISEASE/PHENOMENON

RAYNAUD'S DISEASE

Small arteries and arterioles in extremities undergo vasospasm in response to cold or emotional stress, producing pain and color changes from white to blue to red

Usually affects young, healthy women

No anatomic abnormality seen

RAYNAUD'S PHENOMENON

Cold sensitivity, pain, color changes in skin secondary to an anatomic lesion in the vessel wall

Can be seen with arteriosclerosis, connective tissue diseases (scleroderma, SLE), vasculitis, etc.

LYMPHEDEMA

Any swelling, usually of extremity, caused by increased interstitial fluid

OBSTRUCTIVE LYMPHEDEMA

From tumors, inflammation, surgery, postradiation fibrosis, filariasis, pregnancy, etc.

Rupture of dilated lymphatics can lead to chylous ascites, chylothorax, chylopericardium

LYMPHEDEMA PRAECOX
Swelling of feet and ankles in women 10–25 yr old that may remain localized or progress upward throughout life
Unknown etiology
MILROY'S DISEASE
Similar to lymphedema praecox but present at birth
Mendelian inheritance

VASCULAR TUMORS

IMMUNOHISTOCHEMISTRY AND ELECTRON MICROSCOPY
Endothelial cells: positive for factor VIII–related antigen (most reliable and most specific), vimentin (esp. epithelioid lesions), *Ulex eruopeaus* I lectin, collagen IV
Normal lymphatic vessels will be negative for factor VIII and will not contain Weibel-Palade bodies
Pericytes (smooth muscle and glomus cells): cytoplasmic microfilaments, pinocytotic vesicles, reactivity for actin, vimentin, myosin; desmin positive only in smooth muscle

Reactive Vascular Proliferations

VASCULAR ECTASIAS
Dilatation of preexisting vessels; not neoplasms
NEVUS FLEMMEUS
AKA: nevus telangiectaticus, ordinary birthmark
Dilatation of vessels of middle and deep dermis
Most commonly middle forehead, eyelids, nape of neck
Most regress spontaneously, those of the neck more slowly
NEVUS VINOSUS (PORT WINE STAIN)
Specialized form of nevus flemmeus that grows with child and does not regress; overlying skin becomes thickened
Sturge-Weber syndrome (AKA encephalotrigeminal angiomatosis): port wine stain of face in distribution of trigeminal nerve associated with ipsilateral vascular malformations of the meninges and/or the retina
NEVUS ARANEUS (ARTERIAL SPIDER)
"Spider telangiectasias" with central feeder vessels and radiating smaller vessels; blanch with pressure
Acquired in pregnancy, liver disease, hyperthyroidism
HEREDITARY HEMORRHAGIC TELANGIECTASIA
AKA: Osler-Weber-Rendu disease
Autosomal dominant, vascular anomalies of skin and mucosal membranes, esp. face and mouth
Prone to bleeding (nose bleeds, GI bleeds, urinary bleeds)
Attempts to treat result in formation of satellite lesions

PAPILLARY ENDOTHELIAL HYPERPLASIA
AKA: intravascular hemangioendothelioma, intravascular angiomatosis, Masson lesion
An unusual form of organizing thrombus
Most commonly excised from head, neck, fingers, trunk
Intraluminal papillary growth of plump endothelial cells overlying a thin collagenous core; simulates angiosarcoma
Pleomorphism and mitoses are minimal
Passive seeding into surrounding tissue may occur following rupture; does not signify malignancy
Excision is curative

BACILLARY ANGIOMATOSIS
AKA: epithelioid angiomatosis
Usually HIV-infected patients; appearance similar to Kaposi's sarcoma and pyogenic granuloma
Multiple friable papules, usually dermal or subcutaneous, involving any site on the body; can involve liver, spleen, and lymph nodes as well
Lobular vascular proliferation with rounded vascular profiles and plump, protuberant, often epithelioid endothelium
Mitoses, necrosis common
Neutrophils present, usually in perivascular clusters (microabscesses)
Clusters of bacteria with trilaminar structure consistent with gram-negative Rickettsia-like bacilli; stain with silver stains
Treatment: antibiotics (erythromycin)

PELIOSIS
(See Liver outline)

VASCULAR TRANSFORMATION OF LYMPH NODES
AKA: nodal angiomatosis
Occurs following obstruction of lymphatic outflow

Benign Tumors

Hemangiomas are among the most common soft tissue tumors
Comprise 7% of all benign tumors
Most common tumor in infancy and childhood
Skin is most common site, liver most common internal site
Many seem to be under hormonal control and fluctuate in size with pregnancy and menarche

CAPILLARY HEMANGIOMA
Proliferation of small, capillary-sized vessels lined by flattened endothelium; well defined but unencapsulated
Characteristically bright red to blue
JUVENILE CAPILLARY HEMANGIOMA
AKA: strawberry nevus, cellular hemangioma, nevus vasculosus
Immature form of capillary hemangioma
1/200 live births; 20% are multiple
Most common on head and neck, esp. parotid region
Grow following birth; may become elevated and protrude
Usually reach largest size by 6 months, then regress over years; 75–90% involute by age 7
Early lesions are cellular with plump endothelial cells; mature with age
ACQUIRED TUFTED ANGIOMA
Similar to juvenile hemangioma, but occurring in older age group
VERRUCOUS HEMANGIOMA
Variant of capillary or cavernous hemangioma, the skin over which undergoes reactive hyperkeratosis
Usually lower extremity, childhood
Tendency to recur if incompletely excised
CHERRY ANGIOMA
AKA: senile angioma, DeMorgan's spots
Small bright-red papule with pale halo
Most commonly seen on trunk and extremities

LOBULAR CAPILLARY HEMANGIOMA

AKA: pyogenic granuloma, granulation tissue hemangioma
Rapidly growing, purple-red friable polypoid lesion occurring on skin or mucosal surfaces: gingiva, finger, lips, face, tongue; all ages affected
One third linked to minor trauma
Each lobule has central vessel with numerous smaller vessels in an inflamed edematous stroma; numerous mitoses common
16% recur following excision

GRANULOMA GRAVIDARUM

Specialized form occurring on gingiva during ~1% of pregnancies
Develop in 1st trimester; regress rapidly postpartum

INTRAVENOUS PYOGENIC GRANULOMA

Usually neck or arm
Often mistaken for organizing thrombus

CAVERNOUS HEMANGIOMA

Large, cavernous vascular channels
Skin, usually of upper body; also liver, spleen, pancreas, CNS
May be engorged capillary hemangiomas, but usually larger, less circumscribed, more likely to be deep, don't regress, may be locally destructive
Thrombosis and calcification common
Kasabach-Merritt syndrome: thrombocytopenia and purpura seen in patients with a giant hemangioma, possibly caused by platelet sequestration within tumor
Maffucci's syndrome: combination of multiple cavernous hemangiomas and numerous enchondromas, usually of the fingers

ARTERIOVENOUS HEMANGIOMA

AKA: cirsoid aneurysm, racemose hemangioma
Superficial and deep types
Symptoms related to degree of shunting; deep type tends to have more significant shunting
Usually young individuals; most commonly head, neck, legs
Medium-sized arteries and veins amidst capillary hemangioma
Cure often requires deep surgical excision

VENOUS HEMANGIOMA

AKA: large vessel hemangioma
Similar to cavernous hemangiomas but larger
Smooth muscle of venous wall often disorganized and blends into surrounding tissues
Thrombosis and calcification common

EPITHELIOID HEMANGIOMA

AKA: angiolymphoid hyperplasia with eosinophilia, Kimura's disease, histiocytoid hemangioma, inflammatory angiomatous nodule, pseudopyogenic granuloma
20–40 yr old; female > male; head and neck, esp. around ear
May be multiple, may even be intravascular
Circumscribed, usually subcutis or dermis, but may be deep
Multiple small peripheral vessels around a parent vessel; vascular spaces lined by epithelioid histiocytes, tombstoning into lumen and occasionally forming solid islands; surrounding stroma contains mixed inflammatory cell infiltrate with many eosinophils but also mast cells, plasma cells, lymphoid aggregates, even germinal centers

Controversial as to whether this is reactive or neoplastic
80% respond to radiotherapy; if excised, one third will recur; only one reported case of metastasis

DEEP SOFT TISSUE HEMANGIOMAS

Uncommon

SKELETAL MUSCLE HEMANGIOMA

80–90% before age 30
Most commonly muscles of the thigh
Can be capillary, cavernous, or mixed type; mixed type most likely to recur
May have a significant amount of associated fat
Perineural involvement occurs; does not make malignant
18% will recur following excision

SYNOVIAL HEMANGIOMA

Almost invariably around the knee
Cavernous hemangiomas with myxoid or hyalinized stroma separating the vascular spaces
Overlying synovium is often hyperplastic

ANGIOMATOSIS

AKA: diffuse hemangioma
Multiple lesions involving large areas of the body, often the trunk or an extremity
Proliferation of small- to medium-sized vessels, usually thin walled, diffusely infiltrating the dermis, subcutis, or muscle, accompanied by a lot of mature adipose tissue

LYMPHANGIOMATOSIS

Lymphatic counterpart; two can occur together
Principally children
Three quarters have bone lesions (osteolytic)
Prognosis determined by extent of disease

LYMPHANGIOMA

Much less common than hemangiomas
Most are congenital and represent malformations with obstruction of outflow; rarely may be acquired
Most commonly head and neck, then trunk (axilla), extremities, may be intraabdominal
In mesentery, vessel walls may be thick

CAVERNOUS LYMPHANGIOMA

Congenital/infantile
Large, diffuse, doughy mass, prone to local recurrence
Dilated dermal and subcutaneous lymphatic channels without endothelial atypia

CYSTIC HYGROMA

Large cystic mass, neck or inguinal region, infants, prone to local recurrence
Histology as for cavernous, but grossly dilated spaces

LYMPHANGIOSUM CIRCUMSCRIPTUM

Numerous small vesicles or blebs; any age patient
Deep (subcutaneous) as well as superficial (papillary dermis) dilatation of lymphatics
Overlying papillomatous hyperplasia

LYMPHANGIOMYOMATOSIS

AKA: intrathoracic angiomyomatous hyperplasia
Proliferation of smooth muscle of the lymphatics and lymph nodes in the mediastinum, retroperitoneum, and lungs
Exclusively females; mean age 40 yr
Progressive dyspnea due to chylous pleural effusions
In lung, proliferation of smooth muscle around arterioles, venules, and lymphatics; alveolar septa become thickened

May be part of spectrum of tuberous sclerosis (like angio-myolipomas are) and thus hamartomas rather than true neoplasms

Hemangioendotheliomas

Vascular tumors of intermediate malignancy
Generally greater cellularity and mitotic activity than hemangiomas but lacking features of frank malignancy

INFANTILE HEMANGIOENDOTHELIOMA
Almost always occur before 1 yr of age
TYPE I
Cellular proliferation of small vessels with plump walls occurring in skin
Benign lesions
TYPE II
Freely anastomosing vascular channels, solid areas, mitoses common
More commonly occur in internal sites (e.g., liver)
Can be aggressive; many consider this type to be equivalent to angiosarcoma
Occurrence in multiple sites could represent multifocality or metastases

EPITHELIOID HEMANGIOENDOTHELIOMA
Can occur at any age; male = female; predominantly skin of extremities, liver, and lung
Solitary, slightly painful soft tissue mass often centered about a parent vessel
When vessel present (usually a vein), lumen often filled with tumor and necrotic debris
Epithelial-appearing cells of the tumor cluster in small nests, which do not form vessels but rather have intracellular lumina, frequently confused with mucin vacuoles
Stroma can be myxoid of hyalinized
15% recur; 30% metastasize to local nodes, lung, liver, bone
Significant atypia or high mitotic rate (>1/10 HPF) indicates a more aggressive course
Differential: melanoma, carcinoma, epithelioid sarcoma
INTRAVASCULAR BRONCHOALVEOLAR TUMOR (IV-BAT)
In the lung, this lesion was originally mistaken as an intravascular bronchioloalveolar carcinoma
More common in women
Higher mortality than soft tissue counterpart

SPINDLE CELL HEMANGIOENDOTHELIOMA
Occurs at any age; half of cases less than 25 yr old; male : female = 2 : 1
Small red nodules in the subcutaneous tissue or dermis of the hand (or other distal extremity site)
Cavernous, thin-walled vessels with organizing thrombi, separated by proliferation of spindle cells suggestive of Kaposi's sarcoma but also containing epithelioid endothelial cells with intracytoplasmic lumina; minimal inflammatory response
Spindled cells are often factor VIII negative
Two thirds recur

MALIGNANT ENDOVASCULAR PAPILLARY ANGIOENDOTHELIOMA
AKA: Dabska tumor

Discrete mass or diffuse subcutaneous swelling in the skin of young children
Large, almost cavernous vascular spaces, often without blood cells, with papillary projections containing hyaline cores of basement membrane material and lined by plump cells, which may focally be columnar
Occasional lymph node (LN) metastases, but overall prognosis is good

Malignant Tumors

ANGIOSARCOMA
Rare; <1% of all sarcomas
Most common sites: skin, soft tissue, breast, liver, bone, spleen; soft tissue lesions can arise from major vessels
Predisposing factors: chronic lymphedema, radiation; do *not* appear to arise in benign vascular lesions
Clinically, lesion is poorly defined; lateral extent in subcutaneous tissues often greatly exceeds superficial appearance
Can be very well differentiated; diagnosis based upon irregular channels, occasionally with papillary ingrowth of endothelium; lesion infiltrates rather than merely separating surrounding structures
May have epithelioid or spindle cell areas
CUTANEOUS
One third to one half of all angiosarcomas
Usually elderly; male > female
Most common sites: head and neck (especially scalp), leg, trunk
Half are multifocal
5 yr survival: 12%; prognosis better if smaller than 5 cm
When occur in association with lymphedema (lymphangiosarcoma), almost always women following mastectomy—occurs on arm; this variant is often associated with premalignant proliferation of lymphatics at periphery of tumor; radical excision (e.g., forequarter amputation) only real hope for survival
BREAST
1/2000 of breast malignancies
Always women; usually 20s–30s
Rapidly growing mass diffusely enlarging breast
Deep, infiltrative, usually well differentiated
HEPATIC
Rare
Associated with arsenic, Thorotrast, and polyvinyl chloride exposure, with long latent period

KAPOSI'S SARCOMA
Virally associated if not virally induced
Probably multifocal rather than metastatic process
Angiosarcomatous and fibrosarcomatous elements with numerous mitoses; when occurs in the skin, often a fibrinous exudate below the epidermis
Four clinical settings:
• Classic (chronic): skin of distal lower extremity, males, late adult, indolent course; one third develop a second malignancy
• Lymphadenopathic: African children, sparse if any skin lesions; involves cervical, inguinal, hilar nodes; fulminant course
• Transplant associated: occur in 0.4% renal transplant recipients; relatively aggressive (30% fatal), dramatically improve if discontinue immunosuppression

- AIDS related: 30% of AIDS patients, with predilection for homosexuals; initially small, flat, pink—only later become blue-violet and papular; more aggressive course

HISTOLOGIC STAGES
Patch: flat lesion, circumferential proliferation of many small vessels around a larger central parent vessel
Plaque: elevation of skin, spindle cell component
Nodular: many spindle cells with slitlike vascular spaces; PAS+ hyaline globules, peripheral inflammatory cells

TUMOR STAGING
I   Cutaneous, locally indolent
II   Cutaneous, locally aggressive, ± regional LNs
III   Generalized mucocutaneous or LN involvement
IV   Visceral

Tumors of Other Vascular Components

HEMANGIOPERICYTOMA
Tumor of the pericyte: actin and vimentin positive, desmin and myoglobin negative
Occurs at all ages; peak incidence in 40s
Tumor is painless and therefore often presents clinically only after months or years
Some patients have hypoglycemia, which resolves after removal of tumor
Most commonly thigh or pelvic retroperitoneum; also head and neck, trunk, arm—deep, usually in muscle
Relatively well-defined mass caused by presence of a pseudocapsule, which is very vascular and can cause extensive hemorrhage during surgery
Tumor proper is composed of spindled cells with roundish nuclei; vessels penetrating the lesion have thin walls and irregular contours, often with an antler or staghorn pattern
Each tumor cells is individually surrounded by a reticulin meshwork; important in differentiation from other tumors
May have myxoid stroma, cell palisading, or solid areas; islands of tumor cells may be seen outside pseudocapsule
So many tumors can have a similar "hemangiopericytoma-like pattern" that the diagnosis is essentially one of exclusion: must show negativity for epithelial, smooth muscle, and nerve sheath markers
Differential diagnosis: fibrous histiocytoma (more prominent spindle pattern), synovial sarcoma (not as broad a range of vascular patterns), mesenchymal chondrosarcoma (islands of cartilage)
Prognosis can be difficult to discern; in general, more than four mitoses/10 HPF, necrosis, atypia are worrisome; recurrence is bad sign—most will later metastasize; metastases to lung and bone

INFANTILE HEMANGIOPERICYTOMA
More superficial (subcutis)
Satellite nodules more common
Frequent endovascular proliferation
Increased mitotic activity and focal necrosis do *not* necessarily mean malignancy

ANGIOMYOMA (VASCULAR LEIOMYOMA)
Subcutaneous tissue, usually extremities, particularly lower leg; also arm, head, trunk; female > male

Generally small, slowly enlarging, often painful (one of the five ANGEL painful nodules of the skin with angiolipoma, traumatic neuroma, glomus tumor, eccrine spiradenoma)
Smooth muscle cells forming the tumor mass appear histologically to spread out from thick-walled vessels within or at the edge of the lesion
Myxoid areas, hyalinization, calcification, fat may be seen
Simple excision is curative

GLOMUS TUMOR
(Unrelated to glomus jugulare tumors of the head and neck, which are paragangliomas)
Glomus body is an arteriovenous anastomosis in the skin in which flow is regulated by a polypoid projection into the lumen of the shunt (Sucquet-Hoyer canals), composed of a mixture of traditional smooth muscle cells and glomus cells, specialized epithelial appearing smooth muscle cells; involved in thermal regulation
Tumor seen most commonly subungually in females, but also seen on palm, wrist, forearm, foot, head and neck, tip of spine (glomus coccygeum) and internal organs (stomach, patella, chest wall, bone), where normal glomus structures are not found
Small purple nodules, usually <1 cm, that generally produce intense pain far out of proportion to the size of the lesion, elicited by even mild touch or temperature changes (especially cold)
Radiograph: may see erosion of terminal phalanx
Histology: anastomosing collection of irregular vessels with intervening nests of glomus cells
Glomus cells: rounded cells with sharply demarcated round nuclei, eosinophilic cytoplasm, and poorly defined cell boundaries (can be visualized by PAS staining)
Immunohistochemistry: desmin negative, SMA positive, factor VIII negative
Essentially always benign; complete excision curative (10% recur)

GLOMUS TUMOR PROPER (75%)
Most commonly finger
Well-defined cluster of small vessels, each sheathed by small nests or sheets of glomus cells

GLOMANGIOMA (20%)
Hand, forearm
Seen in patients with multiple or familial lesions
Less well circumscribed
Resemble cavernous hemangiomas with small nests of glomus cells in vessel walls

GLOMANGIOMYOMA (<10%)
Equally divided between upper and lower extremity
Composed of "transforming" glomus cells that have become elongated and more smooth muscle–like; merge with the outer smooth muscle layers of the larger vessels within the mass

GLOMANGIOSARCOMA
Debatable entity
Benign glomus tumor in association with more spindled fibrosarcomatous areas
Few reported cases; no reported metastases

OTHERS
NEOPLASTIC ANGIOENDOTHELIOMATOSIS
Originally thought to be a form of multicentric angiosarcoma
Actually a malignant lymphoma with tropism for vascular lumina

10

SOFT TISSUES

General Information on Sarcomas

In general affect males more frequently than females

Most occur in children under 13 or adults over 50; only a few occur between this age range: synovial sarcoma, alveolar soft part sarcoma, mesenchymal chondrosarcoma, alveolar rhabdomyosarcoma, angiomatoid malignant fibrous histiocytoma, extraskeletal Ewing's sarcoma, epithelioid sarcoma, and clear cell sarcoma

Generally do *not* evolve from benign tumors (exception: malignant schwannoma arising from neurofibroma in von Recklinghausen's disease)

Generally do *not* metastasize to lymph nodes (exception: synovial sarcoma)

Radiation-induced lesions include MFH, extraosseous osteosarcoma, and fibrosarcoma

Classified on a histogenetic basis by the adult tissue that the tumor most closely resembles

Report must include size (esp. > or < 5 cm) and location (subcutis vs. deep soft tissues, compartment)

IMMUNOHISTOCHEMISTRY

Keratin: usually positive in spindled carcinomas, monophasic synovial sarcoma, Merkel's cell carcinomas (perinuclear spot)

HHF-35: muscle actin (smooth and skeletal)

Desmin: smooth and skeletal muscle

S-100: neural crest–derived cells, but also fat, cartilage, myoepithelial cells; only expressed in half of malignant schwannomas

CHROMOSOMAL ABNORMALITIES

del 1p	Leiomyosarcoma
t(2;13)	Alveolar rhabdomyosarcoma
t(9;22)	Myxoid chondrosarcoma
t(11;22)	Ewing's sarcoma, primitive neuroectodermal tumor (PNET)
t(11;22)	Desmoplastic small round cell tumor
t(12;14)	Leiomyoma
t(12;16)	Myxoid liposarcoma
t(12;22)	Clear cell sarcoma
ring 12	Well-differentiated liposarcoma
ring 17	Dermatofibrosarcoma protuberans
t(X;18)	Synovial sarcoma

GRADING AND STAGING

Grading is usually three tiered (sometimes four), with most emphasis placed on necrosis (<15% vs. >15%) and mitotic activity, but also including atypia

Some tumors receive automatic grades (e.g., dermatofibrosarcoma protuberans and well-differentiated liposarcomas are all grade 1, and synovial sarcomas, angiosarcomas, and alveolar rhabdomyosarcomas are all grade 3)

T1 Primary <5 cm
T2 Primary >5 cm

N1 Regional LNs involved
M1 Distant metastases

	T1	T2
N0, Grade 1	IA	IB
N0, Grade 2	IIA	IIB
N0, Grade 3	IIIA	IIIB
N1	IVA	
M1	IVB	

PROGNOSIS

Survival	5 yr	10 yr
Stage I	75%	63%
Stage II	55%	40%
Stage III	29%	19%
Stage IV	7%	3%

Retroperitoneum

One of the more common locations for sarcomas

Most frequent soft tissue sarcomas of the retroperitoneum, in descending order, are liposarcoma, malignant fibrous histiocytoma, leiomyosarcoma, and rhabdomyosarcoma

ADIPOSE TISSUE

LIPOMA

Most common of the soft tissue tumors

Peak incidence in 40s and 50s; rare before age 20

Most often in subcutaneous tissues of back, shoulder, neck

Delicately encapsulated in superficial soft tissue, poorly circumscribed when arise in deeper structures; in muscle, tend to be infiltrative; diffuse form exists that produces massive enlargement of an entire extremity

Most are indistinguishable from adult fat

Areas of infarction, necrosis, calcification, osseous metaplasia can occur

Fibrolipoma/myxolipoma if have increased amounts of fibrous or myxoid tissue, respectively

ANGIOLIPOMA

Well-circumscribed small tumors; occur shortly after puberty

Often painful; subcutis of trunk or extremities

Vascular component prominent at periphery

Hyaline thrombi common in vessels

MYELOLIPOMA
Lipoma with extramedullary hematopoiesis

SPINDLE CELL LIPOMA
Characteristically shoulder or back of neck; rare on legs
45–65 yr; male : female = 9 : 1
Mixture of mature lipocytes and uniform, primitive, bland, S-100 negative spindle cells in a mucinous and fibrous background with frequent mast cells
May have a hemangiopericytic vascular pattern
Distinguish from myxoid liposarcoma by the thick collagen bundles and by the absence of lipoblasts and a plexiform vascular pattern

PLEOMORPHIC LIPOMA
Circumscribed lesion of the back of the neck or shoulder
Usually men; 60s; 1/10 as common as spindle cell lipoma
Lipoma containing hyperchromatic multinucleated (floret) giant cells (with a wreathlike arrangement of nuclei around cell periphery) within the fibrous septa; a few lipoblasts may be present, but still benign

"ATYPICAL LIPOMA"
Term often used to refer to a well-differentiated liposarcoma that arises in the superficial soft tissues (the same tumor occurring in the retroperitoneum or spermatic cord should be called a well-differentiated liposarcoma)
Mature fat, floret-like cells, cellular fibrous septa
Often recur; generally don't dedifferentiate; don't metastasize

HIBERNOMA
Tumor of "brown fat"
Interscapular region, axilla, mediastinum, retroperitoneum
Brown cut surface
Nests of large cells with central nuclei and cytoplasm filled with many small neutral fat vacuoles that do not indent the nucleus

LIPOBLASTOMA
Almost exclusively infants and young children (<3 yr)
Proximal portions of upper and lower extremities; male > female
Well-localized and superficial or diffusely infiltrating soft tissue (latter referred to as lipoblastomatosis)
Numerous lipoblasts, myxoid stroma
Distinguished from myxoid liposarcoma only by patient age, lobular growth pattern, absence of giant cells, less prominent capillary network

LIPOSARCOMA
Located in deep soft tissues, such as retroperitoneum and thigh; also in mediastinum, omentum, breast, axilla
Most occur after age 50
Second most common soft tissue sarcoma in adults, most common sarcoma of the retroperitoneum
Often very large at diagnosis
Diagnostic cell is lipoblast: mononuclear or multinucleated cell with one or more cytoplasmic fat vacuoles that push aside and indent the nuclei ("mulberry cells")
>50% retroperitoneal liposarcomas, regardless of type, recur and often eventually dedifferentiate
Pleomorphic and round cell liposarcomas metastasize in 80–90% of cases; metastases are usually to the lung
Prognosis: 5 yr survival for well-differentiated and myxoid types is 70%; for round cell and pleomorphic is 18%

WELL-DIFFERENTIATED LIPOSARCOMA (25%)
Often mistaken for lipoma; any "lipoma" in the deep soft tissues, esp. the retroperitoneum or spermatic cord, should be diagnosed as a well-differentiated lipo sarcoma
Three subtypes: lipoma like, sclerosing, inflammatory
Grade I by definition; does not metastasize
Treatment: retroperitoneal exenteration

MYXOID LIPOSARCOMA (50%)
Primitive mesenchymal cells in a mucopolysaccharide-rich matrix (hyaluronidase sensitive); mast cells common
Prominent arborizing vascular component (unlike myxoma) with a hypercellular zone around the larger vessels
Few to no mitotic figures
Often associated with chromosomal translocation t(12;16)
When pure, grade I (by definition)
When metastasizes, usually to the lung
Foci of pleomorphic or round cells that increase the cellularity to >25% decrease prognosis

ROUND CELL (LIPOBLASTIC) LIPOSARCOMA (15%)
AKA: cellular myxoid liposarcoma
Similar to myxoid liposarcoma but with >25% cellularity due to a large number of small, nondescript round cells with acidophilic cytoplasm; cells may cluster
Scattered lipoblasts distinguish from Ewing's sarcoma
Moderate mitotic activity
Grade III by definition; more likely to metastasize

PLEOMORPHIC LIPOSARCOMA (10%)
Usually limbs and limb girdle soft tissues
Undifferentiated: tumor giant cells, often huge (>200 μm!)
Often, neutrophils around and within tumor giant cells
Still should be able to find at least focal S-100 positivity
Grade III by definition; aggressive; tends to metastasize

DEDIFFERENTIATED LIPOSARCOMA
When liposarcomas recur, frequently are more poorly differentiated and can look like malignant fibrous histiocytoma, fibrosarcoma, or leiomyosarcoma
>5 mitoses/10 HPF
Don't see lipogenesis in the high-grade component

FIBROHISTIOCYTIC LESIONS

HISTIOCYTOMA
Tight packing of polygonal cells with minimal stroma; inflammatory cells frequently present; fibrosis common in older lesions

JUVENILE XANTHOGRANULOMA
Two thirds present by 6 months of age; rare after 3 yr
Head, neck, extremities; 5–10% are deep
Ovoid-to-spindle cellular histiocytic proliferation with fibrosis, Touton giant cells, foam cells, lymphocytes, eosinophils
Benign

RETICULOHISTIOCYTOMA
GENERALIZED ERUPTIVE HISTIOCYTOMA

BENIGN FIBROUS HISTIOCYTOMA
DERMATOFIBROMA
Middle adult life, limbs, trunk
Superficial cutaneous nodule, red-brown, slowly growing, painless
Interlacing fascicles of slender spindle cells
Foamy histiocytes, giant cells, branching vessels, chronic inflammation
Pseudoepitheliomatous hyperplasia of overlying epidermis

GIANT CELL TUMOR OF TENDON SHEATH (NODULAR TENOSYNOVITIS)

Predominantly tendons of fingers; also knees, hips
Solitary, circumscribed, lobulated, small (0.5–1.5 cm)
Slowly growing, painless
Sheets of rounded or polygonal cells with scattered benign-appearing giant cells, lipid-laden macrophages, and hemosiderin-laden spindled cells
Well-defined fibrous pseudocapsule
Collagenous stroma with cholesterol clefts
Local recurrence (15%), no malignant potential

PIGMENTED VILLONODULAR SYNOVITIS

Exuberant villous, heavily pigmented synovial overgrowth involving the majority of a joint surface, usually knee
Proliferation of surface synoviocytes and chronic inflammatory cells, thickening of synovial membrane, many pigment-laden macrophages, occasional giant cells

CELLULAR FIBROUS HISTIOCYTOMA

Usually adults; deeper (often subcutaneous) soft tissue
Large (~5 cm); pushing margins
Ovoid to spindled cells, granular foamy cytoplasm, collagen, myofibroblasts; may see giant cells, hemorrhage, necrosis
May recur; does not metastasize

BORDERLINE FIBROUS HISTIOCYTOMA

DERMATOFIBROSARCOMA PROTUBERANS

20s–30s, male > female; usually trunk, most commonly shoulder or proximal extremity
Slow, persistent growth
Multinodular, reddish-blue; poorly circumscribed (infiltrative)
Local recurrence 33%, metastases rare
Deep dermis; infiltrates subcutis (dermatofibromas are more superficial)
Highly cellular lesion of well-differentiated, bland spindle cells in *storiform* pattern (interlacing bundles; basket weave); tumor cells insinuate between adipocytes and adnexal structures; myxoid areas accentuate the vascular pattern
Moderate mitotic activity (no prognostic significance), abundant reticulin, hyperchromasia
Do *not* see giant cells, foamy cells, hemosiderin-laden cells
Grade 1 lesion, by definition
Some will undergo fibrosarcomatous transformation or progression to MFH; when this occurs, outgrows rest of tumor

PIGMENTED DERMATOFIBROSARCOMA (BEDNAR'S TUMOR)

Dermatofibrosarcoma protuberans with population of dendritic cells heavily laden with melanin

ATYPICAL FIBROXANTHOMA

Head and neck (60s–70s) or limbs (30s–40s)
Firm, often ulcerated nodule
Predominantly dermal; may involve superficial fat
Marked pleomorphism: "too bad to be malignant"
Should *not* see storiform pattern, necrosis, myxoid degeneration

MALIGNANT FIBROUS HISTIOCYTOMA

Most common soft tissue sarcoma of late adulthood (50–70 yr); second most common sarcoma of retroperitoneum
Mostly a tumor of soft tissues, but can occur in bone
Of soft tissue tumors, half in lower extremities, 20% in upper extremities, 20% in abdomen and retroperitoneum
Osseous tumors usually around knee; also pelvis, arms
Any age, with peak incidence in 60s
Cells show histiocytoid differentiation: lysozyme, factor XIIIa, alpha-1-antitrypsin

Almost all (except angiomatoid) are grade 3; myxoid forms and densely hyalinized forms may be grade 1 or 2
Satellite lesions are common

STORIFORM-PLEOMORPHIC (~70%)

Polygonal histiocytoid cells, often with bizarre prominent oval nuclei, and spindled fibroblasts, myofibroblasts, and smaller undifferentiated mesenchymal cells
Tend to grow in a swirling, cartwheel, storiform pattern
Pleomorphism, giant cells, slitlike vascular spaces common
Metastases present at diagnosis in 50%

MYXOID (MYXOFIBROSARCOMA) (15%)

Loose myxoid stroma constituting >50% of the tumor mass, interspersed with areas of higher cellularity
Abundant plexiform vascular network, scattered giant cells
Distinguished from myxoid liposarcoma by presence of typical MFH growth pattern elsewhere in lesion
Metastases present at diagnosis in 25%
Second best prognosis of the variants (5 yr survival >50%)

GIANT CELL (MALIGNANT GIANT CELL TUMOR OF SOFT PARTS) (10%)

Spindled and polygonal cells arranged in vague nodules
Giant cells are osteoclast-like and are abundant

INFLAMMATORY (MALIGNANT XANTHOGRANULOMA) (5%)

Rare; predominantly in retroperitoneum
Intense inflammatory infiltrate interspersed with, occasionally obscured by, tumor cells
Tumor cells may contain phagocytosed neutrophils
Very aggressive
Differential diagnosis: malacoplakia, sarcomatoid renal cell carcinoma

ANGIOMATOID (<5%)

Clinically and pathologically a completely different lesion
Younger individuals; extremities, well circumscribed
Very cellular areas (round, bland cells) interspersed with hemorrhagic cystlike spaces and chronic inflammatory cells, which may aggregate to form lymphoid follicles
Much better prognosis than other variants: 12% recur, only 5% metastasize; only 1% die of disease

FIBROUS LESIONS

Benign

NODULAR FASCIITIS

AKA: subcutaneous pseudosarcomatous fibromatosis
Often misdiagnosed as fibrosarcoma or liposarcoma
Peak incidence 40 yr
Unclear pathogenesis; probably reactive; some cases associated with trauma
Upper extremities (flexor surfaces), trunk, neck
Rapid growth, small size (2–3 cm), painful
Zonal growth, with hypocellular center and hypercellular periphery
Cellular tissue-culture like spindle cell proliferation (fibroblasts and myofibroblasts) in a myxoid matrix; may have many mitoses, but generally smooth nuclear contours and fine chromatin pattern
Vascular proliferation, lymphocytic infiltration, extravasated red blood cells (RBCs), undulating wide bands of collagen that increase with the age of the lesion
Focal metaplastic bone may be seen

If <3 cm, may regress without treatment
Generally do not recur, even if incompletely excised

CRANIAL FASCIITIS
Children; erosion of skull; may be related to birth trauma

INTRAVASCULAR FASCIITIS
Involves walls of medium-sized vessels

PROLIFERATIVE FASCIITIS
Rare; adults (40–70 yr)
66% occur on extremities
Histology of nodular fasciitis, but with large basophilic cells resembling ganglion cells

PROLIFERATIVE MYOSITIS
Muscles of shoulder, thorax, thigh
Intramuscular variant of proliferative fasciitis
Cellular proliferation of fibroblasts surrounding individual muscle fibers with *very large ganglion-like basophilic cells with vesicular nuclei and very prominent nucleoli*

EOSINOPHILIC FASCIITIS
Superficial soft tissues, usually thighs, often symmetrical
Fibrosing inflammation with eosinophils, lymphocytes, and mast cells
Sometimes associated with myalgias (eosinophilia-myalgia syndrome: caused by a toxin contaminating early preparations of L-tryptophan)

MYOSITIS OSSIFICANS
Solitary, nonprogressive reactive condition, often mistaken for osteosarcoma
Flexors of arm, quadriceps, adductors of thigh, gluteal muscles, soft tissue of hand most common; may not involve muscle
Occurs following trauma; usually young males
Highly cellular stroma associated with new bone with or without cartilage; usually no inflammation
As evolves, becomes zonal with cellular core, intermediate zone of osteoid, peripheral shell of highly organized, calcified bone

ELASTOFIBROMA
Poorly circumscribed; subscapular region (95%) of elderly adults (>55 yr)
More common in women; more common in Japanese; no pain
Densely collagenized lesion with numerous thick, eosinophilic extracellular refractile fibers that stain strongly for elastin

FIBROMA
OVARIAN FIBROMA
NUCHAL FIBROMA
NASOPHARYNGEAL FIBROMA
FIBROMA OF TENDON SHEATH
Usually males, 30–50 yr old
Well circumscribed, lobulated; attached to tendon
Dense fibrous tissue with spindled mesenchymal cells (may be myofibroblasts) and dilated or slitlike channels resembling tenosynovial spaces
Numerous medium-sized vessels
Probably a "burnt-out" giant cell tumor of tendon sheath

KELOID
Hypertrophic scar, thick collagen bands (see Skin outline)

Tumors of Infancy and Childhood

FOCAL MYOSITIS
Inflammatory pseudotumor of skeletal muscle in children

Usually lower extremity; painful
Degeneration/regeneration of muscle fibers with interstitial inflammation and fibrosis

FIBROUS HAMARTOMA OF INFANCY
Tumor-like (benign) condition seen during first 2 yr of life
Usually boys; shoulder, axilla, upper arm
Solitary, poorly circumscribed, dermal to subcutaneous whitish mass with islands of fat
Organoid pattern composed of 1) well-differentiated fibrous tissue, 2) mature adipose tissue, 3) immature cellular areas resembling primitive mesenchyme
Vimentin positive

INFANTILE MYOFIBROMATOSIS
SOLITARY (50%)
Most cases in 1st month of life
Dermal, subcutis, muscle
Whirling pattern of benign fibrous tissue
MULTICENTRIC (50%)
May have extensive visceral involvement
May be fatal

CALCIFYING APONEUROTIC FIBROMA
AKA: juvenile aponeurotic fibroma
Usually child (10–15 yr old), usually hand or wrist (70%); occasionally feet
Nodule or ill-defined infiltrating mass; slow growing, painless
May be attached to tendon; infiltrates fat and muscle
Diffuse proliferation of fibroblasts with focal calcifications
Often have scattered osteoclast-like giant cells
Proliferating cells have chrondrocyte features

GIANT CELL FIBROBLASTOMA
Almost exclusively children <10 yr; usually boys
Superficial soft tissues of back or thigh
Ill-defined proliferation of fibroblasts in collagenized, focally myxoid stroma; hypocellular regions often alternate with hypercellular regions with prominent, thick-walled vessels
Multinucleated cells have floret-like appearance
Cystic or sinusoidal structures (pseudovascular spaces) lined by hyperchromatic giant cells is characteristic feature
May be juvenile version of dermatofibrosarcoma protuberans

Aggressive/Malignant Lesions

FIBROMATOSIS
Proliferation of well-defined fibroblasts, focally very cellular but intermixed with more collagenous areas, with an *infiltrative* growth pattern and tendency to recur
Male predominance
Variety of names, patterns, associations
Uniformity of cells, rarity of mitoses
Superficial
PALMAR (DUPUYTREN'S CONTRACTURE)
Bilateral in 50%; concurrent plantar disease in 10%
Results in fixed painless flexion contractures of digits

PLANTAR (LEDDERHOSE'S FIBROMATOSIS)
Middle of sole of foot; bilateral in 10–25%
Often some degree of pain/paresthesias
Usually present 10 yr earlier than palmar
PENILE (PEYRONIE'S DISEASE)
Usually dorsolateral penis; palpable induration

Deep (Musculoaponeurotic)
DESMOID (ABDOMINAL)
Abdominal wall of women during or following pregnancy
Can be associated with Gardner's syndrome: 45% of Gardner's syndrome patients develop desmoids
"EXTRAABDOMINAL"
AKA: aggressive fibromatoses
Shoulder (22%), chest/back (17%), mesentery (10% [not really "extraabdominal"]), thigh (12%)
Mitoses up to 1 per 5 HPF allowed; must not be atypical
Characteristically have thin-walled, elongated, ectatic vessels
Initial recurrence rate ~50%; rate increases with each successive recurrence
POSTRADIATION

Fibromatoses of Childhood
Fibromatosis coli
Infantile digital fibromatosis
Infantile fibromatosis, desmoid type
Gingival fibromatosis
Hyalin fibromatosis

IDIOPATHIC RETROPERITONEAL FIBROSIS
AKA: Ormond's disease, sclerosing fibrosis, sclerosing retroperitonitis
Ill-defined mass composed of mixed inflammatory cells (lymphocytes and germinal centers, plasma cells, eosinophils) in a cellular fibrous stroma with foci of fat necrosis; mass surrounds the abdominal aorta and displaces the ureters medially
Polyclonal immunoglobin (Ig) production, predominantly IgA
Probably an immunologic hypersensitivity disorder
May be associated with mediastinal fibrosis, sclerosing cholangitis, Riedel's thyroiditis, pseudotumor of the orbit
Results in progressive renal failure from constriction and ultimately obliteration of the ureters

SOLITARY FIBROUS TUMOR
(See Lung outline, under Pleura)

FIBROSARCOMA
Frequency of this lesion decreasing because most are reclassified as other entities, usually malignant fibrous histiocytoma; largely a diagnosis of exclusion
Most common in retroperitoneum, thigh, about the knee
Unencapsulated, infiltrative, soft "fish-flesh" masses
Areas of hemorrhage and necrosis
Classically a "herringbone" pattern of growth
Immunoreactive for vimentin and type I collagen
5 yr survival 41%; 10 yr survival 29%
Prognosis better for more superficial, better differentiated
Congenital fibrosarcomas and those occurring before 5 yr of age are usually on extremities, usually painless, and tend not to metastasize

Often produce hypoglycemia secondary to elaboration of insulin-like substances

SMOOTH MUSCLE

LEIOMYOMA
95% occur in female genital tract
CUTANEOUS LEIOMYOMA
Arise from erector pili muscles
Typically superficial, small, multiple, grouped
GENITAL LEIOMYOMAS
Smooth muscle of superficial subcutaneous tissue of genital areas (nipple, areola, axilla, scrotum, penis, etc.)
VASCULAR LEIOMYOMA (ANGIOLEIOMYOMA)
Smooth muscle of blood vessels
Generally in females, usually legs and feet
Often painful (painful nodules of skin and soft tissue are Angiolipoma, traumatic Neuroma, Glomus tumor, Eccrine spiradenoma, vascular Leiomyoma)
Often multiple vascular profiles
SYMPLASTIC LEIOMYOMA
AKA: bizarre, atypical, apoplectic leiomyoma
An otherwise traditional leiomyoma with scattered cells containing large, atypical nuclei
Almost always uterus or skin
Prognosis determined by mitotic rate (see Uterus outline)

LEIOMYOSARCOMA
Most are in extremities, arising from wall of vessels
Large, soft, tendency for necrosis, hemorrhage, cystic degeneration; when arise from vessel, may be luminal
Fascicular pattern of growth (bundles intersect at right angles, unlike the herringbone pattern of fibrosarcoma); palisading of cigar-shaped, blunt-ended nuclei; mitoses
Often cytoplasmic vacuoles are seen at both ends of nucleus, sometimes indenting it (unlike neural lesions)
Cutaneous and subcutaneous tumors have an excellent prognosis; deeper lesions are more likely to metastasize
Retroperitoneal and/or mesenteric tumors almost always malignant; prognosis worse when >5 cm

LEIOMYOBLASTOMA
AKA: clear cell (epithelioid) smooth muscle tumors
Uncommon in soft tissues; usually seen in stomach
(See GI Tract outline)

STRIATED MUSCLE

Terminology
Myofiber: skeletal muscle cell

Myofibril: array of actin (thin) and myosin (thick) filaments surrounded by sarcoplasmic reticulum; can have many myofibrils per myofiber

Sarcomere: collection of filaments between two Z-bands; the functional unit of the muscle cell

Banding pattern of a sarcomere
- **Z-band:** electron-dense discs; anchor the actin filaments
- **A-band:** central portion of sarcomere containing the thick myosin filaments
- **H-band:** central portion of A band not overlapped by actin filaments
- **M-line:** interfilament bridge at center of A-band
- **I-band:** portion of actin filaments not overlapped by myosin

The term *A-band* stands for anisotropic and I-band for isotropic

Actually, both the A- and I-bands are anisotropic, meaning they can rotate plane polarized light, but the A-band is more anisotropic than the I-band

During sarcomere shortening, the A-band remains the same size; as the Z-bands approach each other, the I-bands and H-bands become shorter

Sarcolemma: cell membrane of a skeletal muscle cell

Sarcoplasmic reticulum: endoplasmic reticulum of a myofiber, specialized for transport and storage of calcium

Transverse tubules: invaginations of the sarcolemma that extend to the sarcoplasmic reticulum of each myofibril of a myofiber, allowing rapid transmission of an electrical stimulus (depolarization)

Connective tissue: epimysium surrounds entire muscle, perimysium separates groups of myofibers into muscle fascicles, and endomysium surrounds each individual muscle cell

Motor unit: refers to a single lower motor neuron (usually in anterior horn of spinal cord) and all of the muscle cells it innervates (<10 for fine motor control, >1,000 for large leg muscles); any given myofiber is innervated by only one neuron (except for the extraocular muscles)

Medial motor neurons tend to control proximal muscles

Muscle Fiber Types

Two "types" of muscle fibers, randomly intermixed within muscles; type determined by pattern of innervation from lower motor neuron; all myofibers in a given motor unit are of the same type; a fiber of one type can be converted to one of the other type by changing the pattern of stimulation (i.e., reinnervation with different nerve)

		Type I	Type II
Color		Red	White
Speed		Slow	Fast
Duration		Prolonged	Quick
Fatigue		Slow	Rapid
Prevalence		1/3	2/3
Use		Postural	Strength
Mitochondria		Numerous	Fewer
Myoglobin		High concentration	Low
Glycogen content		Low	High
Lipid content		High	Low
Metabolism		Aerobic	Anaerobic
ATPase (pH 9.4)		Unstained	Dark
ATPase (pH 4.6) ("reverse ATPase")		Dark	IIA: Light IIB: Intermediate
NADH-TR		Dark	Light

Note: NADH is actually a stain for lipid, and is not as useful as the ATPase reaction because denervation causes both fiber types to stain dark

Type II muscles hypertrophy in response to training or anabolic steroids, and atrophy in response to disuse; type I fibers generally do not vary in size

Nonspecific esterase reaction: stains type I fibers slightly darker than type II, but stains denervated fibers of either type very dark, owing to the diffuse distribution of acetylcholine esterase activity

Alkaline phosphatase reaction: stains regenerating fibers

Histogenesis

Arise from fusion of myoblasts to form a multinucleated syncytium called a *myotube,* which stimulates the formation of myofibrils

When becomes innervated, diffusely distributed acetylcholine receptors become concentrated at motor end plate

Evaluating Muscle Biopsies

When evaluating muscle biopsies, need to first determine whether the changes are neuropathic or myopathic; in chronic conditions, there can be a mixture of these features, making distinction difficult

Myopathic processes will show coexistent degeneration and regeneration

If process is myopathic, determine whether it is inflammatory or noninflammatory: inflammatory processes show neutrophils and mononuclear cells within the muscle and often have an accompanying vasculitis; noninflammatory processes show coagulative necrosis and "ragged-red" fibers

Note: variation in fiber size and internal nuclei are normal at the site of tendinous insertion

REGENERATION
Regenerating fibers tend to have rounded edges, nuclei that may be central, and a prominent nucleolus, and stain strongly with the alkaline phosphatase reaction

RHABDOMYOLYSIS
Diffuse destruction or lysis of skeletal muscle, which may be acute, subacute, or chronic

Cause is often unknown

Massive myoglobinuria can induce renal failure

DISUSE (NONSPECIFIC) ATROPHY
Not caused by denervation

Selective loss of type II fibers

Can also be seen secondary to large doses of steroids

Neurogenic Disorders

DENERVATION

Denervation results in atrophy (loss of myofibrils) of all the fibers in the motor unit associated with the lower motor neuron; loss of individual neurons will show small group atrophy, loss of larger nerves will show large group atrophy

Myofibers become angulated when viewed in cross section, and nuclei aggregate into hyperchromatic clumps

Both type I and type II fibers are lost; type II fibers lost first

Target fibers: central pallor with condensed eosinophilic rim surrounded by normal-appearing muscle; seen in some cases of denervation; probably a transient state

Renervation usually occurs simultaneously with denervation, converting the previously "randomly" distributed type I and type II fibers into fibers of all one type: "type grouping"

WERDNIG-HOFFMAN DISEASE
AKA: infantile spinal muscular atrophy

Autosomal recessive congenital hypotonia with progressive group atrophy usually resulting in death by one year

Loss of lower motor neurons from the anterior horn of the spinal cord with widespread group atrophy

AMYOTROPHIC LATERAL SCLEROSIS
(See also CNS outline)
Onset in 30s–60s
Upper motor neuron loss results in fasciculations
Lower motor neuron loss results in group atrophy
Median survival 3 yr

MYASTHENIA GRAVIS
Disorder of the neuromuscular junction
Autoimmune disease in which antibodies to the acetylcholine receptors at the postsynaptic membrane both block stimulation by acetylcholine and induce receptor downregulation
Increasing muscle fatigue with use; patients usually present with ocular muscle involvement
One third of patients have a thymoma; most of those without have thymic hyperplasia
Mortality in severe cases is caused by respiratory compromise

EATON-LAMBERT SYNDROME
Myasthenia-like syndrome
Two thirds of patients have a small cell carcinoma of the lung

Myopathic Disorders

MUSCULAR DYSTROPHIES
Inherited progressive primary degenerative diseases of skeletal muscle
Great variability in fiber size (compensatory hypertrophy of fibers not yet affected)
Diffuse endomysial fibrosis

DUCHENNE MUSCULAR DYSTROPHY
AKA: progressive muscular dystrophy
1/3,500 live male births; one third represent new mutation
X-linked recessive (affects primarily boys), inherited mutation mapped to defect in the dystrophin gene on chromosome Xp21; this large gene product (430 kD) is absent from affected patients
Involves primarily proximal muscles
Immobilization for even short periods of time can result in contractures
Develop "pseudohypertrophy" of calf muscles
Normal muscle strength at birth; weakness becomes apparent by age 3–4, usually wheelchair dependent at age 10 and bedridden by age 15; death due to involvement of respiratory muscles or heart
Serum creatine kinase levels elevated from birth
Breakdown of sarcolemma with degeneration of the muscle fibers (dark, hyalinized, overcontracted), myophagocytosis, alkaline phosphatase–positive regenerating muscle fibers with prominent nucleoli
Later, endomysial fibrosis and fibrofatty replacement of muscle as degeneration exceeds capacity for regeneration; eventually, near-complete loss of myofibers

BECKER'S MUSCULAR DYSTROPHY
Milder form of Duchenne muscular dystrophy (1/10 as common), with later onset (teens), which is also X-linked and maps to the same locus
Affected individuals usually retain ability to walk into adulthood

LIMB-GIRDLE DYSTROPHY
Group of diseases predominantly affecting the axial muscles

Most are autosomal recessive
Late onset (young adulthood)
Slow but progressive deterioration
Markedly increased numbers of central nuclei, with fiber splitting and dramatic fiber hypertrophy

MYOTONIC DYSTROPHY
1/20,000 live births
Autosomal dominant (linked to chromosome 19q13.2) but with variable penetrance
Syndrome that includes, usually, cataracts, frontal baldness, testicular atrophy, heart disease, and dementia
Onset often in 20s–30s; involves primarily facial and pharyngeal muscles
Myotonia: inability of muscle to relax once contracted
Increased number of central nuclei, many *ring fibers* (circumferential disposition of myofibers on cross section), chains of nuclei, type I fiber atrophy

CONGENITAL MYOPATHIES
Group of disorders that are not progressive but do restrict activity and are complicated by secondary skeletal problems such as kyphoscoliosis
Often present at birth, with hypotonia, decreased deep tendon reflexes, and low muscle mass; with age, motor milestones are delayed
Biopsies reveal that morphologic abnormalities are restricted to the type I fibers, which predominate; type II fibers are decreased in number but structurally normal

CENTRAL CORE DISEASE
Sporadic, autosomal recessive, and autosomal dominant forms
Type I fibers show a central core of lucency running the length of the cell (best demonstrated with the NADH-TR reaction) caused by a loss of membranous organelles, often with disorganization of the surrounding myofibrils

NEMALINE (ROD) MYOPATHY
Inclusions within the type I myofibers of rod-shaped structures, which arise from the Z-bands and are stainable with trichrome stain or with phosphotungstic acid hematoxylin (PTAH)
Probably a group of disorders
Facial, pharyngeal, and neck muscle can be markedly involved
Note: rods can also be seen in muscular dystrophy, denervation atrophy, and inflammation—not specific

CENTRAL NUCLEAR MYOPATHY (TUBULAR MYOPATHY)
Autosomal dominant, recessive, and X-linked varieties
X-linked form presents at birth; autosomal dominant is later onset
Predominance of small, type I fibers with a single, centrally located nucleus (normally, nuclei should be central in <3% of the fibers, unless near site of tendinous insertion)

GLYCOGEN STORAGE DISEASES
Some of these disorders, in particular glycogenosis II (Pompe's disease) and glycogenosis V (McArdle's disease) affect predominantly muscle
(See "Congenital Syndromes" outline)

MITOCHONDRIAL MYOPATHIES
Inherited defects of mitochondrial metabolism
Examples include ATPase deficiency, carnitine metabolism defect, cytochrome deficiencies

INFLAMMATORY MYOPATHIES

Often see perifascicular atrophy, in which the peripheral fibers of a fascicle or group undergo degeneration/regeneration without involvement of the central fibers; often associated with a vasculitis

POLYMYOSITIS/DERMATOMYOSITIS

Idiopathic disorder confined to striated muscle, often with exacerbations and remissions but slow, progressive weakness; ultimately fatal

Patients respond to corticosteroid therapy

May represent a paraneoplastic syndrome in some patients (See "Inflammation and Immunology" outline under "Autoimmune Diseases")

VIRAL MYOSITIS

Neoplasms

MYXOMA

Often a moderately well-circumscribed gelatinous mass deep within muscle, usually of an extremity (esp. thigh), but may be poorly circumscribed and infiltrating

Almost always adults; usually female

Proteoglycan matrix, slightly basophilic, with rare stellate cells; lacks the endothelial cell proliferation of a cardiac myxoma

Excellent prognosis: rarely if ever recurs

RHABDOMYOMA

Cardiac and extracardiac types; cardiac "tumors" are probably hamartomatous rather than neoplastic

Extracardiac are probably true neoplasms and are divided into two types, with some overlap

ADULT TYPE

Oral cavity and vicinity

Large, well-differentiated, plump cells with abundant acidophilic cytoplasm and various amounts of clearing caused by lipid and/or glycogen

Cross striations may be seen in some cells

Differential diagnosis: hibernoma, granular cell tumor

FETAL TYPE (GENITAL TYPE)

Head and neck in children under 3 yr; vulvovaginal in middle-aged women (latter also called *genital rhabdomyoma*)

Cellular, randomly intersecting bundles of immature skeletal muscle fibers, separated by strands of collagen with primitive mesenchymal cells

Lacks mitoses, cambium layer, and infiltrative margins of rhabdomyosarcoma

RHABDOMYOSARCOMA

More common than rhabdomyomas; relatively common soft tissue sarcoma in children

Except for pleomorphic type, 90% occur before age 20

males ≥ females; whites > blacks

Generally at least focally positive for muscle-specific actin, desmin, myosin, myoglobin

MyoD: new antigen: 318 amino acid DNA binding protein that seems to initiate the commitment of undifferentiated mesenchymal cells to myoblasts; present in normal skeletal muscle and in all rhabdomyosarcomas, even those that are desmin negative (another factor needed for complete differentiation appears to be missing)

EM: thick + thin myofilaments, ribosomal-myosin complexes

All are grade III by definition

Chemotherapy, and in some cases radiotherapy, can induce partial differentiation in childhood rhabdomyosarcomas

5 yr survival by surgical stage:

I	Localized; completely excised	82%
II	Microscopic residual or + LN	78%
III	Gross residual tumor	64%
IV	Distant metastases	27%

EMBRYONAL RHABDOMYOSARCOMA (50–60%)

Most commonly head and neck (orbit or nasopharynx), also retroperitoneum, bile ducts, urogenital tract

Generally 3–12 yr old

Poorly circumscribed, white, soft

Rhabdomyoblasts take on many characteristic morphologies:

- Strap cells: elongated cells with one or several nuclei and long extended cytoplasmic processes with cross striations
- Racquet-shaped cells with a single nucleus in expanded end
- Spider cells: giant cells with peripherally arranged PAS+ vacuoles separated by thin strands of cytoplasm
- Broken straw sign: spindled rhabdomyoblast with focal cytoplasmic bend

BOTRYOID RHABDOMYOSARCOMA (5–10%)

Some pathologists consider this a subtype of embryonal rhabdomyosarcoma with grapelike gross appearance, but it occurs in a slightly younger age group (mean age = 7 yr)

Seen in vagina, urinary bladder, nasal cavity, bile ducts

Dense collection of undifferentiated tumor cells immediately beneath the epithelium: Nicholson's *cambium layer*

Favorable prognosis

ALVEOLAR RHABDOMYOSARCOMA (20%)

Generally 10–30 yr old (mean = 23 yr); extremities, perineum, occasionally sinuses

Thin strands of fibrovascular stroma forming nests containing loose clusters of small, round, undifferentiated tumor cells that tend to "float free" in "lumen"

Occasional multinucleated giant cells

80% are associated with t(2;13)(q37;q14)

Solid variant exists in which cells remain better attached

Worst prognosis of all types; any alveolar component imparts the bad prognosis

PLEOMORPHIC RHABDOMYOSARCOMA (<5%)

Tends to occur in individuals over 45 yr (mean age = 50 yr)

Usually extremity, esp. thigh

Large, atypical tumor cells, often giant cells

Difficult to distinguish from liposarcoma or MFH without immunohistochemistry

SPINDLE CELL VARIANT (<3%)

Rare; newly recognized

Alternate Classification

Favorable: botryoid, well-differentiated, embryonal

Unfavorable: alveolar, pleomorphic

ALVEOLAR SOFT PART SARCOMA

AKA: malignant organoid granular cell myoblastoma; malignant nonchromaffin paraganglioma

Deep soft tissues, usually thigh and leg, also head and neck (orbit, tongue); young adults (15–35 yr)

Necrosis and hemorrhage common

Fibrous tissue strands forming nests of large, polygonal, loosely cohesive tumor cells with large vesicular nuclei, prominent nucleoli, granular cytoplasm

Often cells near center of nests loose connection with surrounding cells, forming the alveolar pattern

Mitoses are rare

Probably an immature rhabdomyosarcoma; myo-D positive

Highly malignant, with blood-borne metastases, most commonly to lung; lethal over protracted course of 5–10 yr
Lesion is considered ungradable

PERIPHERAL NERVE LESIONS

NEUROMA
Most occur following trauma (hence, traumatic neuroma)
Often very painful
Non-neoplastic overgrowth of nerve fibers and Schwann cells
Extensive perineural fibrosis common
MORTON'S NEUROMA
Variant caused by repeated mild trauma
Typically interdigital plantar nerve between 3rd and 4th metatarsals; results in shooting pains upon standing
More common in women
Proliferation of Schwann cells and fibroblasts associated with fibrosis, nerve degeneration, endarteritis, and thrombosis of the accompanying artery

NEURILEMOMA (SCHWANNOMA)
Truly encapsulated neoplasm; grows eccentrically along periphery of nerve, compressing it; nerve usually does not penetrate tumor
Almost always solitary
Usually flexor surfaces of extremities, neck, mediastinum, retroperitoneum, posterior spinal roots
Larger lesions may be cystic
Antoni A areas: cellular, spindle cells, often palisading or in an organoid (Verocay bodies) pattern, predominate in smaller lesions
Antoni B areas: tumor cells separated by abundant edematous myxoid stroma; occasional isolated bizarre cells
Blood vessels may be very prominent (fenestrated on electron microscopy [EM]) and are often thick walled
Mitoses can be seen
When arise from spinal nerve root, may have many melanocytes mixed in throughout tumor
Strongly S-100 positive; usually keratin negative
ANCIENT SCHWANNOMA
Degenerative changes seen in "older" schwannomas, including cyst formation, hemosiderin, fibrosis, hyalinization of the vessels, calcification
These degenerative features all favor a benign diagnosis
CELLULAR SCHWANNOMA
Antoni A areas predominate

NEUROFIBROMA
Solitary (90%) or multiple (10%); multiple usually means neurofibromatosis
20–30 yr old most commonly
Tumors generally are *not* encapsulated
Nerve routinely runs through middle of tumor
May have diffuse, tortuous enlargement of nerve: plexiform
Combined proliferation of all nerve elements: Schwann cells, fibroblasts, axons, perineural cells; Schwann cells frequently predominate
Mast cells commonly present throughout stroma
Can have atypia, but should be no mitoses
Vessels are generally thin walled
Usually S-100 and GFAP positive, but often only weakly so

PLEXIFORM NEUROFIBROMA
Classic lesion of von Recklinghausen's disease
Diffuse enlargement of a nerve trunk by a neurofibroma, causing a convoluted "bag of worms" appearance, appearing lobulated on cut section; may become very large
Prone to malignant degeneration: 5–10% of von Recklinghausen's disease patients develop malignant tumors arising in benign neurofibromas, almost always of deep large nerve trunks of neck or extremities

GRANULAR CELL TUMOR
AKA: granular cell schwannoma
Almost always benign
Unknown histogenesis; originally thought to be myoblastic, but presence of S-100 positivity has suggested neural
Most common in the tongue and subcutaneous tissue, but can occur anywhere (any organ); young to middle age
Generally small, firm, gray-white to tan
Nests and sheets of round to polygonal cells with distinct borders, small central nuclei, occasional multinucleation or pleomorphism, scattered mitoses, and a prominent filling of the cytoplasm with PAS+ diastase-resistant granules, which by EM are membrane-bound autophagic vacuoles
When present in the skin of adults, often produce a pseudo-epitheliomatous hyperplasia of the overlying epidermis, simulating squamous cell carcinoma
Because of infiltrative projections at periphery, 10% will recur
MALIGNANT GRANULAR CELL TUMOR
Very rare
Large, rapidly growing, more infiltrative, numerous mitoses
May be very difficult to distinguish from benign counterpart

OSSIFYING FIBROMYXOID TUMOR OF SOFT PARTS
Uncertain histogenesis; probably neural
Adults; male > female
Usually shell of mature bone enclosing bland, round to oval cells; arranged in cords and nests in a myxoid to fibrous matrix with osteoid production
Two thirds are S-100 positive
Recur; generally do not metastasize

MALIGNANT SCHWANNOMA
AKA: neurogenic sarcoma, neurofibrosarcoma, malignant peripheral nerve sheath tumor
50% arise *de novo,* 50% from pre-existing neurofibroma in patients with von Recklinghausen's disease
Most commonly neck, forearm, lower leg, buttock
Cellular spindle cell tumor with abundant mitoses; some extremely bizarre cells may be present; metaplastic tissue present in 15%
Epithelioid and glandular variants exist
S-100 and Leu7 immunoreactive in only 50%
When arises in setting of von Recklinghausen's disease, very fulminant clinical course
MALIGNANT TRITON TUMOR
Malignant schwannoma containing metaplastic skeletal muscle tissue

MISCELLANEOUS

SYNOVIAL SARCOMA
80% arise about the knee and ankle joints of young adults (15–35 yr); male : female = 1.5 : 1

Also seen in shoulder, elbow, hip, retropharyngeal soft tissues, oral cavity, anterior abdominal wall

May be very aggressive or very indolent

Cell of origin unclear; probably primitive mesenchymal cell

Rarely involves synovial membrane or joint

Well circumscribed, firm, grayish pink

Focal calcification frequent

Most show biphasic differentiation with a mixture of epithelial areas (glandular, papillary fronds, or nests of keratinizing squamous epithelium) and a sarcomatous spindle cell stroma

Spindle cells generally have plump nuclei, lobular growth pattern, focally whirled; numerous mast cells common; calcifications common; may have metaplastic bone or cartilage

Reticulin stains can highlight biphasic nature of tumor

May be predominantly or completely epithelial or spindled (monophasic variants)

Keratin reactivity is seen in both the epithelial (strong) and also the spindle cell component

Can also be immunoreactive for CEA, EMA, vimentin

LN metastases present in 10–15% (uncommonly high for a sarcoma)

5 yr survival now approaching 50%; prognosis better for younger age, *tumor <5 cm* (single most important prognostic factor), <15 mitoses/10 HPF, diploid

CALCIFYING SYNOVIAL SARCOMA

Extensive calcification of stroma; most are <5 cm

Better 5 yr survival

EPITHELIOID SARCOMA

Usually extremities (hands, fingers [30%]) of adolescents and young adults (median age 26 yr)

Inconspicuous-appearing spindled and polygonal tumor cells, typically forming small nests with central comedo-like necrosis; may be mistaken for necrotizing granulomas

Unknown histogenesis

Immunoreactive for keratin, vimentin, EMA, occasionally CEA

Favorable prognostic factors: <2 cm, female, few mitoses, no necrosis, diploid

CLEAR CELL SARCOMA

AKA: malignant melanoma of soft parts

Generally arises from large tendons or aponeuroses of extremities

Most commonly feet; usually young adults

Firm, well-circumscribed, gray-white lesion with gritty texture

Pale cuboidal to fusiform cells with large prominent basophilic nucleoli forming nests or interlacing fascicles

Melanin may be present focally

Consistently S-100 positive; may be HMB-45 positive

Slow but relentless progression

PIGMENTED NEUROECTODERMAL TUMOR OF INFANCY (MELANOTIC PROGONOMA)

Occurs in children <6 months old; male = female

Anterior maxilla or other head and neck locations

Neuroblasts and melanoblasts in nests

Invades, but rarely metastasizes

PRIMITIVE NEUROECTODERMAL TUMOR (PNET)

AKA: peripheral neuroectodermal tumor, neuroepithelioma

Sheets of small, round, blue cells, often with rosette-like structures, with salt-and-pepper chromatin pattern

Related to Ewing's sarcoma (same t[11;22] translocation) but cells don't have the clear cytoplasm of Ewing's sarcoma

O-13 antibody to MIC-2 is a marker specific for both PNET and Ewing's sarcoma

(See also Bone and Cartilage outline)

MALIGNANT SMALL CELL TUMOR OF THORACOPULMONARY ORIGIN

AKA: Askin's tumor

Same lesion occurring in the chest wall, probably originating from an intercostal nerve

Mean age 14; female > male

DESMOPLASTIC SMALL ROUND CELL TUMOR

Intra-abdominal (95%) mass with pain, ascites, and often obstruction of the colon, ureter, bile duct, or esophagus

Male : female = 4 : 1; wide age incidence with mean of 21 yr (7–48 yr)

Usually large, multinodular to lobulated mass, often with many small implants

Small, blue cells with round nuclei, dispersed chromatin growing in nests with angulated edges and peripheral palisading embedded in a fibrotic bland stroma; relative amounts of cells and stroma can vary widely

Can see focal necrosis and cyst formation, glandular differentiation, ectatic vessels

EM characteristically shows bundles of intermediate filaments near the nuclei, often entrapping other organelles

Keratin, EMA, desmin (punctate perinuclear stain), vimentin, and NSE positive; LCA, actin, HHF-35, chromogranin negative; usually O-13 negative

>90% show t(11;22)(p13;q12), translocating the C-terminal DNA-binding domain of WT-1 (11p13) to the N-terminus of EWS (22q12)

Poor prognosis: most patients dead of tumor within 5 yr

SACROCOCCYGEAL TERATOMA

Most common teratoma in children; female > male

95% are benign, even when immature elements present

Risk of malignancy increases with age of patient

MESENCHYMOMA

Tumors with two or more mesenchymal elements (not counting fibrous tissue)

Benign and malignant forms exist

Most frequent is angiomyolipoma

OTHERS

Extragonadal germ cell tumors

Extracranial meningiomas

Myxopapillary ependymomas

Extraskeletal Ewing's sarcoma

Phosphaturic mesenchymal tumor

Rhabdoid tumor

11

BONE AND CARTILAGE

NORMAL ANATOMY

Bone and cartilage are composed of a matrix containing a fibrillar protein (collagen) and mucopolysaccharides; in cartilage, the latter predominates; in bone, the matrix becomes mineralized

Epiphysis: endochondral ossification

Metaphysis: also endochondral ossification; supplied by diaphyseal vessels; primary site of Ca and PO_4 exchange

Diaphysis: supplied via Volkmann's and Haversian canals

Epiphyseal plate can act as barrier to tumor spread

Periosteum: bone-forming "membrane" surrounding bone; can become elevated and form new bone perpendicular to surface in primary tumors (Codman's triangle), but also in trauma, hematoma, TB, syphilis, metastases

Osteoblasts: make osteoid; prominent golgi, abundant alkaline phosphatase activity; become osteocytes

Osteoclasts: resorb bone, numerous mitochondria, abundant acid phosphatase activity; can remove bone $100\times$ faster than osteoblasts can make it

In adults, more than 1–2 osteoclasts/cm^2 is abnormal: Paget's, hyperparathyroidism, chronic osteomyelitis, tumor

Parathormone receptors are located on osteoblasts; they secrete factors that activate osteoclasts; osteoclasts by themselves are *not* responsive to parathormone

Osteoid: 90–95% type I collagen

Mineralization: hydroxyapatite: $Ca_{10}(PO_4)_6(OH)_2$

Mineralization normally lags behind osteoid deposition by 12–15 days, leaving a 15 μm rim of unmineralized osteoid

Woven bone: haphazard arrangement of fibers (vs. lamellar); occurs in fibrous dysplasia, high turnover states (healing)

FRACTURES

Healing:
- Hematoma forms
- Organized by influx of vessels
- Absorption of devitalized bone begins at ~3 days
- Intramembranous "pseudosarcomatous" bone growth begins at periosteum of two sides of fracture and grows across the break, forming the primary callus (procallus)
- Primary callus absorbed; replaced by lamellar bone (secondary callus)

Exuberant callus usually means slow healing: infection, poor blood supply, delayed reduction, inadequate immobilization

Sequestrum: dead bone; may be extruded through skin

Involucrum: new bone formed sub-periosteally, which envelops an inflammatory focus (reactive periosteal bone)

Foreign material: (e.g., screws) eventually become isolated from bone by fibrous tissue continuous with periosteum; no foreign body giant cell reaction occurs

NECROSIS

INFARCT

Seen following trauma; also seen in alcoholism, Gaucher's disease, decompression sickness, steroid use, sickle cell anemia, chronic pancreatitis

No radiological abnormalities seen for 1–2 wk

Eventually get absorption with decreased density

Commonly involves the femoral head: aseptic (avascular) necrosis: see "creeping substitution" of new bone for the nonviable bone; eventually get osteochondral collapse and secondary arthritis

Increased incidence of malignancy

OSTEOCHONDRITIS DISSECANS

Articular cartilage and subchondral bone undergo necrosis with separation from the rest of the bone

Usually medial femoral condyle; usually due to trauma

OSTEOMYELITIS

BACTERIAL

70–80% *Staphylococcus aureus,* often penicillin resistant

Also *Klebsiella, E. coli, Proteus, Pseudomonas, Streptococcus,* gonococcus

Sickle cell patients prone to *Salmonella* osteomyelitis

Newborns prone to *Haemophilus influenzae* infection

IV drug users prone to *Pseudomonas* infection

Hematogenous spread: most commonly ends of long bones (blood flow slowest in metaphyses)

Children <1 yr old primarily have epiphyseal involvement

Plasma cell osteomyelitis: abundant plasma cells

Xanthogranulomatous osteomyelitis: many foamy histiocytes

CHRONIC

Cutaneous fistulas; surface may heal, forming an epidermal inclusion cyst

Infection persists as long as dead bone with bacteria remain

Sequestra are cortical

TUBERCULOUS

Formerly children/young adults; now more common in debilitated elderly

Characteristically insidious, chronic, persistent, destructive, and resistant to management

Vertebrae (Pott's disease), hip, knee, ankle, elbow, wrist

Hematogenous spread: metaphysis, epiphysis, synovium

Sequestra are cancellous

SYPHILIS

Periosteal bone proliferation as well as destruction

Vertebrae, hands, feet, Hutchinson's teeth

When congenital, usually epiphyseal

FUNGAL

Blastomycosis, actinomycosis, histoplasmosis

ABNORMALITIES OF PRODUCTION

OSTEOPOROSIS

Decrease in mass of normally mineralized bones

Usually caused by increased absorption

Occurs postmenopausally if no estrogen replacement; also seen in endocrine dysfunctions, neoplasms, immobilization

Compression fractures of spine common

OSTEOMALACIA
"Rickets" in children with open epiphyseal plates (produces a characteristic cup-shaped deformity on x-ray)

Accumulation of unmineralized bone matrix caused by defective mineralization

Decreased rate of mineralization (decreased serum calcium or phosphate, usually due to decreased levels of vitamin D)

OSTEOPETROSIS
AKA: Albers-Schönberg disease, marble-bone disease

Defect in remodeling by osteoclasts (lysosomal defect)

Abnormal bone formation with excess lamellar bone and calcified cartilage

Curable by bone marrow transplantation

Malignant autosomal recessive form with obliteration of marrow cavity and early death from neutropenia/anemia

Adult autosomal dominant form more benign (less severe)

OSTEOGENESIS IMPERFECTA
Disorder of type I collagen synthesis, resulting in brittle bones

Fractures common in the lower extremities, esp. around the knees; leading to short stature

Type I: postnatal fractures, blue sclerae, hearing impairment, autosomal dominant, abnormality of pro-α1 chain

Type II: perinatal lethal; autosomal recessive

Type III: progressive deforming; abnormality of pro-α2 chain

Type IV: postnatal fractures, normal sclerae; autosomal dominant

ACHONDROPLASIA
Autosomal dominant; normal longevity when heterozygous, lethal when homozygous

Premature ossification of epiphyseal plates with normal appositional growth of bones, resulting in short disproportionately wide bones

RENAL OSTEODYSTROPHY
Bone changes and hypocalcemia seen in setting of chronic renal failure due to hyperphosphatemia and secondary hyperparathyroidism

Includes osteitis fibrosa cystica, osteomalacia, occasionally osteosclerosis

HYPERTROPHIC OSTEOARTHROPATHY
New periosteal bone formation at distal ends of long bones, esp. the bones of the hands and feet, with arthritis of adjacent joints and clubbing of the digits

Seen in patients with intrathoracic tumor, usually bronchogenic carcinoma

Clubbing alone can also be seen in cyanotic heart disease, infective endocarditis, inflammatory bowel disease

TUMOR-LIKE LESIONS

PAGET'S DISEASE (OSTEITIS DEFORMANS)
90% of patients >55 yr old; very rare before 40 yr; male = female

More common in England, Australia, northern Europe

Many cases are monostotic and asymptomatic, usually affecting the axial skeleton (lumbosacral spine [70%], pelvis [65%]; also femur, skull); some are polyostotic

May be viral (slow virus): osteoclasts contain viral-like inclusions

Initially lytic, followed by abnormal hyperplasia, thick trabeculae, disjointed and discontinuous lamellae, mosaic of cement lines (scalloped); advances through bone at 1mm/month

Increased incidence of sarcoma (femur, humerus, innominate, tibia, skull)

Fractures are usually transverse

Serum alkaline phosphatase often elevated (increased osteoblastic activity)

OSTEITIS FIBROSA
Chronic hyperparathyroidism induced osteoclastic destruction of bone

When cystic (osteitis fibrosa cystica), also known as von Recklinghausen's disease of bone

Initially see only demineralization; later, reabsorption and fibrosis with bizarre osteoclasts tunneling within scalloped reabsorption cavities

Microfractures lead to hemorrhage and hemosiderin-laden macrophages ("*brown tumor*")

Organization of hemorrhage creates mixture of macrophages, fibroblasts, osteoclasts, collectively forming a "*reparative giant cell granuloma*" (see also ABC)

MYOSITIS OSSIFICANS
Solitary, nonprogressive reactive condition often mistaken for osteosarcoma

Flexors of arm, quadriceps, adductors of thigh, gluteal muscles, soft tissue of hand most common; may not involve muscle

Occurs following trauma, usually no inflammation

Highly cellular stroma associated with new bone, with or without cartilage

As evolves, becomes zonal with cellular core, intermediate zone of osteoid, peripheral shell of highly organized bone

FIBROUS DYSPLASIA
Monostotic type (70%): older children, rib, femur, tibia

Polyostotic type: rarer; can be seen without endocrine dysfunction (25%) or with endocrine dysfunction, skin hyperpigmentation, and precocious puberty (5%; AKA Albright's syndrome)

Fusiform expanding mass arising in cancellous bone with thinning of overlying cortex

Narrow, curved, mis-shapen (Chinese characters) metaplastic bone spicules (without lining osteoblasts) in sea of variably cellular fibrous tissue; with or without giant cells

Cured by resection

OSSIFYING FIBROMA
AKA: osteofibrous dysplasia

Usually involves jaw

Like fibrous dysplasia except osteoblasts line trabeculae, lamellar bone is present, tends to be cortical vs. medullary

Greater tendency to recur

METAPHYSEAL FIBROUS DEFECT
AKA: nonossifying fibroma, "benign fibrous histiocytoma," fibrous cortical defect

Adolescents, usually tibia or lower femur; bilateral in 50%

Eccentric, sharply delimited lesions near epiphysis, often involving epiphyseal disorder

"Nonossifying fibroma" initially used to indicate variant, which is loose and involves medullary space

Cellular storiform fibrous tissue, scattered osteoclasts, foamy macrophages, hemosiderin

Usually asymptomatic—found incidentally; may be painful

Non-neoplastic; no malignant potential; often disappears spontaneously

ANEURYSMAL BONE CYST (ABC)

Patients usually 10–20 yr old

Usually vertebrae or flat bones, also diaphysis of long bones

Often grow rapidly, mimicking a neoplasm

Soft, spongelike mass composed of large, blood-filled spaces without endothelial lining, surrounded by a shell of reactive bone, producing an eccentric, often multicystic expansion of the bone, eroding the cortex, sometimes extending into the soft tissues

Osteoclasts, reactive bone, degenerated calcifying fibromyxoid tissue

ABC-like areas can be seen in chondroblastoma, giant cell tumor, fibrous dysplasia; also nonossifying fibroma, osteoblastoma, chondrosarcoma, hamartoma of chest

20–30% will recur if treated with curettage alone

SOLID ANEURYSMAL BONE CYST

Variant in which no cystic cavities are present

Seen in small bones of hands and feet, jaw, vertebra, sacrum

Spindle cell proliferation with osteoid, new bone formation, and giant cells

Some equate this with a "giant cell reparative granuloma" (see also osteitis fibrosa)

GANGLION CYST OF BONE

Similar to soft tissue counterpart, but much rarer

When found in intraosseous location, close to joint space

Cyst surrounded by zone of sclerotic bone

Gelatinous content and wall of fibrous tissue

Ankle (esp. tibia) most commonly affected

UNICAMERAL BONE CYST

AKA: solitary bone cyst, simple bone cyst

Usually upper humerus or femur; long or short bones

Most occur in males, almost all under 20 yr

Metaphyseal—with time, migrate away from epiphysis

Cyst contain clear or yellow fluid—lined by brown (hemosiderin-stained), well-vascularized connective tissue membrane, often with trapped cholesterol clefts

May see reactive changes; often present following fracture

Curettage and packing is treatment of choice

TUMORS

Characteristic Locations

Epiphysis: chondroblastoma, giant cell tumor

Metaphysis: giant cell tumor, enchondroma, chondrosarcoma, osteosarcoma, osteochondroma, osteoblastoma

Metaphyseal/diaphyseal junction: fibrosarcoma, fibrous cortical defect, chondromyxoid fibroma, fibrous dysplasia, osteoid osteoma

Diaphysis: Ewing's, adamantinoma

Grading

LOW GRADE

Grade I: well differentiated

Grade II: moderately differentiated

HIGH GRADE

Grade III: poorly differentiated

Grade IV: undifferentiated

Staging

T1: confined by cortex

T2: extends beyond cortex

N1: regional lymph nodes involved

	T1	T2
N0, low grade	IA	IB
N0, high grade	IIA	IIB
N1	IVA	IVA

IVB: M1

(Note: there is no Stage III)

Bone Forming

OSTEOMA

40–50 yr old; male : female = 2 : 1

Bosselated lesion composed of dense, mature, predominantly lamellar bone, located usually on the flat bones of skull and face; may protrude into sinuses

May be a reactive rather than a neoplastic process

Seen in patients with Gardner's syndrome

OSTEOID OSTEOMA

Male : female = 2 : 1; 10–30 yr old

Can occur anywhere, most commonly femur, tibia, humerus

Intense, well-localized pain (out of proportion to size of lesion), which is rapidly relieved by aspirin

Usually metaphyseal in long bones, pedicle in vertebrae

85% begin in cortex; 13% in medulla, 2% subperiosteal

Central radiolucent nidus (0.5–1.5 cm; osteoid growing in highly vascular osteoblastic connective tissue with some benign giant cells) surrounded by dense sclerotic bone

High levels of prostaglandins present, perhaps accounting for pain

OSTEOBLASTOMA

AKA: giant osteoid osteoma

Similar to osteoid osteoma, with larger (>1.5 cm by definition) nidus and minimal surrounding sclerotic bone

Most arise in medulla; metaphyseal; male : female = 2 : 1; 10–30 yr

Spine, large bones of legs; may be painless

May be difficult to distinguish from osteosarcoma; presence of infiltrative margin or *cartilage* suggests malignancy

AGGRESSIVE OSTEOBLASTOMA

AKA: malignant osteoblastoma, osteosarcoma resembling osteoblastoma

Atypical cytological features, wide irregular trabeculae lined by epithelioid osteoblasts, nontrabecular osteoid

Differentiation from osteosarcoma: low mitotic rate, osteoid not lacelike, the tumor does not penetrate into surrounding tissues

OSTEOSARCOMA

Most common primary bone malignancy (except hematopoietic)

Male : female = 3 : 2; usually 10–25 yr old (second peak after 40 yr)

Usually metaphyseal (~90%), particularly lower femur, upper tibia, upper humerus

Must identify irregularly contoured osteoid and/or bone produced by tumor cells; commonly anastomosing microtrabeculae

Most arise in medullary cavity and extend along marrow, to cortex, to soft tissues, to epiphysis, to joint; may elevate periosteum (Codman's triangle: new bone made by elevated periosteum); often have satellite nodules (skip metastases)

May destroy preexisting bone or grow around it

Spindle cell tumor; 50% are predominantly osteoblastic, 25% chondroblastic, and 25% fibroblastic; non-osteoblastic patterns can dominate histology—no effect on prognosis

Osteosarcoma cells may be alkaline phosphatase positive, usually vimentin positive, usually make type I collagen

Metastases via blood: lung (98%), other bones (37%), pleura (33%), heart (20%); regional LNs almost never involved

PREDISPOSING CONDITIONS

Note: most arise *de novo*

- Paget's disease: accounts for many osteosarcomas in individuals >50 yr old
- Radiation: 2nd most common post radiation sarcoma (after malignant fibrous histiocytoma); usually 10 yr after radiation—most high grade
- Chemotherapy: children with retinoblastoma (Rb) or other malignancy; increased frequency of osteosarcoma in patients with mutations of the Rb gene
- Benign lesions: fibrous dysplasia, osteochondromatosis
- Foreign bodies: e.g., at site of total hip replacement—rare
- (Trauma: does not cause—merely brings to attention)

THERAPY

Often use preoperative chemotherapy; >90% response associated with good prognosis

Excise entire biopsy tract with specimen

Removal of metastases from lung appears to prolong survival

PROGNOSIS

5 yr survival increased from 20% to 50% with advent of preadjuvant chemotherapy

Good prognosis: jaw or distal extremities; parosteal, periosteal, well-differentiated intramedullary types

Bad prognosis: Paget's, radiation induced (30% 5 yr), multifocal, focal dedifferentiation, telangiectatic

No effect on prognosis: age, sex

Variants/Special Types

WELL-DIFFERENTIATED OSTEOSARCOMA

AKA: intramedullary, central low-grade osteosarcoma

Mostly adults, femur or tibia; very bland

Hypocellular; resembles fibrous dysplasia, but with cortical destruction

Recurrences common, metastases rare

JUXTACORTICAL (PAROSTEAL) OSTEOSARCOMA

Infrequent; occurs in older age group (30s–40s); female > male

Metaphysis of long bones, usually distal femur (70%)

Slow growing—some up to 15 yr

Large lobulated hypocellular mass, with spindle cells in a predominantly fibrous background; tends to encircle the bone; heavily calcified

Very good prognosis if low grade

Late in evolution, may become high grade (dedifferentiate) and penetrate medullary cavity—bad prognosis

PERIOSTEAL OSTEOSARCOMA

Grows on surface of long bones

Upper tibial shaft or femur—usually limited to cortex

Predominantly chondroblastic, usually high grade

Prognosis better than conventional osteosarcoma

OSTEOSARCOMA OF THE JAW

Slightly older (average age 34)

Prominent cartilaginous component

Relatively good prognosis

TELANGIECTATIC OSTEOSARCOMA

Prominent blood-filled cystic formations (resembles an aneurysmal bone cyst)

Malignant stroma in septa separating bloody cysts

Pathologic fractures common

May have more aggressive clinical course

SMALL CELL OSTEOSARCOMA

Often confused with Ewing's or lymphoma, but focally produces osteoid, sometimes mixed with cartilage

Poor prognosis

FIBROHISTIOCYTIC OSTEOSARCOMA

Looks like MFH, especially in soft tissue

ANAPLASTIC OSTEOSARCOMA

Marked pleomorphism—bizarre nuclei

OSTEOSARCOMA IN PAGET'S DISEASE

Occurs in <1% of patients with polyostotic Paget's

Pelvis, humerus, femur, tibia, skull

Usually many osteoclasts

Extremely poor prognosis

Cartilage-Forming

OSTEOCHONDROMA (EXOSTOSIS)

Most common benign bone "tumor" (may be simply aberrant growth of cartilage rather than a true neoplasm)

Young (~10 yr old); male > female; usually asymptomatic

Metaphysis, most commonly lower femur, upper tibia, upper humerus, pelvis

Grows out in direction opposite that of the adjacent joint

Usually ~4 cm, may get larger; larger tumors pedunculated

Lobulated cap of cartilage (covered by fibrous membrane), with mature bone beneath making up the bulk of lesion; active endochondral ossification at interface

Cap rarely exceeds 1 cm; in older lesions, cap may thin out or disappear

Whole lesion may spontaneously regress

If single, malignant transformation in 1–2%

Signs of malignancy: >8 cm, cap >3 cm, irregular cap

Bursa may develop around head—can lead to chondrosarcoma

OSTEOCHONDROMATOSIS

AKA: Ehrenfried's hereditary deforming chondrodysplasia

Multiple lesions; autosomal dominant

Can be associated with Gardner's syndrome

More likely to develop chondrosarcoma (10%)

SUBUNGUAL EXOSTOSES

AKA: Dupuytren's exostoses

Usually located on great toe

Not really osteochondromas; different entity

Invariably benign

CHONDROMA

AKA: enchondroma when in center of diaphysis

Common benign lesions

Radiology: popcorn-like densities

Usually small bones of hands or feet, esp. proximal phalanges; unusual in ribs or long bones

Mature, well-circumscribed lobules of hyaline cartilage, often with foci of myxoid degeneration, calcification, peripheral endochondral ossification; usually *not* painful

In general, cellular myxoid areas should raise suspicion for low-grade chondrosarcoma; however, lesions in the hands (which are often painful) can show cellular myxoid areas as well as double-nucleated lacunae and still behave in a benign fashion

Nonhereditary syndromes of multiple chondromas have risk of malignant transformation (to chondrosarcoma):
- Ollier's disease: predominantly unilateral, associated with ovarian sex-cord stromal tumors
- Maffucci's syndrome: with soft tissue hemangiomas

CALCIFYING ENCHONDROMA
Massive calcification, present in metaphysis of long bones

JUXTACORTICAL (PERIOSTEAL)
Small (usually <3 cm) and well demarcated

Like enchondromas of the hands, these lesions tend to be more cellular with occasional myxoid areas and atypical chondrocytes; may erode and induce sclerosis of contiguous cortex; still behave in a benign fashion

CARTILAGINOUS AND VASCULAR HAMARTOMA (MESENCHYMOMA)
Occurs in chest wall of infants; most are congenital

Not strictly a chondroma

Chondroid areas mixed with spindle areas in an aneurysmal bone cystlike appearance

CHONDROBLASTOMA
Male : female = 2 : 1; usually 10–20 yr old; characteristically painful

Epiphyseal: distal femur, proximal humerus, proximal tibia

Very cellular, occasional scattered collections of giant cells

May have thick, sharply demarcated cell membranes; glycogen in cytoplasm; plump nuclei, characteristically with a longitudinal groove; reticulin fibers surround each cell (immature cartilage) and in small zones calcifies to form a lacy "chicken wire" pattern; S-100 positive

25–50% show areas resembling aneurysmal bone cyst with giant cells

Differential diagnosis: giant cell tumor, chondromyxoid fibroma

Treatment: curettage; may recur

Rarely, may behave aggressively—identical histology

CHONDROMYXOID FIBROMA
Young adults, often long bones (most commonly tibia) or small bones of the feet; may become large

Radiograph: well-defined lytic lesion of the lateral metaphysis, often with a sclerotic margin and thinned overlying cortex

Solid, yellowish to tan; bone is replaced rather than expanded

Large lobules of a hypocellular myxoid to chondroid matrix separated by a highly cellular stroma containing spindled cells and osteoclasts

Occasional pleomorphic giant cells can be seen; mitoses rare

Presence of binucleate or multinucleated cells, or multiple cells per lacunae, suggests a low-grade chondrosarcoma

25% recur if curette; en bloc excision preferred

FIBROMYXOMA
Probably variant of chondromyxoid fibroma; older individuals

CHONDROSARCOMA
Most patients 30–60 yr old; pelvis, ribs, shoulder

Can occur in children; usually extremities

Radiology: osteolytic lesions with spotty calcification, ill-defined margins, expansive thickening of shaft, cortical thickening with areas of perforation or destruction; rarely grows beyond periosteum

Plump, hyperchromatic nuclei, two or more nuclei per cell, two or more cells per lacuna; cells are S-100 positive

Permeation of bone marrow with trapping of lamellar bone

Correlation with radiology essential: atypical cytology OK in lesion of fingers (enchondroma), but rapidly growing lesions of ribs or long bones, which attain a size of >8 cm are invariably malignant, regardless of cytology

Soft tissue implantation at biopsy common; en bloc excision or removal of biopsy tract important

Prognosis generally better than osteosarcoma

Microscopic grade (based on cellularity) important: 5 yr survival 78%, 53%, 22% for grade I, II, III lesions

Recurrences usually of higher grade than primary, and may occur up to 20 yr later

Metastases common, usually to the lung; never LNs

THREE TYPES BY LOCATION:
- Central: located in medullary cavity, usually of long bone
- Peripheral: arise de novo or in pre-existing osteochondroma; often have heavily calcified center
- Juxtacortical (periosteal): shaft of long bone, usually femur

Variants

CLEAR CELL CHONDROSARCOMA
Often proximal femur, proximal humerus

Abundant clear cytoplasm, sharply defined cell borders, with interspersed fragments of lamellar bone

Similar to chondroblastoma; may be malignant counterpart

Usually entirely lytic, slightly expansile, sharply marginated

Behaves in low-grade fashion

MESENCHYMAL CHONDROSARCOMA
10–30 yr old; jaw, pelvis, femur, ribs; 30% arise in soft tissues

Dimorphic pattern: islands of well-differentiated cartilage intermixed with a highly cellular, undifferentiated stroma of small cells, often with a lymphoma or hemangiopericytoma pattern; pleomorphism and/or mitoses rare

Small cells positive for vimentin, Leu7; negative for S-100

Prognosis variable, generally poor

MYXOID CHONDROSARCOMA (CHORDOID SARCOMA)
Can occur in bone or in soft tissue

Looks like chordoma, but is keratin negative

DEDIFFERENTIATED CHONDROSARCOMA
Focus of poorly differentiated sarcomatous element, usually at periphery of an otherwise low-grade lesion

Focal areas may resemble MFH, rhabdomyosarcoma, fibrosarcoma, osteosarcoma

Marked acceleration of clinical course; very bad prognosis

Fibrohistiocytic Lesions

BENIGN FIBROUS HISTIOCYTOMA
(See Metaphyseal Fibrous Defect, earlier)

DESMOPLASTIC FIBROMA
Rare benign to borderline neoplasm; most often long bones, pelvis, and mandible
Radiograph: purely lytic, honeycombed
Mature fibroblasts with abundant collagen
Probably represents osseous counterpart of fibromatosis
Often recurs, doesn't metastasize

MALIGNANT FIBROUS HISTIOCYTOMA
Similar to soft tissue counterpart
Long bones or jaw; mean age 40 yr
Bone infarcts, foreign bodies, irradiation, Paget's, dedifferentiation in chondrosarcoma account for 30%

FIBROSARCOMA
Metaphyseal; 50% in distal femur or proximal tibia
Arises in medulla, destroys cortex, extends into soft tissues
Radiograph: lytic with soap-bubble appearance
If significant pleomorphism present, should diagnose as MFH
May be well differentiated; need radiology to call malignant
Cellular areas, mitoses, hyperchromasia favor malignancy
Survival correlates well with grade

Other Primary Bone Tumors

GIANT CELL TUMOR
AKA: osteoclastoma; however, cells are *not* osteoclasts
Female > male; usually 20s–30s; Asian > western; 95% at metaphyseal-epiphyseal junction growing into epiphysis (after plate closure)
Usually ends of long bones, particularly lower femur, upper tibia, lower radius, humerus, fibula; also sacrum
When occurs in an uncommon site, more likely to be an aneurysmal bone cyst
Radiographically: entirely lytic, expansile, usually without peripheral sclerosis or periosteal reaction (unless it recurs in soft tissue, where it usually is surrounded by an eggshell of ossification)
Variable size; solid, tan to light brown, often hemorrhagic
Giant cells with many central nuclei regularly distributed in a sea of somewhat spindled stromal cells (malignant cells)
Most likely, mononuclear cells arise from mesenchymal cells and then fuse to form giant cells
Mitoses common, but atypia is not
Focal osteoid or bone seen in one third of cases
All potentially malignant: 30–50% recur, 5–10% metastasize
Recurrence rate: 35% for curettage, 7% for en bloc excision
Even 1–2% of low-grade tumors will metastasize
Metastases (usually to lung) occur after surgical intervention
Radiation therapy often induces malignant transformation

EWING'S SARCOMA
<5% of all malignant bone tumors
Children and adults <30 yr; most 5–20 yr old
Usually long bones (femur, tibia, humerus, fibula), pelvis, rib, vertebra, mandible, clavicle; may be extraosseous
Arises in medullary cavity of diaphysis; widens the medulla and thickens the cortex; often extensive, and may involve entire bone; eventually penetrates cortex and invades soft tissues (bad sign); may present as soft tissue lesion because permeation of medullary cavity may be nondestructive and radiographically inapparent
As elevates periosteum and new bone is laid down, an onion-skin layering may be seen about the cortex on x-ray
Gross: white, fleshy
Composed of sheets of small, uniform cells with indented nuclei (if nuclei are spindled, probably not Ewing's) and inconspicuous nucleoli; cell borders may be inapparent; occasional pseudorosettes (necrotic cells in center; no true lumen); strands of fibrous stroma separate tumor into irregular masses
Cytogenetics: reciprocal translocation t(11;22)(q24;q12); the 22q12 locus is known as EWS, a putative tumor suppressor gene
Glycogen usually present (PAS+); vimentin positive; may be keratin positive
Anti-O13: stains Ewing's sarcoma and peripheral neuroectodermal tumors (PNETs); reacts with MIC^2 gene product (~38kD); gene in "autosomal" region of X and Y chromosomes; also expressed in pancreatic islets, ependyma, lymphoblastic lymphoma, some rhabdomyosarcomas; Ewing's is probably a less differentiated form of PNET
Electron microscopy (EM) shows two cell types: large nuclei with open chromatin, small contracted nuclei with hyperchromatic chromatin
All are high grade by definition
25% have multiple metastases at presentation: lungs, pleura, other bones (especially skull), CNS, regional LNs
Becomes more pleomorphic following therapy
Treatment: surgery and radiation: 5 yr survival 5–8%; multidrug chemotherapy has increased to 75%

CHORDOMA
Arises from remnants of fetal notochord; malignant
Most frequent in 40s and 50s, but can occur at any age; male > female
Usually within vertebral bodies, intervertebral discs, sacrum 50% sacrococcygeal (older patients), 35% spheno-occipital (children), 15% cervicothoracolumbar spine
Slow-growing tumor; destroys bone, compresses structures
Gelatinous, soft, areas of hemorrhage, may have bone/cartilage
Cells grow in cords and *lobules* separated by a mucoid matrix
Physaliferous cells: very large tumor cells with bubbly cytoplasm (some glycogen) and vesicular nuclei
Mitoses scant or absent
May simulate renal cell carcinoma
EM: mitochondrial-endoplasmic reticulum complexes
Immunohistochemistry: S-100, vimentin, keratin, EMA positive; CEA negative
Repeated local recurrences, often for decades; can focally dedifferentiate; eventually fatal
Metastases late in course: skin, bone
Treatment: surgery, radiation
CHONDROID CHORDOMA
Abundant cartilaginous component
Usually spheno-occipital
Better prognosis than ordinary chordoma
Keratin stain usually only focally positive

ADAMANTINOMA
Predominantly tibia; also femur, ulna, fibula; diaphysis or metaphysis; counterpart in jaw is referred to as ameloblastoma (see Head and Neck outline)

Poorly defined lytic lesion with marked sclerosis outlining single or multiple lucent areas; may extend to soft tissues

Various microscopic patterns: fibrous dysplasia-like spindle cell component surrounding solid nests of usually basaloid cells with palisading at periphery but occasionally squamoid or tubular formations are seen; stroma probably reflects mesenchymal differentiation of epithelial tumor cells

Low-grade malignancy: local recurrences, occasional LN metastases

MISCELLANEOUS OTHER TUMORS

PLASMA CELL MYELOMA

Most common primary tumor of bone (30%)

Skull, spine, ribs

See hematolymphoid outline

MALIGNANT LYMPHOMA

Patchy, cortical and medullary, diaphyseal and metaphyseal

Most are large cell lymphomas, although Burkitt's can occur, as can Hodgkin's disease

EOSINOPHILIC GRANULOMA

(See Hematolymphoid outline)

VASCULAR TUMORS

- Hemangioma: common (12% at autopsy); probably malformation; skull, vertebrae, jaw can be clinically significant
- Massive osteolysis (Gorham's disease): reabsorption of whole or multiple bones and filling of residual spaces with heavily vascularized fibrous tissue; not a true neoplasm; unknown etiology
- Hemangiopericytoma: usually pelvis
- Epithelioid (histiocytoid) hemangioendothelioma: often rich in eosinophils, often prominent inflammatory component; protracted clinical course
- Angiosarcoma

PERIPHERAL NERVE TUMORS

Neurilemoma: predilection for mandible

Metastases

Most common of all malignant tumors of bone (25–30 × more common than primary bone tumors)

80% are metastatic from breast, lung, prostate, thyroid, or kidney; 50% patients with these tumors will have bone metastases

70% involve axial skeleton, 30% extremities (usually from lung)

Usually osteolytic, may be osteoblastic (prostate, breast, carcinoid) or mixed

Generally does not destroy vertebral disc (unlike osteomyelitis)

Most are painful; local radiation effective for pain relief in 80%

ARTICULAR AND PERIARTICULAR DISEASES

ARTHRITIS

Functional failure of the joint with pain and limitation on range of motion; may be a primary inflammatory lesion, but inflammation may also be minimal or purely secondary

Cartilage injury presents as loss of chondrocytes from lacunae, vertical or horizontal clefts within the cartilage (collagen injury), and/or depletion of proteoglycan from the matrix, resulting in decreased basophilia

Cartilage proliferation/repair can be both intrinsic (islands of chondrocytes within the matrix) or extrinsic (new cartilage formation at the cartilage/bone interface)

Bone injury includes focal necrosis, microfractures, subchondral sclerosis, and development of subchondral cysts

Reactive synovium is often hyperplastic with increased cellularity and papillary projections into the joint space

Loose bodies: fragments of bone or cartilage that become detached into the joint space; may continue to grow by surface apposition; centers eventually necrose and calcify

OSTEOARTHRITIS

AKA: degenerative joint disease

Disease of elderly, usually involving joints symmetrically

Most common sites: metatarsophalangeal joint of big toe, hip, knee

Damage to the cartilage and the underlying bone common, with areas of complete cartilage loss and a "polishing sclerosis" (eburnation) of the exposed bone

Marginal bony outgrowths (osteophytes) are commonly seen

Divided into primary and secondary:

- Primary: usually elderly women; affects "normal" joints; often asymptomatic
- Secondary: any age; affects previously damaged or congenitally abnormal joints; often involves weight-bearing joints

RHEUMATOID ARTHRITIS

Usually women, 30s–40s

Initially involves small joints of hands and feet, then later wrists, elbows, knees; extension of disease is usually symmetric

Acute inflammatory infiltrate composed predominantly of neutrophils seen in acute effusions

Chronic disease shows marked proliferation of the synovium, often including rheumatoid nodules (seen in 25%: palisading histiocytes surrounding an irregular area of fibrinoid necrosis), lymphocytes, and many plasma cells, which extends over the articular surface to form the characteristic "pannus," destroying the underlying cartilage, occasionally leading to fibrous or osseous fusion of the joint

Hyperplastic synovium also seen outside the joint proper

Most likely an autoimmune disease: most patients have autoantibody against the Fc portion of IgG (rheumatoid factor)

JUVENILE RHEUMATOID ARTHRITIS

AKA: Still's disease

Different disease than adult rheumatoid arthritis

Joint involvement more commonly acute, limited to one or a few joints, more commonly involves the knees, and is preceded by a febrile illness with generalized lymphadenopathy and hepatosplenomegaly

Rheumatoid factor often not present

AVASCULAR NECROSIS

Most commonly seen in the femoral head following infarction

Collapsed avascularized segment of bone results in secondary arthritis

GOUT

Hyperuricemia leading to deposition of sodium urate crystals in joint and viscera (most patients have uric acid stones in the kidneys)

Recurrent attacks of acute gouty arthritis usually involve the lower extremities (especially big toe), usually monoarticular

Examination of aspirated fluid (in ethyl alcohol; crystals are water soluble) can show birefringent, needle-shaped crystals

Granulomatous response to crystals seen in tissue sections

In chronic disease, large deposits (tophi) of urate crystals and chronic inflammatory cells in and around joints produces "tophaceous gout"

90% of cases are primary; secondary causes include increased nucleic acid turnover (leukemia), enzyme deficiency (Lesch-Nyhan syndrome: deficiency of hypoxanthine-guanine phosphoribosyltransferase), decreased renal secretion

PSEUDOGOUT
AKA: calcium pyrophosphate crystal deposition disease; chondrocalcinosis

Deposition within joints of chalky-white calcium pyrophosphate crystals (small, rhomboid, weakly birefringent)

Most commonly affects knees, then ankles, wrists, hips, elbows

ANKYLOSING SPONDYLITIS
AKA: rheumatoid spondylitis; Marie-Strümpell disease

HLA-B27 associated inflammation of the axial skeleton, always involving the sacroiliac joints and variably involving the hips and shoulders

Occurs most commonly in young men

INFECTIOUS ARTHRITIS
Suppurative: usually gonococci, staphylococci, streptococci, *Haemophilus influenzae*

Tuberculous: most commonly spine (Pott's disease); also hip in children, knees in adults; organisms usually not demonstrable in the bone

Lyme disease: caused by spirochete *Borrelia burgdorferi;* pathology similar to rheumatoid arthritis, with additional onion-skin thickening of arterioles

BURSITIS
Clinical syndrome with pain, erythema, and swelling of one of the bursae associated with muscles, tendons, or joints

More common in men than women

Usually occurs in setting of chronic trauma, or less commonly infection, but may be a complication of rheumatoid arthritis

Thick wall, chronic inflammation, fibrinous exudate, focal vascular proliferations; may calcify

BAKER'S CYST
Herniation of synovium of knee into the popliteal space

Wall is lined by synovium

Seen as a complication of increased intra-articular pressure caused by degenerative joint disease or rheumatoid arthritis

GANGLION
Occur about joints (usually hands, feet) or in soft tissue; can cause pain, deformity, weakness, partial disability

Fibrous-walled cyst (no epithelial lining), usually 1–2 cm diameter, containing a clear fluid, often mucinous

Etiology unclear: herniations of synovium or, more likely, mucinous degeneration of fibrous connective tissue

On rare occasion, may communicate with joint space or erode into bone

MORTON'S NEUROMA
Swelling of an interdigital nerve of the foot, usually between the 3rd and 4th metatarsal, usually in a woman, resulting in shooting pains upon standing

Proliferation of Schwann cells and fibroblasts associated with fibrosis, nerve degeneration, endarteritis, and thrombosis of the accompanying artery

PIGMENTED VILLONODULAR SYNOVITIS
Locally aggressive "tumor" of the synovium of the hand (swelling of tendon sheath) or knee (effusion), usually affecting only a single joint

Proliferation of polygonal cells in a collagenous background, with scattered giant cells and often significant hemosiderin deposition

Variable amounts of nonspecific chronic inflammation accompanies the proliferation

Probably similar entity to giant cell tumor of tendon sheath occurring in association with a joint

May recur locally

(See also Soft Tissues outline, Fibrohistiocytic Lesions)

PRIMARY SYNOVIAL CHONDROMATOSIS
Lobulated overgrowth of cellular cartilage without an associated inflammation, often fragmenting into the joint space, creating many loose bodies

Chondrometaplasia of synovium occurs, often atypical

Can also see cartilage proliferation secondary to osteoarthritis or loose bodies, but it is not atypical

12

HEMATOPOIETIC ONTOGENY

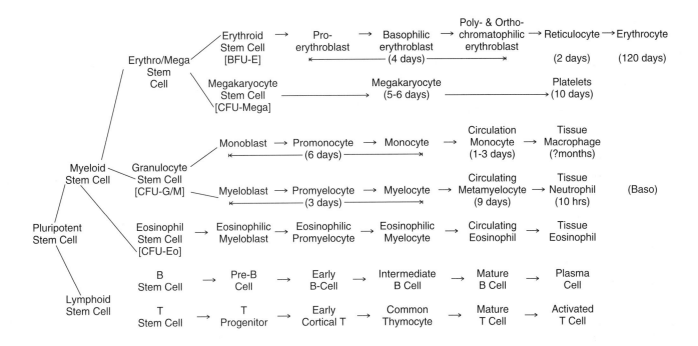

Marker Changes with Ontogeny

B CELLS

Lymphoid Pluripotent Stem Cell	B Lymphoid → Stem Cell	Early Pre-B →	Middle Pre-B →	Late Pre-B →	Early B Cell →	Virgin Intermediate → B Cell	Mature B Cell →	Pre- Plasma →	Plasma Cell
CD34 TdT	CD34 TdT HLA-DR	CD34 TdT HLA-DR CD19	-cd34- TdT HLA-DR CD19 CD10	-tdt- HLA-DR CD19 CD10 CD20	HLA-DR CD19 CD20 CD21	HLA-DR CD19 CD20 CD21	HLA-DR CD19 CD20 -cd21- CD25	HLA-DR CD19 CD20	HLA-DR
	Heavy: Light:	Rearranged	—	Expressed Rearranged	IgM Exp.	IgM,IgD	IgM,IgD,IgX		

Note: Separate lineage exists for which all cells are CD5⁺ (peritoneal B cells vs. CD5⁻ B cells in lymph nodes and spleen)

93

T CELLS

Lymphoid Pluripotent Stem Cell	→	T Lymphoid Stem Cell	→	T Lymphoid Progenitor	→	Early Cortical Thymocyte	→	Common Thymocyte	→	Mature Medullary Thymocyte	→	Mature T Cells	→	Activated T Cell
CD34		CD34		CD34				CD1a						
TdT		TdT		TdT				TdT		TdT				
		CD7		CD7		CD7		CD7		CD7		CD7		CD7
				CD2		CD2		CD2		CD2		CD2		CD2
				CD5		CD5		CD5		CD5		CD5		CD5
								CD3(cyto)		CD3		CD3		CD3
								CD4+CD8						

CD4, CD8, neither, both

CD25

β:		Rearranged		—		TcR$_{\alpha\beta}$		TcR$_{\alpha\beta}$
α:				Rearranged		TcR$_{\alpha\beta}$		TcR$_{\alpha\beta}$

Note: Separate lineage, beginning after T-lymphoid progenitor, of CD4⁻,CD8⁻ γδ-T cell (epidermis and intestinal epithelium) vs the αβ-T cell of lymph nodes and spleen

Cluster Designation/Clusters of Differentiation

Identified immunologically: Cell surface markers were identified by monoclonal antibodies. Those that consistently recognized the same subsets of cells (clustered) were felt most likely to be reacting with the same molecule.

	Synonyms	Cell Types	MW (kD)	Function
CD1a	T6, Leu6, Na1-34	Early T, LC	49	MHC-I–like
CD1b	WM-25, 4A76	Early T, LC	43	MHC-I–like
CD1c	L161, M241	Early T, LC	45	MHC-I–like
CD2	T11, Leu5	Pan-T, NK	50	CD58 receptor, sheep RBC binding (rosette)
CD3	T3, Leu4, UCHT1	Pan-T (mature)	26,20,16	Associated with TcR
CD4	T4, Leu3a	Helper/Inducer T	60	MHC-II receptor, HIV receptor
CD5	T1, Leu1, UCHT2	Pan-T, B-cell CLL	67	Present on subset of B cells
CD6	T12, TU33, T411	T, rare B	100	
CD7	Leu9, OKT-16, WT1	Early + mature T, NK	40	IgM Fc receptor
CD8	T8, Leu2, UCHT4	Suppressor/cytotoxic T, NK	32	MHC-I binding (2 chains)
CD9	ALB-6, J2	Pre-B, M, Plt	24	
CD10	J5, CALLA	Pre-B, pre-T, some mature B, G	100	Neutral endopeptidase
CD11a	LFA-1 α chain	Leukocytes	180	Adhesion (see CD18); binds CD54 (ICAM)
CD11b	Mo1, Mac1, Leu15	NK, M, G, T-suppressor	155	C3bi (CR3) receptor (see CD18)
CD11c	LeuM5, L29	M, G, NK, hairy cell leukemia cell	150	Cell adhesion (see CD18)
CDw12	M67	M, G, Plt	90–120	
CD13	My7, LeuM7	Myeloid	150	Aminopeptidase N
CD14	Mo2, My4, LeuM3	M, Mac, LC, immature G	55	
CD15	My1, LeuM1	G, M, Mac, Reed-Sternberg cells		
CD16	Leu11	NK, G, Mac	50–65	Fc$_\gamma$III receptor
CDw17	GO35	G, M, Plt		Lactosylceramide
CD18	M232, MHM23	Leukocytes		β-chain for LFA-1 (CD11a,b,c)
CD19	B4,Leu12	Pan-B (not plasma cells)	95	Ig-like
CD20	Leu16, L26, B1	Pan-B (not plasma cells)	37/32	Calcium channel
CD21	B2	B in blood, mantle zone	140	C3d (CR2) and EBV receptor
CD22	4KB-128, Leu14	Pan-B (cytoplasm + surface)	135	Homologous to myelin associated gp
CD23	Blast-2, Leu20	Mantle zone B, activated M, Eos	45–50	Fcε receptor
CD24	BA-1	Pan-B, plasma cells, G	41	
CD25	Tac, IL-2R	Activated T, B, M	55	α chain of IL-2 receptor
CD26	134-2C2	Activated T	120	Dipeptidylpeptidase IV
CD27	VIT14, OKT18a	T subset	55	
CD28	KOLT2	T subset, plasma cells	44	
CD29	K20	Many cells	130	Integrin β1-chain, platelet GPIIa
CD30	Ki-1, Ber-H2	Act T, B, Reed-Sternberg cells	105–120	
CD31	SG134	Plt, M, G, B	140	Platelet GPIIa
CD32	C1KM5, 41H	M, G, B, Eos, basophils	39	Fc$_\gamma$II receptor
CD33	My9, LeuM9	Immature myeloid	67	
CD34	My10	Progenitors, vascular endothelium	105–120	
CD35	To5	G, M, B	160–250	CR1, C3b receptor
CD36	SF1, gp90	M, Plt, B	90	Platelet gpIV
CD37	HD28	B, (T, M)	40–52	

	Synonyms	Cell Types	MW (kD)	Function
CD38	T16, Leu17	Act T , Act B, NK, plasma cells	45	
CD39	AC2, OKT28	B subset, (M)	70-100	
CD40		B, carcinomas	50	Homologous to NGF receptor
CD41	CLB-thromb7, J15	Platelets, megakaryocytes	123,110	Platelet gpIIb/IIIa
CD43	Leu22, L60	T, G, M, NK, brain		Leukosialin, altered in Wiskott-Aldrich
CD44	Pgp-1	RBC, many WBC, brain	80-95	Lymphocytes homing receptor, memory marker?
CD45	LCA, T200, Leu18	T , B, G, M	180–220	Memory marker?
CD45RO	UCHL-1	T, myeloid cells	205–220	
CD51		Platelets	125/25	Vitronectin receptor alpha chain (see CD61)
CD54	Leu54, My13	Many cells	90	Cell adhesion (ICAM-1)
CD56	NKH1, Leu19	NK, activated lymphocytes	220/135	Isoform of N-CAM
CD57	Leu7, HNK1	NK, T subset, B subset	110	
CD58	G26	Leukocytes, epithelial		LFA-3, ligand for CD2
CD61		Megakaryocytes, platelets	110	β3 chain for CD41 and CD51
CD64		M	75	Fc$_\gamma$1 receptor
CD68	EMB11, KP-1	M, Mac	110	
CD69	Leu23	Act B, Act T, Act M, NK	32/28	
CD71	T9, OKT9, VIP-1	Proliferating cells	95	Transferrin receptor
CD74		B, M	41/35/33	MHC-II invariant chain

G: granulocytes; M: monocyte; LC: Langerhan's cells; NK: natural killer cells; CLL: chronic lymphocytic leukemia; Plt: platelet; Mac: macrophage; Eos: eosinophils; Act: activated; ICAM: intercellular adhesion molecule; N-CAM: neural cell adhesion molecule.

GENERAL

DEVELOPMENT

"Blood islands" appear in yolk sac in 3rd wk of development
~3 months: migrate to liver (major hematopoietic site until birth)
Spleen, lymph nodes (LNs), thymus contribute in the 2nd and 3rd trimesters
Bone marrow becomes active at ~4 months
Full term: bone marrow main site; liver nearly inactive
All marrow is active until puberty
By 18 yr, active marrow is restricted to ribs, vertebrae, pelvis, skull, epiphyses of humerus and femur; rest becomes fatty and inactive
Marrow output can increase seven- to eight–fold if needed
When needed, extramedullary hematopoiesis reappears first in liver, then spleen, then lymph nodes (LNs), never thymus

GROWTH FACTORS

GM-CSF: granulocyte/macrophage colony stimulating factor; made by T cells, fibroblasts, endothelial cells
Erythropoietin: red cell maturation
Interleukin (IL)-3: (AKA multi-CSF); growth factor for trilineage myeloid stem cell; made by T cells

BONE MARROW

Normal

Cellularity: 90% for young children, 50–60% for adults, 40–50% after 60 yr of age
60% granulocytic; 20% erythroid; 10% lymphocytes and monocytes; 10% unidentifiable
Myeloid (M) : erythroid (E) ratio 3 : 1 (based on spacing of red cell clusters)
Maturation: ~75% of myelocytic elements should be mature neutrophils, ~75% erythroid elements should be normoblasts
Early granulocytic precursors usually located next to bone spicules
Abnormally located granulocytic precursors can be a clue to preleukemic state; paratrabecular lymphoid aggregates can indicate a lymphoma
Megakaryocytes: normally 3–5 per 40× field
Macrophages: if you notice them, there are too many
Lymphocytic aggregates can be seen; increase in number with age; more prominent in AIDS, rheumatoid arthritis, interleukin (IL)-2 therapy
Iron: stored in macrophages: one iron-positive cell per 40× field is normal, 2 is increased, <1 is decreased; children under 14 yr have no stainable iron
30–40% of normoblasts have ferritin granules (sideroblasts); iron overload → ring sideroblasts (ruptured mitochondria)

Non-neoplastic Lesions

SEROUS DEGENERATION

AKA: gelatinous transformation
Extremely malnourished patients (kwashiorkor, cachexia, AIDS)

NECROSIS

Seen in tumors (metastatic and primary), sickle cell anemia, infectious processes, systemic lupus erythematosus (SLE), anorexia nervosa
Generalized bone pain
Aspirates tend to be gelatinous
Marrow replaced by amorphous granular eosinophilic debris

GRANULOMATOUS INFLAMMATION

Fungus, TB, Mycobacterium avium-intracellulare (MAI), viral infections (e.g., mono), sarcoidosis
Also seen in Hodgkin's and non-Hodgkin's lymphomas
No etiology can be found in 80%
Lipid granulomas common—loosely spaced macrophages with fat vacuoles—giant cells seen in 5%

AIDS

Generally hypercellular with plasmacytosis
Serous degeneration, elevated reticulin
May have opportunistic infection, even without granulomas (scattered macrophages are enough to get special stains)
Lymphocytic aggregates, both paratrabecular and non-paratrabecular
Patients may develop a myelodysplastic picture

SPLEEN
- Normally 150 g, ~12 cm long
- Functions: filtration, immune, source of lymphoreticular or hematopoietic cells, storage for platelets
- In an unstimulated spleen, see two layers of lymphocytes around central arterioles: central T-zone area (white pulp) and peripheral marginal zone (B and T cells); when stimulated, germinal centers form: get three layers—germinal center, mantle zone, and marginal zone

CONGENITAL ANOMALIES
- Complete absence (rare)
- Abnormal lobulation
- Accessory spleens—usually near hilum
- Hyposplenia
- Polysplenia

HYPERSPLENISM
- Seen in minority of patients with splenic enlargement
- Features:
  - Enlarged spleen (usually secondary to another problem)
  - Sequestration/loss of circulating RBCs, platelets, white blood cells (WBCs), or some combination
  - Correction following splenectomy

Disorders of White Pulp

REACTIVE FOLLICULAR HYPERPLASIA
- Common among children and adolescents
- Acute infections, idiopathic thrombocytopenic purpura (ITP), rheumatoid arthritis, acquired hemolytic anemia, chronic hemodialysis, Castleman's disease

REACTIVE NONFOLLICULAR LYMPHOID HYPERPLASIA
- Expansion of white pulp without formation of germinal centers
- Viral infections, graft rejection, angioimmunoblastic lymphadenopathy with dysproteinemia (AILD)

CHRONIC LYMPHOCYTIC LEUKEMIA
- Only leukemia that consistently and selectively involves the white pulp—irregular involvement

MALIGNANT LYMPHOMAS
- Cannot distinguish nodular from diffuse in the spleen
- Small cleaved, mixed small cleaved and large, and small noncleaved generally remain confined to white pulp
- Small lymphocytic, mantle cell, marginal zone cell, large cell, Hodgkin's, and cutaneous T-cell lymphoma (CTCL) will bleed out into the red pulp as well

Disorders of the Red Pulp

CONGESTION (1–5 kg)
- Hemolytic anemias
- Gamna-Gandy bodies: organized, fibrosed old hemorrhages with hemosiderin and calcium

INFECTION
- Infectious mononucleosis, acute septic splenitis

LEUKEMIAS
- Often diffusely infiltrate the red pulp, making the white pulp barely discernible
- Chronic myelogenous leukemia (CML): polymorphous infiltrate with eosinophilic myelocytes
- Myeloid metaplasia (agnogenic or secondary): all three cell lines present for agnogenic, secondary may be limited to a single cell line
- Hairy cell leukemia (see later under Other Leukemias)

SYSTEMIC MASTOCYTOSIS
- Often relatively tight clusters of cells with clear cytoplasm and surrounded by fibrosis

HISTIOCYTIC PROLIFERATIONS
- Granulomatous inflammation, Gaucher's disease, Langerhans' cell histiocytosis, malignant histiocytosis

Ceroid histiocytosis: accumulation of foamy macrophages laden with waxy material, predominantly sphingomyelin; seen most commonly in ITP and CML

Other Non-neoplastic Conditions
- Inflammatory pseudotumor: spindle cell proliferation infiltrated by plasma cells, lymphocytes, eosinophils, and histiocytes; may be symptomatic
- Hyaline perisplenitis: collagenous thickening of capsule (sugar coating); no symptoms or sequelae
- Spontaneous rupture: always caused by pathology (mononucleosis, malaria, typhoid fever, CML, acute splenitis); can result in seeding of peritoneal cavity with spleens (splenosis)
- Peliosis: widespread, blood-filled cystic spaces, sometimes occurring independently of peliosis hepatis; usually patients with chronic wasting diseases (TB, carcinoma)

Tumors
- Benign: hemangiomas, lymphangiomas, splenic hamartoma (nodular lesion composed exclusively of red pulp elements), lipomas, fibromas, osteomas, chondromas
- Malignant: hemangiosarcomas

THYMUS
Normal
- Embryologically derived from the 3rd and occasionally 4th pair of pharyngeal pouches
- Thymus weighs 10–35 g at birth, grows to maximum size at puberty (20–50 g), and then atrophies with replacement by fibrofatty tissue
- Cortical and medullary regions; epithelial cells and lymphocytes (mostly T [medullary are mature, cortical are immature], some B)
- Hassall's corpuscles: concentric aggregates of keratin surrounded by keratinized epithelial cells; found in the medulla
- Parathyroids (arise from same pouches) may become entrapped in the thymus

Non-neoplastic Lesions

CONGENITAL THYMIC HYPOPLASIA
- Seen in a variety of congenital immunodeficiency syndromes, including reticular dysgenesis, severe combined immunodeficiency disease, ataxia-telangiectasia, DiGeorge syndrome
- Thymus most commonly completely absent; a fibrous mass may be present in its place

ACQUIRED THYMIC HYPOPLASIA
- Can occur in the young following severe stress, irradiation, chronic malnutrition, or associated with cytotoxic drugs or glucocorticoids

THYMIC HYPERPLASIA
- Difficult to evaluate by weight; therefore, use presence of lymphoid follicles within the thymus (thymic follicular hyperplasia) as indicator of hyperplasia
- Germinal centers are located primarily in the medulla
- Most frequently encountered in myasthenia gravis (MG, seen in 85% of patients with MG, more common in younger)

Tumors

THYMOMA
- Neoplasm of thymic epithelial cells; most common tumor of the anterior mediastinum
- Mean age = 50 yr; incidence increases with age
- Associated with myasthenia gravis, hematologic cytopenias, hypogammaglobulinemia, collagen vascular diseases

Because the thymus can be present in atypical locations (e.g., neck), the thymomas can also be present
Most (90%) are benign
Lobulated, weakly encapsulated (80%), gray-yellow-tan
Soft to firm; may have hemorrhages; cysts common
May be lymphocyte rich or lymphocyte poor
Epithelial component may be normal looking with poorly defined cell borders or may be oval to spindled
Spindled pattern is more commonly associated with red cell aplasia; it is usually *not* associated with myasthenia gravis
Tumor cells are keratin, Leu–7, and CEA positive

MALIGNANT THYMOMA (TYPE I)
10% of thymomas
Histologically identical to benign thymoma but with invasion beyond the capsule or with lymphatic or hematogenous spread

THYMIC CARCINOMA (TYPE II MALIGNANT THYMOMA)
Thymic epithelial cells are cytologically malignant

RED CELL PATHOLOGY

ERYTHROPOIETIN
Stimulates red cell commitment (serum level: 0.01 nM)
Glycoprotein (18.4 kD protein plus 18 kD sugars)
Believed to originate in kidney—may be enzyme
Responds to tissue oxygen tension, dependent on blood flow, hemoglobin (Hg) concentration, Hg saturation
Occasionally excessively produced in renal cell carcinoma, cerebellar hemangioblastomas, hepatic carcinomas, adrenal adenomas, and uterine leiomyomas

HEMOGLOBINS
α-globins: 2/chromosome 16 (141 amino acids); also, ζ-gene
$\beta, \delta, ^A\gamma, ^A\gamma^G\gamma, \gamma$-globins: chromosome 11 (146 amino acids); γ: Ala vs. Gly at amino acid 136
Embryonic: ε_4 (Gower 1); $\zeta_2\varepsilon_2$ (Portland); $\alpha_2\varepsilon_2$ (Gower 2)
Fetal: 75% HgF ($\alpha_2\gamma_2$), 25% HgA ($\alpha_2\beta_2$)
Adults: 96% HgA($\alpha_2\beta_2$), 3% HgA$_2$($\alpha_2\delta_2$), 1% HgF($\alpha_2\gamma_2$)

ANEMIAS

Blood Loss

ACUTE
Initially, there is no change in the hematocrit
Maximum hemodilution occurs at 48–72 hr
Plasma proteins replaced more quickly, then red cells
When blood loss is internal, iron can be reclaimed
Reticulocyte count can reach 10–15% within 1 wk

CHRONIC
Anemia occurs when the rate of blood loss exceeds regenerative capacity, which is usually limited by availability of *iron*
Results in iron deficiency anemia (see later)

Increased Hemolysis

Premature destruction of RBCs in the body, with retention of iron and expansion of marrow erythron, usually with increased number of circulating reticulocytes
Manifestations: hemoglobinemia, methemalbuminemia, jaundice, hemoglobinuria, hemosiderinuria:
• Hg bound by α2-globulin (haptoglobulin), preventing excretion in urine; cleared by reticuloendothelial system
• Some metabolized, releasing unconjugated (indirect) bilirubin; jaundice
• When haptoglobulin depleted, free Hg oxidized to metHg and both excreted in urine; red brown
• If renal excretion capacity exceeded, metHg binds to albumin: methemalbuminemia: blood red-brown
• Metabolization of some by renal tubular cells results in hemosiderosis with shedding of these cells in urine
Marrow: increased number of normoblasts, with pressure atrophy of the inner cortical bone and new bone formation on the outside, esp. in the ribs and facial bones
Chronicity: pigment gallstones, hemosiderosis, extramedullary hematopoiesis

HEMOGLOBINOPATHIES

SICKLE CELL ANEMIA
Mutation of Glu to Val at amino acid 6 of beta chain
8% of black Americans are carriers (heterozygous) = sickle cell trait (40% Hg is HgS): protection against malaria
Deoxy-HgS "crystallizes," leading to hemolysis (anemia) and to obstruction of small vessels (vaso-occlusive crisis)
Sickling is initially reversible, but with repeated episodes, membrane damage occurs, resulting in irreversible sickling
HgSC and HgSD have sickle cell anemia, but less severe
Not apparent at birth: HgF persists 1–2 yr
Spleen: initially enlarged, then focal scarring with calcium and hemosiderin deposits (Gamna-Gandy bodies); get functional autosplenectomy: predisposes to *Salmonella* (osteomyelitis), *Streptococcus pneumoniae, Haemophilus influenza* infections
Prenatal diagnosis possible by restriction fragment length polymorphism (RFLP) using *Mst*II

HEMOGLOBIN C DISEASE
Mutation of Glu to Lys at amino acid 6 of beta chain
HbC only one fourth as prevalent as HbS
Splenomegaly, mild anemia
Target cells common

THALASSEMIA
Decreased synthesis of α or β chains, leading to excess of other chain; chain excess contributes to pathology
$\alpha\alpha/\alpha$- is silent carrier
$\alpha\alpha/$-- or α-/α- is alpha thalassemia minor (trait): hypochromic microcytic; same seen in beta thalassemia minor (β^0/β or β^+/β)
Beta thalassemia minor accompanied by increased HgA$_2$ and HgF
Complete absence of alpha (HgBarts—see later) is fatal
Most beta thalassemias caused by point mutations, most commonly leading to aberrant splicing; most alpha thalassemias caused by gene deletions
Beta thalassemia major (complete absence [β^0] or reduced synthesis [β^+] genes) results in decreased production but also active hemolysis because excess alpha precipitates as Heinz bodies, causing 70–85% of precursor cells to be destroyed in the marrow (ineffective erythropoiesis)

OTHER HEMOGLOBINS
HgD Los Angeles: mutation of Glu 121 to Gln in beta chain
HgM: His to Tyr at iron binding site of alpha or beta chain
Iron stabilized in ferric state—cannot bind oxygen
HgH (β_4): see in --/-α thalassemia major, unstable, precipitates forming inclusions
HgBarts (γ_4): results in hydrops fetalis

UNSTABLE HEMOGLOBINS
Riverdale-Bronx: Gly to Arg at residue 6 of beta chain
Gun Hill: deletion of 5 amino acids from beta chain

OTHER HEREDITARY HEMOLYTIC DISORDERS
HEREDITARY SPHEROCYTOSIS
Autosomal dominant; 1/4,500; 20% caused by new mutations
Red cells spheroidal in shape—more fragile
Manifests at birth or later; severe in infants; children/adults may compensate
Splenic enlargement is characteristic (500–1,000 g)
Cholelithiasis occurs in 40–50%
Defect in spectrin—many different types
Hemolytic crisis: fever, nausea, vomiting, jaundice
Aplastic crisis: usually triggered by parvovirus; worse anemia, loss of reticulocytes
Splenectomy prevents destruction—"curative"

HEREDITARY ELLIPTOCYTOSIS (OVALOCYTOSIS)
Autosomal dominant; 1/4,000–5,000
Anemic and non-anemic varieties exist; most patients have only mild anemia

HEREDITARY STOMATOCYTOSIS
RBCs have a slitlike central zone of pallor on wet smears
Autosomal dominant
Red cells have an increased permeability to sodium and potassium, and increased active transport of these ions
• Overhydrated form (hydrocytosis):
   Stomatocytes seen even on dried smears
   Excess of ions and water; decreased MCHC
   Increased osmotic fragility
   Absence of band 7.2b (stomatin) from RBC membranes
• Dehydrated form (desiccytosis):
   Dried smears show target cells rather than stomatocytes
   Increased mean corpuscular hemoglobin concentration
   Decreased osmotic fragility

G-6-PD DEFICIENCY
Glutathione (GSH) prevents injury by exogenous oxidants
Glucose-6-P-dehydrogenase (G-6-PD; X-linked) is enzyme in hexose monophosphate shunt that produces GSH
Many G-6-PD variants; two clinically significant
• G-6-PD A⁻: mutant enzyme has shorter life than RBC
   Hemolytic crisis affects older cells
   Present in 10% of American blacks
• G-6-PD Mediterranean: enzyme has lower activity throughout life—hemolytic crisis can be disastrous
Defect protects against malaria
Antimalarials (e.g., primaquine, quinacrine) can trigger hemolytic crisis
Hg oxidizes to metHg and precipitates in the cytoplasm, clumps (Heinz bodies) attach to cell membrane and increase osmotic fragility—Heinz bodies removed in spleen, decreasing size of RBCs and tendency to form spherocytes

OTHER ENZYME DEFICIENCIES
Other pentose phosphate shunt enzymes
Glycolytic enzymes (e.g., pyruvate kinase)

ACQUIRED HEMOLYTIC DISORDERS
PAROXYSMAL NOCTURNAL HEMOGLOBINURIA (PNH)
Chronic intravascular hemolysis, worse at night in 25%
Abnormal sensitivity of RBCs to complement-mediated lysis because of a deficiency of the membrane glycoprotein decay accelerating factor (DAF)
Similar defect seen in platelets and granulocytes; defect is in a multipotent stem cell
Significant risk of progression to leukemia

AUTOIMMUNE HEMOLYTIC ANEMIAS (AHA)
Warm Antibody AHA:
• Polyclonal IgG, does not fix complement, active at 37°C
• Primary (60%) or secondary to lymphoma, neoplasm, drugs, SLE
• RBCs sequestered in spleen, leading to splenomegaly
• Hemolysis is extravascular, usually in the spleen
Cold Agglutinin AHA:
• Monoclonal IgM, fixes complement, agglutinates in cooler parts of body
• Acute (Ab titers rise following mycoplasma pneumonia or mononucleosis) or chronic (lymphoma)
• RBCs sequestered in liver
• Hemolysis is extravascular, usually in spleen
Cold Hemolysin AHA:
• AKA: paroxysmal cold hemoglobinuria (PCH)
• Massive intravascular hemolysis, complement dependent, following exposure to cold
• IgG autoantibodies against P-blood group antigens; bind complement at low temperatures
• Occurs following infections (mycoplasma, measles, mumps)

MECHANICAL HEMOLYSIS (MICROANGIOPATHIC)
Schizocytes: sheared RBCs (helmet cells, burr cells)
• Prosthetic cardiac ball valves
• Advanced atherosclerosis
• Small vessel thrombi—diffuse intravascular coagulation (DIC)
• Hemolytic uremic syndrome
• Malignant hypertension
• Thrombocytic thrombocytopenic purpura (TTP)
• Ulcerative colitis

ISOANTIBODY ASSOCIATED
Transfusion mismatch; complement-mediated destruction

DRUG INDUCED, INFECTIONS, HYPERSPLENISM

Diminished Erythropoiesis

NUTRITIONAL DEFICIENCY
PERNICIOUS ANEMIA (MEGALOBLASTIC ANEMIA)
B₁₂ malabsorption caused by genetic defect (juvenile) or chronic atrophic gastritis with loss of parietal cells, resulting in decreased intrinsic factor activity
Three autoantibodies associated with disease:
• Blocks binding of IF to B₁₂ (75% patients)
• Binds to IF and IF-B₁₂ complex (50%)
• Binds to parietal cell brush border (85–90%)
Marrow: nests of darkly staining megaloblasts (immature nuclei, mature cytoplasm, larger than erythroblasts)

Myelin degeneration in dorsal and lateral tracts of spinal cord

In acquired form, also see atrophic glossitis and atrophic gastritis with intestinal metaplasia

In folate deficiency, get all of above changes except CNS

IRON (Fe) DEFICIENCY

Most common nutritional disorder in the world

Normal total body iron stores: male = 3.5 g, female = 2.5 g

Normally, 80% of total body Fe functional, 80% of that in Hg 20% in storage form as ferritin (protein-iron complex) or hemosiderin within reticuloendothelial cells and in the liver

Iron is transported as ferritin, bound to transferrin (76 kD divalent for Fe), which is normally one third saturated

Iron reserves depleted before serum levels drop

Iron deficiency leads to hypochromic microcytic anemia

Bone marrow:
- Increased erythropoietic activity
- Sideroblasts and stainable iron absent

Low iron levels also depletes iron from enzymes, resulting in oxidation of membrane proteins and decreased plasticity of the RBCs leading to *poikilocytosis*

Plummer Vinson syndrome: microcytic hypochromic anemia, atrophic glossitis, esophageal webs

May take months to see response from iron supplements

INTESTINAL MALABSORPTION

BONE MARROW FAILURE (APLASTIC ANEMIA)

Normochromic, normocytic anemia, usually with neutropenia and thrombocytopenia

Pure red cell aplasia rarely seen, although some association exists with thymoma

Marrow is hypocellular; replaced by fat and fibrous stroma

50% of cases are idiopathic

Other causes: Fanconi's anemia (autosomal recessive; associated findings: renal hypoplasia, absent or hypoplastic thumbs or radii, hyperpigmentation of skin, microcephaly), whole body irradiation, dose-related or idiosyncratic drug reactions, postinfectious

Can also see in tumors metastatic to the marrow (myelophthisic anemia), diffuse liver disease, chronic renal failure, endocrine disorders

POLYCYTHEMIA

ERYTHROCYTOSIS

Relative polycythemia caused by hemoconcentration

Total red cell mass is not increased

Seen in dehydration, vomiting, burns, electrolyte imbalance, and "stress polycythemia" (Gaisböcks syndrome)

POLYCYTHEMIA VERA

Absolute increase in red cell mass (usually accompanied by increase in white cell count, and esp. platelet count) with a low erythropoietin level

Etiology appears to be related to increased sensitivity of myeloid stem cells to erythropoietin

Male > female, 40–60 yr old, whites > blacks

Marrow usually hypercellular, but not always

Reticulin increased in areas of megakaryocyte cellularity

Hyperviscosity of blood often leads to infarction of, most commonly, heart, spleen, kidney

20% develop peptic ulcers

30% die from thrombosis (usually brain), 10–15% from hemorrhage (often GI), 2% from acute myeloblastic leukemia (AML)—15% if irradiated

15–20% of long-term survivors (>10 yr) undergo transition to myeloid metaplasia with myelofibrosis

Associated with del20q11

SECONDARY POLYCYTHEMIA

Usually normal white cell and platelet counts

Caused by increased production of erythropoietin

APPROPRIATE

High altitude living

Carboxyhemoglobin

Chronic obstructive or other pulmonary disease

Right-to-left circulatory shunts (septal defects)

Low-output cardiac failure

Hemoglobinopathies (high oxygen affinity)

INAPPROPRIATE

Erythropoietin-secreting malignancies: renal cell carcinoma, cerebellar hemangioblastoma, hepatoma, adrenal adenoma, uterine leiomyoma

Hydronephrosis and renal cysts

ERYTHROLEUKEMIA

AKA: DiGuglielmo's syndrome, erythromyeloblastic leukemia

See later (M6 AML)

Marked anemia, leukopenia

If survive initial phase, gradual transition to immature myeloblastic leukemia

Course: months to 2 yr, ending in death

LYMPH NODE PATHOLOGY

Non-Inflammatory

INCLUSIONS/LESIONS:

Nevus cells: in capsule, usually axillary nodes

Thyroid follicles: marginal sinus of midcervical node; usually represent metastatic papillary carcinoma

Ectopic thymus: supraclavicular LNs—differential diagnosis is from metastatic epidermoid carcinoma

Salivary gland tissue: common in high cervical nodes; if becomes neoplastic, usually get Warthin's tumor

Müllerian epithelium: endosalpingiosis, endometriosis; decidual reaction may simulate carcinoma

Breast tissue: normal mammary lobules in axillary LN

Adipose metaplasia: up to 10 cm, external iliac and obturator groups most common

Silicone lymphadenopathy: this is a side effect of breast reconstruction, nonbirefringent material in sinuses, giant cells

Proteinaceous lymphadenopathy: like amyloid, but it isn't

Hyaline material: esp. aortoiliac region, may become calcified, no clinical significance

Infarction: painful swelling, necrosis, perinodal inflammation and granulation tissue

Vasculitis: systemic vasculitides, AILD

Hemangioma/lymphangioma: usually represent extension from primary soft tissue lesion

Epithelioid hemangioma

METASTATIC TUMORS
Upper cervical: oropharynx, nasopharynx
Midcervical: thyroid, salivary glands, pharynx, larynx
Supraclavicular: lung, breast (left: stomach, pancreas, prostate, testis)
Axillary nodes: breast, melanoma, lung
Inguinal: external genital organs, melanoma of legs—rarely internal pelvic organs or testis

Acute Lymphadenitis

Focal: usually direct drainage of infected areas
Generalized: viral, bacteremic, exotoxic diseases
Nodes: swollen, gray-red, engorged; large germinal centers with many mitoses; lymphocytes may penetrate capsule
Histiocytes with particulate debris
When pyogenic in origin, may see necrosis
Neutrophils frequently present

Chronic Lymphadenitis

FOLLICULAR HYPERPLASIA
B cells stimulated
Large germinal centers with "blasts" bulging against well-demarcated mantle zone—follicles expand at expense of mantle zone
Plasma cells, histiocytes, rare neutrophils in paracortex
Follicles vary in size and shape (vs. lymphoma)

NONSPECIFIC REACTIVE
May be limited to cortex or throughout
Follicles usually remain polarized; may coalesce
More florid in children

TOXOPLASMOSIS
AKA: Piringer-Kuchinka's syndrome
Typically posterior cervical nodes, younger woman
Triad (not all three always present):
• Follicular hyperplasia, numerous mitoses, nuclear debris
• Small, epithelioid (non–sarcoid-like) granulomas, both within and at periphery of germinal centers—no giant cells
• Monocytoid B-cell distention of marginal/cortical sinuses and paracortex
Rare to find organism: serological testing
Differential diagnosis: lymphocyte predominant Hodgkin's (don't get granulomas)

RHEUMATOID ARTHRITIS OR SJÖGREN'S DISEASE
30–80% show generalized lymphadenopathy
Hyperplasia involves cortex and medulla with intense interfollicular plasmacytosis and numerous Russell bodies
Hyperplasia otherwise unusual in elderly
Identical changes in Sjögren's, Felty's syndromes
Longstanding rheumatoid arthritis (RA) increases risk for lymphoma
Juvenile rheumatoid arthritis: above features plus neutrophils

SYSTEMIC LUPUS ERYTHEMATOSUS
Predominantly cervical adenopathy: cortical follicular hyperplasia with interfollicular plasmacytosis
Often sharply circumscribed areas of paracortical necrosis with none or few neutrophils

NECROTIZING LYMPHADENITIS (KIKUCHI'S)
Most common in Japan and Asian countries
Usually young women, painless cervical lymphadenopathy
Focal, well-circumscribed, paracortical necrotizing lesions
Scattered fibrin deposits
Collections of large mononuclear cells
Scant numbers of neutrophils and plasma cells
Electron microscopy (EM): tubuloreticular inclusions, intracytoplasmic rodlets

CAT-SCRATCH DISEASE
Primary cutaneous lesion with enlarged regional LNs
Early: follicular hyperplasia, histiocytic proliferation
Intermediate: granulomatous changes
Late: large abscesses with central stellate necrosis, neutrophils, and palisading histiocytes

LYMPHOGRANULOMA VENEREUM
Sexually transmitted: *Chlamydia*
Tiny necrotic foci; enlarge to form large stellate abscesses
Langhans' giant cells, fibroblasts, fistula tracts common

KIMURA'S DISEASE
Follicular hyperplasia, interfollicular eosinophilia, proliferation of thin walled vessels
LN changes accompany similar lesions in soft tissues

SYPHILIS
Generalized lymphadenopathy in secondary, localized in primary and tertiary
Primary: capsular and pericapsular inflammation, fibrosis, diffuse plasma cell infiltrate, proliferation of blood vessels with endothelial swelling and inflammation, epithelioid histiocyte clusters, occasional sarcoid-like granulomas
Secondary: florid follicular hyperplasia, large clusters of epithelioid histiocytes, sarcoid-like granulomas
Look for spirochetes in wall of blood vessels

CASTLEMAN'S DISEASE
AKA: giant LN hyperplasia, LN hamartoma, angiofollicular mediastinal LN hyperplasia, follicular lymphoreticuloma
Male = female; 8–70 yr old
Two major histological types:
• Hyaline vascular (angiofollicular)
　Large follicles with vascular proliferation
　Hyalinization in center of follicles
　Onion-skin layering of lymphocytes at follicle periphery
　Prominent interfollicular stroma, plasma cells
　Lymphoid subtype: expansion of mantle zone with small regressed germinal centers
　Polyclonal Ig production (vs. lymphoma)
• Plasma cell type
　Diffuse interfollicular plasma cell proliferation
　Deposition of amorphous acidophilic material in follicles (probably fibrin and Ig)
Two major clinical presentations:
• Solitary form
　Mass, usually mediastinal; also neck, lung, axilla, mesentery, retroperitoneum, extremities
　Round, well circumscribed, up to 15 cm
　90% hyaline vascular type (asymptomatic)
　10% plasma cell type (fever, anemia, elevated erythrocyte sedimentation rate [ESR] and Ig)
　Treatment: surgical excision
• Multicentric (systemic) form
　Patients tend to be older
　Generalized lymphadenopathy; may involve spleen
　Nearly always plasma cell type
　Poor long-term prognosis
Some association with spindle cell sarcoma development, presumably from vessels

PROGRESSIVELY TRANSFORMED GERMINAL CENTERS
Large (2–3 × normal) centrally located follicles without follicle centers

Indistinct margin with surrounding mantle zone (mantle cells infiltrate into follicles)

May be seen concurrently or as an antecedent to lymphocyte predominant Hodgkin's disease

AIDS-RELATED LYMPHADENOPATHY

Most commonly, see "florid reactive hyperplasia"

"Follicle lysis": collapse of the central portions of the germinal centers with invagination of mantle lymphocytes

May see advanced lymphocyte depletion (regressed germinal centers)

DIFFUSE (PARACORTICAL) HYPERPLASIA

Expansion of T-cell regions with effacement of follicles

Hypertrophy of endothelium—pseudolymphomatous

Seen in drug reactions (Dilantin), following smallpox vaccination, chronic dermatitis, viral infection

POSTVACCINIAL VIRAL LYMPHADENITIS

Usually 1–10 wk postvaccination, usually supraclavicular

Diffuse or nodular paracortical expansion, immunoblast proliferation, vascular proliferation, sinusoidal dilatation, mixed cellular infiltrate (eosinophils, plasma cells, mast cells)

Immunoblasts may simulate Reed-Sternberg cells

INFECTIOUS MONONUCLEOSIS

Variable, nonspecific effacement of nodal architecture with infiltration of the trabeculae, capsule, and perinodal fat by immunoblasts and numerous plasma cells

Distinction from lymphoma: sinusoidal distribution of large lymphoid cells, increase in plasma cells, and vascular proliferation

DERMATOPATHIC LYMPHADENITIS

AKA: Lipomelanosis reticularis of Pautrier

Lymphadenopathy secondary to itching and scratching dermatidities (psoriasis, mycosis fungoides [MF], etc.)

Sometimes no identifiable cutaneous lesion can be found

Pale yellow LNs, often with black periphery (clumps of melanin)

Expansion of the T-dependent paracortical zone by a proliferation of the interdigitating reticulum S-100+ histiocytes with folded nuclei (Langerhans' cells), compressing the follicles against the capsule

SINUS PATTERN

"SINUS HISTIOCYTOSIS"

Seen in nodes draining cancer

Prominence of sinusoids—distended with histiocytes

SINUS HISTIOCYTOSIS WITH MASSIVE LYMPHADENOPATHY

AKA: Rosai-Dorfman disease (1969)

(See Histiocytoses)

LIPOPHAGIC REACTIONS

Accumulation of phagocytosed fat in histiocytes

Many types:

- Mineral oil ingestion: asymptomatic, periportal and mesenteric LNs, common (70% of all patients)
- Whipple's disease: mesenteric nodes; poorly formed granulomas with lipid in the macrophages and PAS+ particles in the cytoplasm; electron microscopy (EM) shows bacilliform bodies within the histiocytes; associated with intestinal malabsorption
- Lymphangiography: lipophagic granulomas may persist for months; neutrophils and then eosinophils common

VASCULAR TRANSFORMATION OF LYMPH NODE SINUSES

Subcapsular and interfollicular sinuses with blood-filled endothelial-lined spaces, variable fibrosis, and extravasated erythrocytes

Secondary to extranodal venous outflow obstruction

Vascular proliferation follows the sinuses (unlike Kaposi's)

PREDOMINANTLY GRANULOMATOUS PATTERN

SARCOIDOSIS

Diagnosis is always one of exclusion; rule out TB, atypical mycobacteria, fungus, leprosy, syphilis, *Leishmania,* brucella, etc.

Black : white = 10–15 : 1 (in U.S.)

Lung (90%), LNs, eyes, skin most commonly affected

Often some degree of anergy—deficient peripheral T-cell response; central T-cell response still seems to work

Erythema nodosum often precedes or accompanies

Functional hypoparathyroidism is the rule

Noncaseating granulomatous inflammation in nodes/skin, with scattered Langhans' giant cells

Necrosis is absent or limited to small central fibrinoid focus

Schaumann bodies, asteroid bodies, and calcium oxalate crystals in cytoplasm of giant cells; none are specific

- Schaumann: round, concentric laminations, with Fe, Ca
- Asteriod: crisscrossing collagen fibers

Kveim test: 60–85% show granulomatous intradermal reaction following inoculation with extract of human spleen involved with sarcoidosis

Etiology unclear—mycobacteria or virus suspected

Two thirds recover with minimal sequelae; 20% have some permanent loss of pulmonary function; 10% will die of cardiac, CNS involvement or progressive pulmonary fibrosis

TUBERCULOSIS

Lymph nodes may become adherent to each other: matting, similar to that seen in metastatic carcinoma

Scrofula: matted cervical lymphadenopathy

Scrofuloderma: scrofula forms draining sinus to skin

Small epithelioid granulomas to large caseous masses

Must demonstrate organisms

ATYPICAL MYCOBACTERIOSIS

Typically lateral middle neck nodes of a child

Similar to TB with more of a suppurative component

FUNGAL INFECTIONS

Suppurative or granulomatous

Histoplasmosis: can cause widespread nodal necrosis and marked diffuse hyperplasia of sinus histiocytes

Sporotrichosis: may be suppurative

CHRONIC GRANULOMATOUS DISEASE

Genetically determined enzymatic defect—cannot digest some microorganisms

Granulomas with necrotic, purulent centers

OTHERS/MIXED PATTERN

MUCOCUTANEOUS LYMPH NODE SYNDROME (KAWASAKI'S)

Usually children; more common in Japanese

Fever, cervical lymphadenopathy, pharyngeal and conjunctival inflammation, erythematous skin rashes

Fatalities usually secondary to coronary arteritis

LN: fibrin thrombi in smaller vessels, patchy infarcts

LEPROSY

Large, pale, round histiocytes; no granuloma formation; minimal necrosis

MESENTERIC LYMPHADENITIS

AKA: Masshoff lymphadenitis

Caused by *Yersinia*

Benign, self limited, may simulate appendicitis clinically

LN: capsular thickening and edema, immunoblasts, plasma cells in cortical/paracortical region, germinal centers

ANGIOIMMUNOBLASTIC LYMPHADENOPATHY WITH DYSPROTEINEMIA (AILD)

Polyclonal proliferation of immunoblasts and plasma cells
Adults and elderly—fever, anemia, polyclonal hyper-Ig
27% occur after drug administration, particularly penicillin
Systemic (spleen, liver, LNs, bone marrow . . .)
LN: partial obliteration of nodal architecture by eosinophils, plasma cells, immunoblasts, some giant cells and proliferation of postcapillary venules, with amorphous eosinophilic interstitial deposits of a PAS+ material (probably cellular debris); no germinal centers
Bone marrow (BM): involved in 50–70%; usually focal, may be diffuse; increased reticulin in involved areas
Treatment: steroids ± combination chemotherapy
75% of patients die; ability to achieve remission single most important prognostic factor
Appearance of clones of tightly packed immunoblasts is bad sign—progress to immunoblastic sarcoma (usually T cell) and death

HODGKIN'S LYMPHOMAS

General

40% of all lymphomas in the U.S. (much less in Orient)
Age: major peak in 20s, minor in 60s
Male preponderance (especially in 5–11 yr olds) except for nodular sclerosing
Generally starts with involvement of a single node or group of contiguous nodes (most commonly cervical and/or supraclavicular), rather than generalized lymphadenopathy
Fever, night sweats, weight loss common (alters stage)
Patients have predisposition to opportunistic infections
Microscopic typing should be done *before* treatment; necrosis, fibrosis, cellular changes alter histologic appearance
May see only focal involvement of a LN early—don't type for this or only extranodal involvement unless NS type
Noncaseating granulomas may be seen in involved and uninvolved nodes and organs (10%)
Vascular invasion present in 6–14%
Skin, GI, CNS, Waldeyer's ring are rarely involved; if they are, probably a non-Hodgkin's lymphoma (NHL)
Increased incidence in HIV, NHL, familial
Unusual in setting of natural immune deficiency or suppression
Almost never see leukemic transformation
When spleen involved (40%), usually exclusively white pulp; multiple randomly distributed nodules 1–20 mm diameter
Treatment: radiation for Stage I/II or chemotherapy + x-ray therapy (XRT) for Stage III/IV

REED-STERNBERG (R-S) GIANT CELL

Common feature of all Hodgkin's lymphomas
Classically binucleate or bilobed central nucleus with large acidophilic central nucleoli surrounded by clear halo
Variants: mononuclear (Hodgkin's cell), mummified cell, lacunar cell, L/H cell
Requirement of Reed-Sternberg cell for initial diagnosis is "absolute" (less strict for lymphocyte predominant [LP] Hodgkin's or recurrent disease)

Classic Reed-Sternberg cell:
 +: CD15 (Leu-M1), CD30: (Ki-1), CD25 (IL-2R)
 −: CD45 (LCA), pan-B, S-100, keratin, EMA
40% T-cell, 20% B-cell, 40% neither
Rearrangements of immunoglobulin genes and of T-cell receptor genes have been variably reported

Spread

Generally see a well-behaved spread of disease through contiguous LN groups, (especially NS and LP); <5% show noncontiguous spread
May have direct extension into perinodal tissue
85% of Stage I/II disease are above diaphragm
Spleen: if >400 g, almost always positive
Liver: if positive, spleen and retroperitoneal LNs positive

Staging: (Ann Arbor System)

I: Single LN region
 I_E: Single extralymphatic organ or site
II: Two or more LN regions on same side of diaphragm
 II_E: Localized extralymphatic site and LN on same side
III: LN regions on both sides of diaphragm
 III_E: III plus involvement of extralymphatic site
 III_S: III plus splenic involvement
 III_{ES}: III plus extralymphatic site and spleen
IV: Diffuse or disseminated involvement of one or more extralymphatic organs, ± LN involvement
 A: Asymptomatic
 B: With fever, sweats, weight loss (>10% body weight) in 6 months preceding diagnosis
 Liver:
 • "indicative": Reed–Sternberg (R-S) variants in proper milieu
 • "suggestive": atypical histiocytes or reticular cells
 BM: "strongly suggestive": focal/diffuse fibrosis in proper milieu

Prognosis

• Clinical stage
• Pathologic stage:
 • Extranodal involvement bad (esp. if distant rather than by direct spread)
 • Degree of splenic involvement: ≥5 nodules poor prognosis
 • Bulky disease unfavorable (mediastinal or abdominal)
• Age: >50 yr unfavorable
• Sex and race: black males have worse prognosis than white females
• Microscopic type: LP and NS best, mixed cellularity (MC) intermediate, lymphocyte depleted (LD) worst (less important with current treatment protocols)
When recurs within radiation portal, frequently has altered histology: more malignant cells and fibrosis; original histology present outside radiation portal
70–90% advanced stage go into complete remission; one third relapse, one third of which are salvageable: net 75% cure rate
Increased risk of developing acute nonlymphocytic leukemia (0.5–2%/yr; cumulative risk: 3.3–10%); NHL (4–5% at 10 yr), esp. Burkitt's-like lymphoma; solid tumors in radiation field (13%/10 yr)
Other risks: pneumococcal sepsis, azospermia (100%), amenorrhea, hypothyroidism (6–25%)

Microscopic Types (Rye Classification)

NODULAR SCLEROSIS (60%)

Most common type in U.S. by far
Distinct clinically and histologically from the other types

Typically, neck or mediastinum of young female; mediastinal involvement is almost always present

Usually presents in Stage I or II; 11 yr median Stage I survival

Broad, well-organized (birefringent) collagen bands separating lymphoid tissue into well-defined nodules

Fibrosis often vasculocentric

Lacunar cell: large (40–50 μm) cells with abundant, clear cytoplasm (artifactual contraction from formalin fixation) and multiple convoluted nuclei with nucleoli smaller than classic R-S cell

Can see microabscesses with areas of necrosis surrounded by R-S variants; mummified cells also seen

Cell types present can vary widely, and can include clumps of foamy macrophages, neutrophils, mast cells, etc.

EM: collagen fibers and myofibroblasts

Three subtypes based on cellularity of nodules: LP, MC, LD, with correspondingly increasing numbers of classic R-S cells, decreasing lymphocytes, lacunar cells, and prognosis

Differential diagnosis: peripheral T-cell lymphoma with sclerosis, agnogenic myeloid metaplasia (osteosclerosis with extramedullary hematopoiesis), nasopharyngeal carcinoma

OBLITERATIVE TOTAL SCLEROSIS

Obliterative nonbirefringent fibrosis of nodules with sparse residual cells (usually lacunar cells)

CELLULAR PHASE

Minimal to no sclerosis but all other components present

This histology common in relapses

Traditionally, worse survival than when collagen present

A nodular cellular variant exists

SYNCYTIAL VARIANT

Sheets and cohesive clusters of lacunar variants; can simulate carcinoma

LYMPHOCYTE PREDOMINANT (5%)

Typically younger patient; usually presents in Stage I

Usually high cervical nodes in young male (<35 yr old)

Inguinal LN 2nd most common site (1st for nodular type)

Almost never involves spleen, liver, BM, mediastinum

Usually remains in isolated site unless progresses to another form of Hodgkin's disease (HD) (62% progress)

Other LNs may show progressive transformation of the germinal centers

Lymphocytic and histiocytic forms

Diffuse and nodular forms; LN architecture effaced

Eosinophils, plasma cells, and fibrosis scanty or absent

Very few Reed-Sternberg cells; see many of the "L/H" (popcorn) variant, with folded multilobed nucleus; too many R-S cells suggest transition to mixed cellularity

Malignant cells are B cells (really is a follicular B-cell lymphoma): monoclonal Ig, LCA+, CD20+, CD30−, CD15−

Prognosis increases with abundance of lymphocytes and presence of pseudonodules

Differential diagnosis: Well-differentiated lymphocytic lymphoma, mononucleosis, malignant melanoma, progressive transformation of germinal centers

MIXED CELLULARITY (30%)

Generally middle aged patient, usually presents as Stage II or III

Median survival 5 yr, even for Stage I

This category used by some to include all types that don't fit neatly into LP, NS, or LD, including partial node involvement

Often represents disease in transition between LP and LD

Large numbers of eosinophils, plasma cells, and atypical mononuclear cells admixed with classic Reed-Sternberg cells (which tend to be numerous; may be CD15−)

Differential diagnosis: Lennert's lymphoma (diffuse mixed T-cell ML with excessive histiocytes)

INTERFOLLICULAR HODGKIN'S DISEASE

Frequently paracortical

Usually on a background of florid reactive follicular hyperplasia

"WITH EPITHELIOID HISTIOCYTES"

Common

Scattered cohesive clusters of histiocytes to frank granulomas

LYMPHOCYTE DEPLETED (5%)

Generally older individuals, usually men; extremely rare in children

Present as febrile illness with pancytopenia, hepatomegaly, and no peripheral lymphadenopathy

Usually presents in Stage IV

Predominance of R-S cells, disorderly fibrosis, lymphocyte depletion, and absence of R-S variants (lacunar cells)

Necrosis more common than in other types

Highest incidence of vascular invasion

Differential diagnosis: large cell NHL, MF

"DIFFUSE FIBROSIS TYPE"

Decreasing number of cells secondary to heavy deposition of disordered, nonbirefringent collagen

>90% have marrow involvement

Median survival = 39 months

"RETICULAR" TYPE

Numerous diagnostic Reed-Sternberg cells

Sarcomatous and nonsarcomatous subtypes, based on appearance of R-S cells

<25% have BM involvement

Median survival = 10 months

MALIGNANT NON-HODGKIN'S LYMPHOMAS

General

Normal maturation of follicular center B cells to immunoblast proceeds through 1) small cleaved cell, 2) large cleaved cell, 3) small noncleaved cell, 4) large noncleaved cell

Nucleoli normally present in noncleaved cells

Staging essentially same as for Hodgkin's lymphomas

Marrow involvement may be diffuse, interstitial, focal paratrabecular, or focal nonparatrabecular

In contrast to epithelial tumors, hematopoietic tumors tend to have single, nonrandom alterations and/or balanced translocations

NON-HODGKIN'S LYMPHOMAS (VS. HODGKIN'S)

Multiple distinct diseases

Show more variable, noncontiguous spread

Involve peripheral LNs and mesenteric LNs

Frequently present in extranodal sites

Tend to arise from B cells (most common) or prethymic or thymic T cells

CHILDHOOD LYMPHOMAS
Lymphoblastic lymphoma and Burkitt's are almost exclusively childhood lymphomas

Diffuse large cell and diffuse large cell immunoblastic lymphomas occur in both children and adults

Classifications

RAPPAPORT CLASSIFICATION (1966)
First popularly used system

Divided growth patterns into nodular and diffuse; cell types into well differentiated, poorly differentiated (cleaved follicular center cells), histiocytic (large cells), and undifferentiated (round; between lymphocytic and histiocytic)

LUKES-COLLINS CLASSIFICATION (1973)
Based on proposed cell of origin; follicular center cells, cleaved or uncleaved; immunoblasts; B or T cells

KIEL CLASSIFICATION (1973)
Similar to Lukes-Collins

WORKING FORMULATION FOR CLINICAL USE (1982)
Intended to establish a common language of communication between pathologists and clinicians, rather than to represent specific disease entities

An individual patient can progress from one histologic type to another
- Low grade: small lymphocytic, follicular small cleaved, follicular mixed
- Intermediate grade: follicular large cell, intermediate cell, diffuse small, mixed, or large cell
- High grade: immunoblastic, lymphoblastic, small non-cleaved

CURRENT
Monoclonal antibodies and gene rearrangement studies have shown that patterns formerly thought to represent different diseases are actually part of the same process

New classification scheme is emerging based on immunophenotype and genotype of the malignant cells

This outline uses a modified version of the Working Formulation, incorporating new information from immunophenotyping

Clinical Grades

CLINICALLY LOW-GRADE LESIONS
Indolent clinical course despite disseminated disease

Long survival with or without aggressive therapy

May be controlled by therapy, almost never cured

Nondestructive growth, well differentiated cytologically

CLINICALLY HIGH-GRADE LESIONS
Aggressive course: untreated, death in 1–2 yr

Aggressive therapy can induce complete remission ("cure") in up to 50%

Destructive growth pattern, cellular atypia

Autonomous, will grow in culture, invade privileged sites

Staging
Same as for Hodgkin's Disease

Overview by Immunophenotype

	B Cell CD19/ CD20	T Cell				
		CD5	CD43	CD23	CD10	bcl
Small lymphocytic	+	+	+	+	–	-
Follicular	+	–	–	+/–	+	2
Mantle cell	+	+	+	–	+/–	1
Marginal zone	+	–	+/–	–	–	-
Burkitt's	+	–	–	–	+	-

Follicular Lymphomas

In the Working Formulation, the predominantly small cleaved and mixed cell types are low grade, and the predominantly large cell type is intermediate grade

Nodular pattern of growth

Arise from follicular center cells: B cells (CD19+, CD20+); CD10+ (most), CD5–

Comprise 50% of adult non-Hodgkin's lymphomas

Usually elderly (median age 60–65); unusual under 40 (especially small cleaved type); uncommon in blacks

Generally present with disseminated involvement (Stage III or IV), except for children (higher frequency of Stage I or II)

Distinction from reactive follicular hyperplasia:
- Effacement of LN architecture
- Filling of sinuses and capsular infiltration
- Numerous follicles with minimal variation in size/shape, evenly distributed at a high density throughout the cortex and medulla of the node
- Poorly defined follicle borders, no polarization, no mantle
- Monomorphic cells within follicles—few mitoses
- Minimal phagocytosis
- Atypical cells in interfollicular regions

Amorphous, eosinophilic material may be present extracellularly in follicles (PAS+, diastase resistant)

Interfollicular regions may show plasmacytosis

Often accompanied by T cells (30–60%), which are usually CD4+

Signet ring lymphoma: variant with prominent intracellular Ig (usually IgG or LCs, vs. IgM of Russell bodies in lymphoplasmacytic malignancies)

Marrow: focal, relatively well-defined lymphoid aggregates, commonly paratrabecular, with increase in reticulin; may be more "mature" than main lesion; follicular center cell lymphomas tend to be paratrabecular, large cell lymphomas frequently are nonparatrabecular

Peripheral blood may be involved (buttock cell), esp. in small cleaved (BM involvement prerequisite)

Splenic involvement in 50%

Hepatic involvement in 50% (portal triads, encroaching on limiting plate without plasma cells; same as for diffuse lymphoma)

>80% have t(14;18)(q32;q21) translocation, juxtaposing the *bcl*-2 oncogene (chromosome 18) next to the Ig heavy chain gene (chromosome 14)

bcl-2 expression absent in reactive follicles, but is expressed in *other* low-grade lymphomas

With time, tendency to progress from small cell (SC) → mixed cell (MC) → large cell (LC)

Rarely, blastic transformation with conversion to leukemic phase—median survival 2 months

WITH OR WITHOUT SCLEROSIS
More common in retroperitoneal and inguinal LNs

Both broad bands and fine reticular pattern

Presence (independent of amount) means better prognosis

WITH OR WITHOUT DIFFUSE AREAS
As disease progresses, becomes diffuse, but one follicle is enough to still call it follicular

No alteration in prognosis, except, perhaps, for large cell

FOLLICULAR, PREDOMINANTLY SMALL CLEAVED
AKA: nodular poorly differentiated lymphocytic lymphoma

40–50% of all follicular lymphomas

Cells slightly larger than normal lymphocytes, with cleaved nuclei with prominent indentations and infoldings
Predominantly small cleaved: <20% large cells in nodules
Mitotic rate low, lower than mixed or predominantly large cell
Marrow: involved in 50–60%
Spleen: evenly distributed, well-defined, similarly sized tumor nodules eccentrically placed in white pulp (B-cell area); essentially every follicle involved
Usually asymptomatic
Tend to relapse when off chemotherapy
Median survival, 7 yr

FOLLICULAR, MIXED SMALL CLEAVED AND LARGE CELL

AKA: nodular mixed cell type lymphoma
40–50% of all follicular lymphomas
Large cells comprise 20–50% of cells in follicles (5–10/high power field [HPF])
Large cells 2–3× diameter of normal lymphocytes; round to oval vesicular nuclei with one to three peripheral basophilic nucleoli
BM involved in 25–50%
Spleen: involvement same as for SC variant
When untreated, labile clinical course, but more rapid mitotic rate makes more responsive to aggressive chemotherapy, and can do better than SC subtype; survival strongly dependent on complete vs. partial response

FOLLICULAR, PREDOMINANTLY LARGE CELL

AKA: nodular histiocytic lymphoma
10–15% of follicular lymphomas
>50% cells in follicles are large cells
BM involvement in <15%
Spleen: when involved, large irregular tumors of unequal size, randomly distributed throughout parenchyma
Cells are poorly mobile and rarely involve peripheral blood
Tend to be localized at time of presentation, but have more aggressive clinical course than other follicular lymphomas
Tend to progress to diffuse growth pattern—similar clinical course to diffuse large cell

Other Low-Grade Lymphomas

SMALL LYMPHOCYTIC

AKA: well-differentiated lymphocytic lymphoma
Low-grade lymphoma in the Working Formulation
Typically middle-aged to elderly
Prolonged evolution, scanty symptoms, good survival
Most have blood and bone marrow involvement, as well as other organs, at presentation (Stage IV); marrow involvement is usually *not* paratrabecular
B-lymphocytes (surface IgM, IgD, CD19+, CD20+) but 70% express T-cell marker CD5; most are also CD23+, CD10−
1% are T-cell neoplasms
Chromosomal abnormalities likely: most common trisomy 12 (30%; 50% of chronic lymphocytic leukemia [CLL] type) or 13q−(25%)
LN: effacement by monotonous small lymphocytes with clumped chromatin, inconspicuous nucleoli, few mitoses; PAS+ inclusions may be present in nuclei or cytoplasm; capsular invasion frequently present

Proliferation centers: collections of blasts and prolymphoblasts, seen in 60%, may cause pseudofollicular appearance (focally less basophilia); distinguish from follicles by round nuclei, poor demarcation, no compression of surrounding reticulin fibers
Some larger cells with vesicular nuclei may be present; no prognostic significance—don't confuse with LP Hodgkin's
Splenomegaly in 25%: predominantly white pulp (asymmetric nodules, sometimes coalescing), extending into red pulp
Hepatomegaly in 15% (portal); sinusoidal involvement in CLL
Richter's transformation to large cell lymphoma or transformation to prolymphocytic leukemia may occur: accompanied by fever, weight loss, rapid LN enlargement, and a poor clinical course; cells have same surface markers as original lymphoma

CONSISTENT WITH CLL
Lymphoma represents tissue manifestation of leukemia
Frequently see absolute lymphocytosis
BM involved in 100% (focal or diffuse)—usually not paratrabecular
A percentage will progress to systemic involvement (CLL)

PLASMACYTOID
AKA: immunocytoma
Usually associated with monoclonal gammopathy
30–50% have BM involvement, usually paratrabecular
Frequently accompanied by increased number of tissue mast cells
If most cells are plasma cell–like, more likely to be myeloma
IgM or heavy chain producers tend to be lymphomas; IgG or light chain producers tend to be myelomas
If IgM dysproteinemia present, Waldenstrom's macroglobulinemia (hyperviscosity, cryoglobulinemia, Coombs positive hemolytic anemia)
Russell bodies: cytoplasmic Ig inclusions
Dutcher bodies: "nuclear" Ig inclusions

MANTLE CELL LYMPHOMA

AKA: mantle zone lymphoma, intermediate lymphocytic, centrocytic lymphoma
Not part of the Working Formulation; most were best classified as diffuse small cleaved lymphoma
Middle age to elderly (median = 58 yr); male:female = 3:1
B-cell lymphoma (most have sIgM, 50% also have sIgD; CD19+, CD20+)
50–90% have T-cell markers CD5 and CD43 (Leu22); CD23−
Immunophenotype most closely matches the B cell of primary lymphoid follicles and the mantle-zone B cells of secondary lymphoid follicles
Usually see t(11;14)(q13;q32), which juxtaposes oncogene *bcl*-1 (chromosome 11; gene AKA PRAD-1 for parathyroid adenomatosis-1) with the Ig heavy chain (chromosome 14)
Lymphadenopathy in 75%, B symptoms in 40%
95% Stage III or IV at presentation
BM involved in 76%; blood 21%—median survival 3 yr
Mixture of small round and small cleaved lymphocytes
Generally modest mitotic rate
Naked benign germinal centers (i.e., no mantle zone) surrounded by malignant cells
Scattered large cells may be present
Nodular and diffuse forms; diffuse behaves poorly

Nodular configuration may be obvious or be represented only by occasional small germinal centers

Spleen: residual germinal centers with marked expansion of mantle zones—massive splenomegaly (>1 kg) can result

Often occur in extranodal sites; when occurs in GI tract, distinct entity: *multiple lymphomatous polyposis* (straddles the muscularis mucosae but does not involve mucosa)

Most behave in a low-grade fashion, but others are more aggressive

MARGINAL CELL LYMPHOMA
Not part of Working Formulation

B-cell malignancy: CD19+, CD20+; CD5−, CD23−, CD10−

30–35% are EMA positive

No rearrangements of the *bcl*-1 or *bcl*-2 genes

Cell of origin is unclear

Strong association with autoimmune disorders

Tend to be indolent lymphomas, but can transform to a large cell lymphoma, which behaves much more aggressively; include low or high grade in diagnosis

MUCOSA-ASSOCIATED LYMPHOID TISSUE (MALT) LYMPHOMAS
AKA: MALTomas

Includes the marginal-zone lymphoma of nonlymphoid tissue

Most common sites: salivary gland, GI tract

Tend to remain localized for long periods before progressing

Early lesions are probably antigen driven (e.g., *Helicobacter pylori* in the stomach) and are reversible by removal of the antigen; later, with dissemination, become antigen independent and, although usually indolent, are no longer reversible

Lymphoepithelial lesions common (distinguishing feature), as are reactive follicles with germinal centers

Nodular and diffuse forms

Cells can be small cleaved (centrocyte-like), monocytoid, or plasmacytoid

Nodular form: perifollicular distribution, then may infiltrate lymphocytic cuff (mantle zone pattern) or may colonize germinal centers (follicular colonization)

Monotypic Ig expression seen (in frozen section material)

MONOCYTOID B-CELL LYMPHOMA
AKA: parafollicular B-cell lymphoma

Male : female = 1 : 2; median age 60–65

Present commonly with enlarged peripheral LNs, usually around the parotid, often involving the parotid; frequently localized at presentation (Stage I or II), 10–20% of patients have Sjögren's disease

Extranodal presentation in 37%: salivary gland, breast, stomach, thyroid, soft tissue, bladder

Cells: small lymphocytes with bland, ovoid nuclei and abundant pale cytoplasm (similar to hairy cells)

LN: sinusoidal and interfollicular/mantle pattern *or* diffuse

Spleen: red pulp; BM: paratrabecular; liver: sinusoidal

Diffuse Lymphomas

Account for 50% of adult and nearly all childhood NHLs (if include lymphoblastic and small noncleaved)

More heterogeneous group than follicular; greater variability in immunophenotype and clinical behavior

In the Working Formulation, all three types are considered to be intermediate grade

May be T cell or B cell

Marrow involvement still frequently focal ("follicular")

If untreated, uniformly fatal within 2 yr

Each may occur with or without sclerosis; prognostic significance is unclear

All respond to combination chemotherapy

Some (esp. of the large cell type) represent progression from follicular lymphoma and are thus follicular center cell in origin; progression often accompanied by a mutation in p53

DIFFUSE, SMALL CLEAVED CELL
AKA: diffuse poorly differentiated lymphocytic lymphoma

Generally B cell

Most of these have been reclassified as either mantle cell lymphomas or marginal cell lymphomas

2 yr survival ~40% (vs. 80% for any follicular component)

DIFFUSE, MIXED SMALL AND LARGE CELL
AKA: diffuse mixed cell type lymphoma

Generally use this classification when 20–50% of the cells are "large"; criteria vary

Includes the diffuse counterpart of the follicular center cell origin (B cell) as well as some peripheral T-cell lymphomas

(See also Peripheral T-cell Lymphomas, later)

WITH EPITHELIOID CELL COMPONENT

DIFFUSE, LARGE CELL
AKA: diffuse histiocytic lymphoma, reticulum cell sarcoma

Occurs in both children and adults, mostly the latter (median age 57 yr)

Not uncommonly seen in setting of AIDS

Grows as large bulky fleshy mass; may resemble carcinoma

Greater tendency for extranodal presentation (40%), including digestive tract, skin, skeletal system

~50% limited to one side of diaphragm (vs. 90% for follicular)

Large cells with vesicular nuclei, subtle peripheral nucleoli

BM/liver involvement less common

When liver/spleen involved, usually large tumor masses rather than smaller nodules

50–60% B cell, 5–15% T cell, 5% histiocytic, 30–40% no markers (most B cell by gene rearrangement)

Associated with translocations involving the *bcl*-6 gene

Rapid progression, poor prognosis if untreated, but aggressive chemotherapy can yield good results

Distinguishing these from immunoblastic lymphomas may be academic

Median survival: 1–2 yr

CLEAVED CELL
Often accompanied by minority of small cleaved cells as well

NONCLEAVED CELL
More common

Vesicular nucleus, but usually with small nucleoli

Difficult to distinguish from B-cell immunoblastic (nuclei more central in latter)

Generally higher mitotic rate than cleaved cell form

T-CELL RICH B-CELL LYMPHOMA
AKA: pseudo-peripheral T-cell lymphoma

Diffuse B-cell lymphoma, sometimes evolving from previous follicular lymphoma, in which >75% of the cells are actually reactive T cells with normal helper : suppressor ratio obscuring the large malignant B cells

Male > female; generally in 60s

Despite the generally high stage of presentation and progression to a diffuse lymphoma, these patients tend to have an indolent course, perhaps because the large number of T cells represents a host response

HISTIOCYTE RICH B-CELL LYMPHOMA
Similar to T-cell rich B-cell lymphoma but with numerous nonepithelioid histiocytes

May be a variant of T-cell rich B-cell lymphoma

High-Grade Lymphomas

LARGE CELL, IMMUNOBLASTIC
PLASMACYTOID
AKA: B-cell immunoblastic sarcoma (some actually T cells)

Immunoblast: large vesicular eccentric nucleus, single prominent central nucleolus, thick nuclear membrane; cells may be binucleate

Intracytoplasmic Ig

Most common lymphoma to arise in setting of immunodeficiency, Hashimotos, Sjögren's, SLE (30%)

Marrow involved in 25% at diagnosis

Disseminates early, poor prognosis (median survival 14 months)

CLEAR CELL
AKA: T-cell immunoblastic sarcoma (some are B cells)

(Note: See also peripheral T-cell lymphomas)

Less common than plasmacytoid

Irregular nuclei, fine chromatin, small but distinct nucleoli, "water-clear" cytoplasm, interlocking plasma membranes (cohesive)

Involves initially paracortical region

Usually *not* preceded by an abnormal immune disorder

Children and adults; may coexist with mycosis fungoides

Generalized lymphadenopathy, polyclonal hyper-Ig

Marrow involved in ~33% at diagnosis

POLYMORPHOUS
AKA: pleomorphic histiocytoid lymphoma

Most of these are Ki-1 positive and have been reclassified as anaplastic large cell lymphoma (see later)

WITH EPITHELIOID CELL COMPONENT
AKA: transformed lymphoepithelioid T-cell lymphoma, transformed Lennert's (see later)

T-cell lymphoma of adults, mostly

74% are Stage IV at presentation

Effacement of lymph node architecture, plasma cells, eosinophils, proliferation of small vessels with plump endothelial cells

May have Reed-Sternberg–like cells

Small atypical lymphocytes between histiocytes

Splenic involvement (this variant) similar to Lennert's

LYMPHOBLASTIC
Usually children and adolescents (accounts for one third of childhood NHLs); also adults

Anterior mediastinal mass in 50–80% (thymic region)

Cerebrospinal fluid (CSF) and skin involvement not uncommon

Untreated: rapid dissemination, leukemia, death in months

Gross: soft, white, foci of hemorrhage and necrosis

Diffuse, monomorphic pattern of lymphocytes (round nuclei with "delicate" convolutions, fine chromatin, small nucleoli, and high mitotic rate); focal "starry sky" areas

Lymphocytes express terminal deoxynucleotidyl transferase (vs. other lymphomas) and usually (80%) have T-cell markers (CD7, ± CD2), some are pre-B (intracytoplasmic μ), some B, some granulocytes; often are O13+

In LN, predominantly paracortical

T-cell tumors: usually male, always mediastinum

May be a tumor of thymocytes (primitive T-cell precursors)

Commonly progress to marrow involvement—acute lymphoblastic leukemia (especially T-cell type)

In about 50% of cases, convolutions cannot be identified

Differential diagnosis: small lymphocytic, LP Hodgkin's, small noncleaved

CONVOLUTED CELL
NON–CONVOLUTED CELL

SMALL NONCLEAVED CELL
AKA: diffuse undifferentiated lymphoma

Cells intermediate in size between lymphocytes and histiocytes

Usually positive for B-cell markers (sIgM, CD19, CD20); CD5−, CD23−

BURKITT'S
Endemic in equatorial strip of Africa

Most cases occur in children; mean age 10 yr

Presentation: Africa (younger), jaw; U.S. (older), ileum

Peripheral lymphadenopathy rare

Bulky, fleshy tumors, ± necrotic areas

Microscopy: monotonous small (10–25 μm) round cells (several prominent basophilic nucleoli) creating a dark "sky" with "stars" of non-neoplastic macrophages; high mitotic rate; may have follicular areas

Numerous fat vacuoles in cytoplasm (Oil Red O positive)

EM: abundant ribosomes, lipid inclusions, no glycogen, nuclear pockets/projections

BM involvement late, leukemia rare

Responsive to chemotherapy (esp. African), 50% relapse

Strong association with Epstein-Barr virus [EBV] (95% of African type; 20% of non-endemic type; 30% in AIDS patients)

Usually CD10+

Consistently see translocation of c-*myc* from chromosome 8q24 to the Ig heavy chain genes (90%) on chromosome 14q32 or the Ig light chain genes on chromosome 2p13 (kappa) or 22 (lambda)

PLEOMORPHIC (NON-BURKITT'S)
Occurs in older age group (mean 34 yr)

Larger tumor cells, more pleomorphic nuclei and cells than in Burkitt's, well-defined cytoplasm rim, large eosinophilic nucleoli, binucleate and multinucleate

GI involvement less common, marrow involvement more common than Burkitt's type

Usually CD10−; c-*myc* gene rearrangements rare, but *bcl*-2 is rearranged in 30%

More aggressive clinical course

PERIPHERAL T-CELL LYMPHOMAS
All are diffuse; adults (rare <20 yr)

Constitute 30% of diffuse aggressive lymphomas in U.S.

Frequently classified as large cell immunoblastic or diffuse mixed in the Working Formulation

Most patients have generalized lymphadenopathy, most Stage IV (involvement of skin, liver, peripheral blood, lungs), B-symptoms common

15% small irregular, 40% mixed cell type, 43% large cell

<2% are small lymphocytic (well-differentiated lymphocytic lymphoma [WDL]); tissue equivalent of T-CLL

Small cells (slightly larger than normal lymphocytes): condensed chromatin, irregular nuclei, small nucleoli, may have abundant pale cytoplasm

Large cells: vesicular nuclei, prominent eosinophilic nucleoli

Both small and large cells show marked nuclear pleomorphism, lobulation, occasionally multinucleation

Often inflammatory background: neutrophils, eosinophils, macrophages, plasma cells

Skin involvement common—restricted to dermis

Peripheral blood involvement only after skin involvement

Cells contain at least one pan-T marker (CD2,3,4,7) but lack the markers of immature T cells (CD1a, TdT)

64% CD4+, 12% CD8+, 8% CD4+CD8+, 16% CD4−CD8−

Most have α/β T-cell receptors

γ/δ VARIANT

Male >> female, usually younger adults

Marked hepatosplenomegaly, minimal lymphadenopathy

Usually CD4− and CD8−; CD3+, CD2+, CD16+

Aggressive course; relapses common, usually fatal

LYMPHOEPITHELIOID CELL LYMPHOMA

AKA: Lennert's lymphoma

Probably just a pattern and not a distinct entity

Atypical large and small lymphocytes with a conspicuous epithelioid cell component, singly or in clusters, and a proliferation of vessels with plump endothelium, numerous plasma cells and eosinophils

Patients are middle age to older, with generalized lymphadenopathy, often involving Waldeyer's ring, and hepatosplenomegaly and B symptoms

Most are CD4+

Spleen usually shows multiple randomly distributed nodules of varying size; collarettes of epithelioid histiocytes seen in marginal zone

May undergo blastic transformation to immunoblastic malignant lymphoma

T-CELL LYMPHOMA RESEMBLING AILD

Preponderance of postcapillary venules

May even get hypergammaglobulinemia

Background of atypical lymphocytes, absent in AILD

AILD may simply be a well-differentiated form of this disease

ANAPLASTIC LARGE CELL LYMPHOMA

AKA: Ki-1 lymphoma

Almost all are CD30+ (but not all)

Usually CD2+, CD5+ (T cells), CD45 (LCA) positive; usually LeuM1 (CD15) negative

Caution: embryonal carcinoma and some melanomas are also CD30+

CLASSIC TYPE

Usually presents in younger individuals, often involving skin, but may be seen in both children and adults

Histologically, may mimic carcinoma, sarcoma, or malignant histiocytosis

"Packman" nuclei common: large lobated to horseshoe-shaped nuclei with pseudoinclusions

Tumor cells often also positive for CD4 and EMA

Erratic clinical course—long remissions ± chemotherapy

Commonly show t(2;5)(p23;q35), esp. when occurring in younger individuals

Small cell and histiocyte-rich variants exist

PRIMARY CUTANEOUS TYPE

Closely related to lymphomatoid papulosis (this is the malignant counterpart)

Usually need clinical progression beyond the skin to make this diagnosis

Usually EMA−; don't see t(2;5)

ADULT T-CELL LEUKEMIA/LYMPHOMA

Associated with human T-cell leukemia virus (HTLV-I)

Distinct clinical/pathological entity, although some consider this a variant of peripheral T-cell lymphoma

Male = female; median age 40 yr; acute to subacute course

Most common in southwestern Japan, southeastern U.S.; the majority of the U.S. cases occur in blacks

Probably long period between exposure to HTLV and development of disease

Histology varies: pleomorphic, medium-sized cell, mixed large and small cells are most common types, but also can get large cell or small cell variants

Generalized lymphadenopathy, hepatosplenomegaly, leukemia; CSF involvement common

Skin: can have epidermotropism with large Pautrier's microabscesses

Hypercalcemia and bone lesions caused by hormonal activation of osteoclasts rather than direct tumor involvement

Markedly pleomorphic lymphoid cells in the peripheral blood with multilobated nuclei

Cells are CD4+, IL2R+ (CD25+)

All present in Stage IV—prognosis poor, independent of histologic type; even with aggressive chemotherapy, median survival is less than 1 yr

Miscellaneous Lymphomas

CUTANEOUS T-CELL LYMPHOMA (CTCL)

AKA: mycosis fungoides, Sézary syndrome

Most cases have "helper" T-cell characteristics: CD4+, IL2R−(CD25−)

Sézary syndrome refers to triad of erythroderma, lymphadenopathy, and atypical lymphocytes in the peripheral blood

Lymphocytes frequently show "cerebriform" appearance, although this may be lost in later stages

Initially skin involvement, but later progresses

Early disease progresses through various "stages":

• Premycotic erythematous/eczematoid: focal oval or round, circumscribed red flat macules

• Patch: coalescence of macules into patches with scaling and intense pruritus, purple brown discoloration; some lesions may spontaneously regress

• Plaque: palpable discrete, indurated papules that may arise in erythematous zones or de novo, may heal centrally while progress peripherally (T1-2)

• Tumor: large elevated nodules >1 cm in diameter; may erode and ulcerate

SKIN

Acanthosis or atrophy, focal parakeratosis

Exocytosis of atypical lymphocytes

Pautrier's microabscesses (also seen in adult T-cell leukemia/lymphoma—almost pathognomonic)

Clusters of atypical lymphocytes in superficial dermis

Increased numbers of Langerhans' cells

May see mucinous degeneration of outer hair shafts

LYMPH NODES: THREE PATTERNS

Nonspecific (rare): only reactive follicular hyperplasia

Frank malignancy: partial or total replacement by monomorphic infiltrate of atypical lymphocytes, ± coagulative necrosis

Dermatopathic lymphadenopathy (80%): paracortical expansion by proliferating histiocytes with racket-shaped granules on EM (Langerhans' cells)

STAGING

TNM

T Skin involvement
   T0   Suspicious lesions
   T1   Plaque stage: <10% body surface
   T2   Plaque stage: >10% body surface
   T3   Tumors
   T4   Generalized erythroderma
N Nodal involvement
   N0   None palpable, normal histology
   N1   Palpable, normal histology
   N2   Not palpable, abnormal histology
   N3   Palpable, abnormal histology
M Visceral involvement (seen in 70% at autopsy)
   M0   Absent
   M1   Present (Stage IVB)
Spleen (50%), lung (45%), liver (40%), BM (2%)
Clinical staging:

	T1	T2	T3	T4
N0	IA	IB	IIB	IIIA
N1	IIA	IIA	IIB	IIIB
N2	IVA	IVA	IVA	IVA
N3	IVA	IVA	IVA	IVA

ANGIOCENTRIC IMMUNOPROLIFERATIVE LESIONS

BENIGN LYMPHOCYTIC VASCULITIS (GRADE I)

Angiocentric mononuclear infiltrate (lymphocytes, plasma cells, immunoblasts) which involves vessel walls but without vascular destruction, luminal compromise, or necrosis

Most commonly lungs and skin

Treatment: chlorambucil more successful than steroids

May progress to more aggressive forms of AIL

LYMPHOMATOID GRANULOMATOSIS (GRADE II)

AKA: polymorphic reticulosis, lethal midline granulomas

Commonly involve nose, lung, paranasal sinuses, nasopharynx; also skin, kidneys, CNS, GI tract

Atypical angiocentric *angiodestructive* lymphoreticular infiltrate with *necrosis,* often extensive

Mixed infiltrate: lymphocytes, plasma cells, immunoblasts, histiocytes, ± eosinophils

Initially felt to be only locally invasive, but many progress to large cell immunoblastic lymphoma; prognosis worsens with increasing numbers of large lymphocytes and decreasing numbers of inflammatory cells

Many patients respond to treatment (radiation if localized)

ANGIOCENTRIC LYMPHOMA (GRADE III)

Neoplastic nature of angiocentric infiltrate usually obvious at presentation—atypia in both small and large cells

If large cells predominate, fulfill criterion for immunoblastic

Vascular infiltration, destruction, extensive necrosis

Discrepant histology at different sites common

Primarily extranodal; may involve nodes—always diffuse

In spleen, periarterial

Lymphokine production by abnormal T cells may induce a hemophagocytic syndrome

LYMPHOMAS IN IMMUNODEFICIENCY

PRIMARY (GENETIC) IMMUNODEFICIENCIES

Increased incidence of malignancies, esp. lymphomas

Ataxia telangiectasia: 10% die from lymphomas, usually B-immunoblastic sarcoma

Wiskott-Aldrich syndrome: 10% die from lymphomas, both HD (50% LD type) and NHL

X-linked recessive lymphoproliferative syndrome (immunodeficiency to EBV): Burkitt's, immunoblastic

POST-TRANSPLANT LYMPHOPROLIFERATIVE DISEASE

4–6% renal transplant patients develop malignancies: skin tumors, malignant lymphoma, Kaposi's, cervical carcinoma

Lymphoma frequency 350× general population (higher in cardiac transplant patients)

Initially a polyclonal B-cell hyperplasia; later evolves into a B-cell lymphoma, often retaining a polyclonal phenotype; etiology may be similar to MALT lymphomas

50% involve CNS (vs. 1% for general population)

30% involve the allograft

Pleomorphic, rapid clinical course; must remove the graft

AIDS

Malignancies: Kaposi's sarcoma, malignant lymphoma

Usually extranodal, involving GI tract, CNS, BM, heart

Usually NHL, usually diffuse large cell (B cell)

OTHERS

Rheumatoid arthritis, Sjögrens, Hashimoto's, and group of "atypical immunoproliferative processes," including AILD

OTHER

COMPOSITE

Patient has two distinct lymphomas at same anatomic site

Most common: Hodgkin's and follicular small cleaved or diffuse large cell

More likely, less differentiated is a blastic form of other

LARGE CELL LYMPHOMA WITH FILOPODIA

AKA: microvillous lymphoma of B-cell origin; probably same as "Anemone cell tumor," "porcupine cell tumor"

Large cell lymphoma with sinus growth pattern; CD45+

By EM, abundant filiform cytoplasmic projections

MALIGNANT ANGIOENDOTHELIOMATOSIS

Systemic lymphoma with marked tropism for blood vessels

Usually B-cell phenotype

Involves skin and CNS most commonly

PLASMA CELL DYSCRASIAS

General

AKA: monoclonal gammopathies, paraproteinemia

Need two components:
- Uncontrolled proliferation of plasma cells or related cell
- Abnormally elevated blood and/or urine levels of a homogeneous Ig and/or one of its constituent chains

Free light chains are small enough to be effectively excreted in urine (Bence Jones proteins)—may occur alone or in combination with any hyper-Ig syndrome

MULTIPLE MYELOMA (60%)

AKA: plasma cell myeloma

Multiple masses of immature plasma cells scattered primarily throughout the skeletal system

Peak incidence 50–60 yr; male > female (slightly)

More common in longstanding chronic infections

Patients present with unexplained anemia, proteinuria, infections (impaired immunity)

Later, bone pain, fractures, renal failure
Generally: 3 g Ig/100 ml serum or 6 mg Ig/100 ml urine

IgG, 60%	IgM, 10–15%	Light chains
IgA, 15–20%	IgD/IgE, rare	only, 5–10%

IgD secretors have more aggressive clinical course
Most are CD19–, CD20–, CD38+
10% show systemic amyloidosis
X-ray: multiple destructive bone lesions, initiating in medullary cavity and eroding cortex, forming sharply punched out defects (1–4 cm)—"soap bubble"

Vertebrae, 66%	Femur, 28%
Ribs, 44%	Clavicle, 10%
Skull, 41%	Scapula, 10%
Pelvis, 28%	

Soft tissue lesions may appear later: spleen, liver, kidneys, lungs, LNs: fleshy, red-brown masses
Mature to very immature plasma cells, binucleate and trinucleate, Russell bodies
Plasma cells may account for 15–90% of cells in marrow; patchy or diffuse involvement
Myeloma nephrosis (60–80%): abnormal interstitial plasma cell infiltrate plus distal tubule and collecting duct casts
Rarely, nonsecreting variant (no serum protein peak)
Survival: 1–2 yr without treatment
Bad prognosis: serum β_2 microglobulin >4 ng/μl, extensive or diffuse marrow involvement, highly immature plasma cells or anaplastic conversion, plasma cell leukemia
Patients have increased risk of developing other cancers

SOLITARY MYELOMA (3–5%)
AKA: solitary plasmacytoma
Two types: bone (see multiple myeloma) or soft tissues (lungs, oronasopharynx, nasal sinuses)
Peak incidence 40–50 yr old; male > female
50% have monoclonal protein in urine and/or serum; but level generally <2 g/100 ml, and nonmonoclonal Ig normal
For those with bone involvement, 50% of those with dysproteinemia and 25% of those without progress to multiple myeloma; therefore, may be early stage of same disease
For those without bone involvement, only 10–20% progress to multiple myeloma

PLASMA CELL LEUKEMIA
Plasma cells in peripheral blood (>20% or absolute plasma cell count >2000)
Variant of multiple myeloma
Usually small numbers of leukemic cells
Tissue involvement rare

WALDENSTROM'S MACROGLOBULINEMIA (5%)
AKA: plasmacytoid lymphoma
Monoclonal gammopathy generally (85%) occurring in a setting of a lymphoproliferative disorder
Rare before 60 yr of age
Diffuse marrow infiltration by plasma cells, plasmacytoid lymphocytes, and lymphocytes (all from same clone); cells do not form tumor masses or produce lytic lesions
Lymphocytes commonly contain Dutcher bodies (intranuclear inclusions)
Similar infiltrate may be seen in LNs, spleen, liver
Usually IgM, rarely IgG or IgA
Symptoms: weakness, fatigue, weight loss
In 90%, total protein in serum >6.5 g/100 ml; IgM 1–3 g
IgM >15% of all Ig (usually 5%)

Bence Jones proteins found in 20–30%
Mean survival: 2–5 yr

HEAVY CHAIN DISEASE
Rare; only heavy chains are produced
Can get hepatosplenomegaly and soft tissue tumors
Can get at any age, although median age is 61
ALPHA
Children
Two patterns:
- Massive infiltrate of lamina propria of intestine with villous atrophy, malabsorption, diarrhea; abdominal LNs involved; AKA: Mediterranean lymphoma (see GI outline)
- Similar infiltrate in respiratory tract
GAMMA
Elderly
More like malignant lymphoma than myeloma—no lytic lesions
May be associated with TB, rheumatoid arthritis, autoimmune
Course: months to years
MU
Rare; usually seen in patients with CLL

MONOCLONAL GAMMOPATHY OF UNDETERMINED SIGNIFICANCE (MGUS) (30%)
Ig peak in blood, but no apparent associated cellular proliferation
Seen in ~3% of people over 70 yr; most are asymptomatic
Bence Jones proteins generally *not* seen

MYELODYSPLASTIC SYNDROMES

Heterogeneous group of stem cell disorders with abnormal hematopoiesis and varying potential to evolve into AML (one third will ultimately progress)
Older individuals (60–75 yr), male > female, present with fatigue
50% hypercellular, 25% normocellular, 25% hypocellular
May see increased reticulin
Abnormal localization of immature precursors (ALIP) may be seen—may indicate increased risk of progression
A picture identical to myelodysplastic syndrome can be seen in patients with AIDS
CYTOGENETICS
May also be seen in chromosome deletion syndromes:
- 5q – : Refractory anemia–like picture; does not progress
- 7q – : Presents at 6–8 months; leukemia by 3–6 yr
50% of all patients have some chromosome deletion, most commonly 5q– (good prognosis), then 8+ (intermediate prognosis), 7– or 7q– (poor prognosis); also see 20q–, 12p–, abnormalities of 17, y–

REFRACTORY ANEMIA
<1% blasts in peripheral blood, <5% in marrow
Hypercellular marrow with erythroid hyperplasia and/or dyserythropoiesis
Normal granulocytes and megakaryocytes

REFRACTORY ANEMIA WITH RINGED SIDEROBLASTS (RARS)

Refractory anemia plus ≥15% of nucleated RBCs are ringed sideroblasts (iron in mitochondria)

Marked increase in erythroid precursors

Significant iron accumulation in macrophages

REFRACTORY ANEMIA WITH EXCESS BLASTS (RAEB)

Cytopenia affecting two or more cell lines

1–5% blasts in peripheral blood, 5–20% in marrow

Hypercellular marrow with erythrocyte or granulocyte hyperplasia

Dysgranulopoiesis, dyserythropoiesis, and/or dysmegakaryocytopoiesis

RAEB IN TRANSFORMATION (RAEB-T)

5–30% of blasts in peripheral blood, 20–30% in marrow

Auer rods may be present

60% progress to AML with median survival of 6 months

CHRONIC MYELOMONOCYTIC LEUKEMIA

Hypercellular marrow with increase in both monocytic and granulocytic lines

Monocytes: $>1 \times 10^9$/L, often with mature granulocytosis

<5% blasts in peripheral blood, 5–20% in marrow

CHRONIC MYELOMONOCYTIC LEUKEMIA IN TRANSFORMATION (CMML-T)

5–30% blasts in peripheral blood, 20–30% in marrow

LEUKEMIAS

General

Diffuse (begins focally) replacement of the bone marrow (rarely, older patients with AML or acute lymphoblastic leukemia [ALL] may present with hypocellular marrow)

Abnormal numbers and forms of immature WBCs in peripheral blood

Widespread infiltrates in the liver, spleen, LNs, and other sites throughout the body

Symptoms, complications, and death arise from anemia, thrombocytopenia, and loss of normally functioning leukocytes

Acute leukemias present aggressively: WBC <10K in 50%, >100K in 10%

Chronic leukemias are insidious, often detected only on routine physical exam

Beyond acute or chronic, typing of the leukemia is better done on smears of peripheral blood or marrow aspirate

Leading cancer killer of children <15 yr in U.S.

Rate of cell growth actually slower than normal, but get accumulation caused by apparent block in differentiation

PRIMARY CHANGES

BM replacement can erode cancellous and cortical bone

Myelofibrosis may be present: ALL > AML >> CLL or CML

Lymphadenopathy common, esp. in lymphocytic

Splenomegaly common, especially in CML (generally <2.5 kg in CLL, <1 kg in monocytic); firm parenchyma; expansion of red pulp

Hepatomegaly, esp. in CLL

SECONDARY CHANGES

Anemia (Note: as marrow recovers, fat cells regenerate first, then erythroids (in islands, often with dyserythropoietic changes), granulocytes, megakaryocytes)

Hemorrhages and hematomas, most frequently in brain

Infection

Vascular sludging/infarcts

Chloroma (Granulocytic Sarcoma)

Extramedullary tumor mass composed of myeloblasts with or without neutrophil promyelocytes

More common in children

Undifferentiated, intermediate, and differentiated types

Look for eosinophilic myelocytes; increase in number with increasing differentiation of lesion

Frequently misdiagnosed as large cell lymphoma

May be isolated or associated with AML, CML, agnogenic myeloid metaplasia, polycythemia vera; may predate AML or be first evidence of relapse

Associated with subperiosteal bone (esp. of the skull, sinuses, sternum, ribs, vertebrae, pelvis), LNs, skin

If occurs within orbit (common) usually presents with proptosis

Gross: fresh-cut surface is often green (peroxidase)

ACUTE LYMPHOBLASTIC (LYMPHOCYTIC) LEUKEMIA (20%)

Most frequent cancer in children <15 yr (peak age = 4yr)

Generalized lymphadenopathy, splenomegaly, hepatomegaly

80% are of B-cell origin; most are pre-B (CD19+ but often CD20 and Ig −); prognosis is best for the pre-B phenotype

High levels of terminal deoxynucleotidyl transferase

Intense therapy induces remission in >50%

Often treatment makes cells smaller—more like lymphocytes

Cytogenetic abnormalities seen in 60%:

- Good prognosis: hyperdiploidy (seen in 25–30%)
- Poor prognosis: Philadelphia chromosome (15% adults, 5% children); t(1:19) (20–25%)

SUBTYPES

- L1 (85%): small cells predominate, homogenous, little cytoplasm, round regular nuclei, nucleoli not visible; some cells up to twice size of small lymphocytes
- L2 (13%): features of L1 and L3; nuclei have clefts; nucleoli present, more cytoplasm—T or B cell; adults
- L3 (1–2%): homogeneous population of large cells (3–4× size of small lymphocytes), round nuclei, prominent nucleoli, abundant deeply basophilic cytoplasm; leukemic form of Burkitt's lymphoma (cells have t(8;14) translocation)

CHRONIC LYMPHOCYTIC LEUKEMIA (25%)

Most common leukemia in adults >60 yr; male:female = 2:1

Extremely uncommon among Asians

Defined as >15K lymphocytes/mm³ with ≤10% blasts

4–15K = early low count CLL, subleukemic CLL

Usually B cell, with weak sIg but also CD5+; rare cases (2%) of T cell (see later)

Generalized lymphadenopathy (65%), splenomegaly (40%), hepatomegaly (25%)

Homogenous population of small mature lymphocytes

Reticulin increased in 25%

Often associated with small lymphocytic lymphoma

With therapy, survival of 10–15 yr not uncommon

T-CELL CLL

Rare; accounts for <2% of all cases of CLL

Circulating cells may (60%) show cytoplasmic azurophilic granules (large granular lymphocytes), suggesting T-CLL

Beta-glucuronidase and acid phosphatase activity almost always elevated (rarely elevated in B-CLL)

CD3+, usually CD8+ (suppressor T-cell); CD56−; clonal rearrangement of T-cell receptor gene(s)

If CD4+, usually a prolymphocytic variant (see later)

Lymphocytosis may range from 3K to 500K; white count may remain stable for years

Cutaneous involvement may be seen, but without epidermal involvement

May get neutropenia, pure red cell aplasia, hypogammaglobulinemia caused by production of gamma interferon

NK-CELL CLL

Even more rare than T-cell CLL; comprise only one fifth of the non–B-cell CLLs

Cells usually CD2+ but CD3−; CD16+, CD56+; usually CD4−, CD8−

No rearrangements of the T-cell receptor genes are seen

PROLYMPHOCYTIC

Larger, predominantly immature lymphocytes

Usually older males

Usually B cell (80%) with strong sIg expression

Remainder are T cell (20%); usually CD4+ (as well as CD2+, CD3+, CD5+)

Markedly elevated WBC with >55% prolymphocytes

Usually massive splenomegaly without lymphadenopathy

Generally low mitotic rate

More aggressive clinical course than typical CLL

INTERMEDIATE (CLL/PROLYMPHOCYTIC LEUKEMIA)

10–55% prolymphocytes in blood

Transformation

PROLYMPHOCYTOID (DEDIFFERENTIATION) (5%)

Increase in prolymphocytes to >20% of marrow or blood lymphocytes

Often focally in BM, surrounded by well-differentiated lymphocytes

Prominent, single eosinophilic nucleoli

RICHTER'S (LARGE CELL TRANSFORMATION) (3–10%)

Pleomorphic, usually B-immunoblastic lymphoma; occasionally Hodgkin's disease

Increased symptoms, frequent lymphopenia, downhill course

Lymphoma cells usually not seen in peripheral blood

Staging

	Rai Staging	Median Survival
0	Lymphocytosis only	150 months
I	Lymphadenopathy	101 months
II	Enlarged liver or spleen, ± LNs	71 months
III	Anemia ± organomegaly	19 months
IV	Thrombocytopenia, ± organomegaly	19 months

	Alternate Staging	Median Survival
A	Enlargement of 1 or 2 of spleen, liver, cervical LNs, axillary LNs, inguinal LNs	Same as gen popul.
B	3 or more	7 yr
C	Anemia or thrombocytopenia	2 yr

ACUTE MYELOCYTIC (MYELOBLASTIC) LEUKEMIA (40%)

>30% blasts (Note: for M3–5, include promyelocytes and promonocytes when counting blasts)

Most common leukemia in the 15–59 yr age group

Etiology may be linked to oncoviruses

Azurophilic granules (appear at promyelocyte stage) are modified primary lysosomes

Myeloperoxidase stain distinguishes myeloblasts from lymphoblasts

Esterases: naphthyl AS-D chloroacetate esterase (NCE) specific for myeloids; alpha-naphthyl acetate esterase (ANE) specific for monocytes

Auer bodies: red, rod-shaped abnormal lysosomes (derived from primary granules) principally seen in myelocytic leukemias (also some monocytic)

Remissions can be achieved, but in general are short lived

All *trans*-retinoic acid can induce differentiation to various degrees

Presence of Philadelphia chromosome (3%) is a bad prognostic sign

SUBTYPES

M0: *Minimally differentiated:* no myeloperoxidase staining; <3% blasts

M1 (20%): *Myeloblastic without maturation:* blasts without Auer rods or granules (≥30% of non-erythroid cells in marrow are myeloblasts)

M2 (30%): *Myeloblastic with maturation:* many blasts (≥30%), but some maturation to promyelocytes (>10%) or beyond, few monocytic elements (<20%); 20–25% have t(8;21)

M3 (5%): *Promyelocytic:* mostly promyelocytes with many Auer rods (Faggot cells: numerous Auer rods, like sticks in a fireplace) and peroxidase-positive granules; frequently present in diffuse intravascular coagulation (DIC); microgranular (hypogranular) variant exists without Auer rods; >90% show t(15;17)

M4 (30%): *Myelomonocytic:* both myeloid (M2) and monocytic elements (20–80% monocytic elements in marrow, or serum lysozyme level >3× normal); present with leukocytosis

• M4EO: myelomonocytic with bone marrow eosinophilia; 100% have inversion of chromosome 16; better prognosis than standard M4

M5 (10%): *Monocytic:* monoblasts and monocytes >30%; must confirm diagnosis with fluoride-inhibited esterase reaction; urine/serum lysozyme usually elevated; present with gingival infiltration; 30% have abnormality of chromosome 11

• M5A (poorly differentiated): ≥80% monocytic elements are blasts

• M5B (differentiated): <80% monocytic elements are blasts

M6 (5%): *Erythroleukemia:* erythroid elements constitute >50% of the cells and have bizarre multilobated nuclei; ≥30% of non-erythroid elements are blasts

M7 (5%): *Megakaryoblastic:* immature and abnormal megakaryocytes (≥30% in aspirate or circulating); myelofibrosis usually present

CHRONIC MYELOCYTIC LEUKEMIA (15%)

90% have Philadelphia chromosome (Ph′: translocation from 22q11 to 9q34, forming chimeric protein c-*abl/bcr* [breakpoint cluster region])

Ph′ negative CML has worse prognosis than Ph′ positive (different disease)
White count invariably elevated, usually >100K
Huge spleens common
BM: usually less than 5% myeloblasts
Mostly neutrophils with scattered myelocytes and promyelocytes; increased number of basophils typical
Leukemic cells usually have markedly decreased alkaline phosphatase activity
2–3 yr course without treatment
May develop myelofibrosis late in course
Treatment induces 2–5 yr remission, usually followed by blast crisis (usually myeloblasts, but 30% are immature B cells) and death

OTHER LEUKEMIAS
HAIRY CELL LEUKEMIA
AKA: leukemic reticuloendotheliosis
Most commonly male (may be young, but median age 50)
Insidious onset with massive splenomegaly, no lymphadenopathy, usually pancytopenia
Hairy cell: 10–14 μm, clear to lightly basophilic cytoplasm with numerous delicate cytoplasmic projections, perinuclear halo (formalin artifact); delicate nuclear chromatin
Marrow: usually hypercellular (may be hypocellular) with loosely packed hairy cells (vs. tight packing in lymphomas); reticulin invariably increased; erythroid hyperplasia common
Spleen: disease of red pulp; diffuse infiltration by monotonous population of small mononuclear cells, usually with invasion into vascular walls (subendothelial)
Contain tartrate resistant acid phosphatase (TRAP)
EM: 50% have ribosome-lamella complex
Monoclonal B lymphocytes, CD5−, CD19+, CD20+, CD10−, IgM+, IL2R+, *CD11c+, CD25+*
Two types:
• Leukopenic (WBC <3K)
    Most common form in U.S.
    Reticulin almost always increased
• Nonleukopenic (WBC >3K)
    Most common form in Japan
Treatment: splenectomy, alpha-interferon, deoxycoformycin
Differential diagnosis: mastocytosis
HISTIOCYTIC LEUKEMIA
Controversial whether or not this exists
STEM CELL LEUKEMIA
Highly acute, extremely immature
Rapidly fatal (months)
ERYTHROLEUKEMIA
AKA: DiGuglielmo's syndrome, erythromyeloblastic leukemia
(See M6 AML)
Marked anemia, leukopenia
If survive initial phase, gradual transition to immature myeloblastic leukemia
Course: months to 2 yr, ending in death

MEGAKARYOCYTES/PLATELETS

Normal Hemostasis
Vasoconstriction at the site of endothelial injury
Platelet adhesion, degranulation, aggregation (primary hemostasis)

• Promoted by exposed subendothelial connective tissue, thromboxane A_2, ADP, thrombin
• Inhibited by prostacyclin, ADPase, anticoagulants (heparin)
Later, platelet plug undergoes a "viscous metamorphosis" caused by activation of ADP and thrombin (secondary hemostasis)

Thrombocytopenia

DECREASED PLATELET PRODUCTION
APLASIA
MYELOPHTHISIC ANEMIAS
Metastatic carcinoma, leukemia
FOLATE OR VITAMIN B_{12} DEFICIENCY
DILUTION BY MULTIPLE TRANSFUSIONS

ABNORMAL PLATELET ACTIVITY
BERNARD-SOULIER SYNDROME
Inherited deficiency of platelet membrane glycoprotein required for platelet-collagen interaction
THROMBASTHENIA
Defective platelet aggregation in response to ADP, collagen, epinephrine, or thrombin
FANCONI'S ANEMIA
WISKOTT-ALDRICH SYNDROME
ASPIRIN ABUSE

INCREASED PLATELET DESTRUCTION
DRUG REACTIONS
Seen with quinine, quinidine, chloramphenicol, alkylating agents, antimetabolites, thiazide diuretics, methyldopa
MECHANICAL INJURY
Prosthetic valves, microangiopathic anemia, malignant hypertension
HYPERSPLENISM
Normally, spleen sequesters 30–40% of platelets; when enlarged, can increase to 90%
ISOIMMUNE THROMBOCYTOPENIA
Seen in neonates and post-transfusion
Most platelets contain specific antigens
PL^{A1}-negative mothers with PL^{A1}-positive fetus create antibodies; similar to Rh disease
IDIOPATHIC THROMBOCYTOPENIC PURPURA (ITP)
AKA: autoimmune thrombocytopenia
• Acute ITP:
    Children, usually following viral infection
    Believed that viral antigens adsorbed onto platelets
• Chronic ITP:
    Adults, usually women
    Primary or associated with another autoimmune disorder
    Appears related to antibody production against platelet surface antigens
    Spleen: usually normal size, congested sinuses, enlarged follicles, megakaryocytes often found in sinuses, masses of agglutinated platelets
    BM: mild increased numbers of megakaryocytes, may have increased numbers of plasma cells
    Hemorrhages in skin, epicardium, GI tract, urinary tract
    70–80% patients markedly improve following splenectomy

THROMBOTIC THROMBOCYTOPENIC PURPURA (TTP)
Thrombocytopenia, microangiopathic anemia, fever, transient neurologic deficits, and renal failure
Widespread microthrombi in arterioles, capillaries, venules
More common in young females (30s)
Once invariably fatal, but many survive now with therapy
Treatment: steroids, splenectomy, exchange transfusions

DISSEMINATED INTRAVASCULAR COAGULATION (DIC)
AKA: consumption coagulopathy, defibrination syndrome
Acquired thrombohemorrhagic disorder secondary to a variety of diseases
Activation of clotting and thrombolytic cascades, with consumption of platelets, fibrin, and coagulation factors
Major initiating mechanisms are release of tissue factors and widespread damage to endothelium
Thrombi found (in order of frequency): brain, heart, lungs, kidneys, adrenals, spleen, liver

Thrombocythemia

PRIMARY THROMBOCYTHEMIA
AKA: essential, idiopathic
Increased number and size of megakaryocytes in BM, with peripheral thrombocytosis
Closely related to polycythemia vera, but lacks necessary red cell mass
Marrow is normal to hypocellular with mildly increased reticulin staining

MEGAKARYOBLASTIC LEUKEMIA
AKA: M7 AML
Related to acute myelofibrosis

MYELOFIBROSIS

MYELOID METAPLASIA
AKA: myelofibrosis; when etiology unknown: "agnogenic" or "primary"
Appearance of extramedullary hematopoiesis (in agnogenic form) or malignant myeloid cells in another organ, usually spleen, with fibrosis in the marrow
Primarily adults (mean age 60 yr); younger age when follows polycythemia vera or CML
Hepatosplenomegaly secondary to extramedullary hematopoiesis
Spleen weight usually ~2 kg
Normal to increased neutrophil alkaline phosphatase activity (decreased in 90% patients with CML)
Marrow: three stages: hypercellular, patchy fibrosis, and obliterative myelosclerosis; degree of fibrosis does not always reflect duration of disease
Hypocellular marrow with condensed nuclear chromatin; megakaryocytes tend to persist but are dysplastic
Osteosclerotic changes present by x-ray in 40%
Extramedullary hematopoietic tumors not uncommon
Indolent, prolonged clinical course: median survival 10 yr

ACUTE MYELOFIBROSIS
AKA: acute myelosclerosis, malignant myelosclerosis, acute myelodysplasia with myelofibrosis

Little to no RBC poikilocytosis, no splenomegaly
Marrow: hyperplasia of all three lines (usually most notable in megakaryocytes) with a significant left shift—*panmyeloid* disorder
Nuclear chromatin more open (vs. agnogenic)
Increased reticulin fibers—may be dense
Closely related to acute megakaryoblastic leukemia
Rapid clinical course: median survival 2 yr

HISTIOCYTOSES

GLYCOGEN STORAGE DISEASES
(See Congenital Syndromes outline)

HEMOPHAGOCYTIC SYNDROME
Associated with both viral (EBV, cytomegalovirus [CMV], adenovirus) and bacterial infections, as well as some peripheral T-cell lymphomas
When occurs in children, high mortality rate
Generally peripheral pancytopenia
BM: pink areas at low power, containing collections of mature histiocytes, many showing phagocytosis of erythroid cells (both mature and nucleated)—phagocytosis often more prominent on smears
Frequently decreased erythroid and granulocyte precursors
Spleen: may be enlarged with prominent histiocytic infiltrate
Coagulation abnormalities in most patients
Unlike histiocytic medullary reticulosis, cells have low nuclear:cytoplasmic ratio and abundant cytoplasm with large vacuoles

SINUS HISTIOCYTOSIS WITH MASSIVE LYMPHADENOPATHY
AKA: Rosai-Dorfman disease (1969)
Massive, painless, bilateral cervical LN enlargement; mean age 20 yr
Nodes matted by perinodal fibrosis
Dilatation of lymphatic sinuses with architectural effacement
Numerous histiocytes with large vesicular nucleus and abundant clear lipid–containing cytoplasm
Lymphocytophagocytosis common
Capsular and pericapsular inflammation/fibrosis
Histiocytes S-100 positive, KP-1 (CD68) positive
May involve extranodal sites (30%): eyes, ocular adnexae, upper respiratory tract, skin, CNS; spleen and BM spared

LANGERHANS' CELL HISTIOCYTOSIS
AKA: histiocytosis X, differentiated histiocytosis, Langerhans' cell granuloma, Hashimoto-Pritzker's (self-limited, congenital)
Proliferation of Langerhans' cells: antigen-presenting "histiocyte" with irregular nuclei containing prominent grooves and folds, and abundant acidophilic cytoplasm; occasionally multinucleated
S-100, Leu-6 (CD1a), sialylated Leu-M1, and vimentin positive; usually LCA, EMA, Leu-M1 negative
Langerhans' cells of histiocytosis X are CD4 positive (normal Langerhans' cells are not)

EM: Birbeck's granule (intracytoplasmic, pentalaminar, rod-like tubular structure with a periodicity and a dilated terminal end: tennis racket)

Variable numbers of eosinophils, lymphocytes, plasma cells, neutrophils are present

Necrosis not uncommon

LN involvement (sinus distention with Langerhans' cells and eosinophils) can occur alone or as a part of a systemic disease

Marrow involvement late—generally focal with granulomatous appearance

UNIFOCAL LANGERHANS' CELL HISTIOCYTOSIS

AKA: eosinophilic granuloma

Benign—usually children and young adults; male > female

Usually in bone: skull, jaw, humerus, rib, femur

Asymptomatic to bone eroding with pain, pathologic fractures

May spontaneously heal by fibrosis

Very radiosensitive—excellent prognosis

No systemic involvement

Must follow to rule out early presentation of multiple form

MULTIPLE BONE LANGERHANS' CELL HISTIOCYTOSIS

AKA: polyostotic EG, Hand-Schüller-Christian Disease

Onset usually before age of 5

Fever, seborrhea-like rash, frequent otitis media, upper respiratory infections

50% have granulomatous involvement of posterior pituitary stalk or hypothalamus → diabetes insipidus

30% have orbital granulomas with exophthalmos

Good prognosis: spontaneous remission in half; other half respond to chemotherapy

MULTIPLE ORGAN EOSINOPHILIC GRANULOMA

Involves skeleton, skin, lungs

Poor prognosis for young (<18 months), hepatomegaly, anemia, marrow involvement, hemorrhagic skin lesions

Aggressive form of multiple bone eosinophilic granuloma

ACUTE DISSEMINATED LANGERHANS' CELL HISTIOCYTOSIS

AKA: progressive differentiated histiocytosis, Letterer-Siwe disease

Progressive systemic proliferation of differentiated histiocytes

Infants and children under 3 yr—may be present at birth

Initially fever, then diffuse maculopapular eczematous skin rash; then splenomegaly, hepatomegaly, lymphadenopathy, cystic lesions in skull, pelvis, long bones

Cells are mature, abundant cytoplasm, occasionally multinucleated

EM: occasional Langerhans' granules (rodlike tubular structures)

Minimal erythrophagocytosis

Infants <6 months generally rapid downhill course

Older children: 1–2 yr without treatment, a little better with aggressive therapy

HISTIOCYTIC MEDULLARY RETICULOSIS

AKA: malignant histiocytosis

When in marrow and blood, "leukemic reticuloendotheliosis"

Progressive systemic proliferation of somewhat immature, morphologically atypical histiocytes and/or precursors

Usually children and young adults

Patient usually acutely ill when first seen

Fever, lymphadenopathy, constitutional symptoms early

Lymphadenopathy, hepatomegaly, splenomegaly, skin involvement common

Anemia, leukopenia, thrombocytopenia, increased serum ferritin

Erythrophagocytosis common, plasma cells common

Infiltration of capsule rare—individual cells

Lysozyme (muramidase), alpha$_1$-antichymotrypsin positive

Usually rapidly fatal (two thirds die within months)

TRUE HISTIOCYTIC LYMPHOMA

Very rare: only six well-documented cases in the literature

All cases are male

No common histologic features

Need markers and absence of T or B rearrangements

SYSTEMIC MASTOCYTOSIS

Round to spindled, monotonous, polygonal cells with inconspicuous nuclei, clear or granular cytoplasm, well-defined cell outlines; granules stain with Giemsa, toluidine blue, Leder

Scattered eosinophils usually present

Median age: 75 without skin lesions; 45 with

LN: partial or complete effacement

Spleen: always involved:
• Ill-defined granuloma-like nodules grossly, scattered throughout parenchyma
• Angiocentric fibrotic nodules with small clusters of mast cells embedded within

Skin: urticaria pigmentosa

Osteoblastic and osteoclastic lesions

Marrow: most frequent noncutaneous site (90%); increased reticulin, focal (more common) or diffuse involvement; any distribution, both monocellular and polycellular (eosinophils, lymphocytes, histiocytes) lesions

Horny et al. classification:

Type	Marrow involvement	Uninvolved marrow	Associations
I	Focal	Normal	Urticaria pigmentosa
II	Focal	Granulocytic hyperplasia	Myeloproliferative disorders
III	Diffuse	—	Mast cell leukemia

Types II and III have more aggressive course than type I

13

GASTROINTESTINAL TRACT AND PERITONEUM

Disorders Common to all Levels of the GI Tract

CARCINOID TUMORS

Tumors of APUD (amine precursor uptake and decarboxylation) cells

All are potentially malignant tumors

More carcinoid tumors occur in the GI tract than elsewhere

60–80% occur in "midgut", that is, appendix or ileum; 10–20% in "hindgut" (mostly rectum), 10–25% in "foregut" (stomach or proximal duodenum)

Tumors in appendix and rectum are rarely malignant, despite extensive local spread

Tumors in the duodenum tend to be low grade and may be associated with Zollinger-Ellison syndrome (gastrinoma) or neurofibromatosis (somatostatinoma)

Tumors in ileum, stomach, and colon are frequently malignant

Most common malignant tumor of the small bowel

Gastric and ileal lesions are frequently multicentric

By convention, 0.1 mm is division between microcarcinoid (hyperplasia) and carcinoid (neoplasia); submucosal invasion warrants diagnosis of carcinoid regardless of size

Usually small, well-defined submucosal elevations, often yellowish in color, covered by a flattened mucosa, which may ulcerate or form a polypoid projection

Monotonous round cells with pale pink cytoplasm, minimal mitotic activity or pleomorphism; infiltrating tumor cells induce a desmoplastic response

Growth pattern tends to vary with location: trabecular or microglandular in the foregut and hindgut, solid nests or insular in the midgut

All are argyrophilic (Grimelius stain); midgut carcinoids are also usually argentaffilic (Fontana-Masson)

Immunoreactive for keratin, CEA (apical or luminal), NSE, chromogranin, synaptophysin, Leu7, serotonin

Usually S-100 negative except in the appendix

Often are multihormonal by special stains

Indicators of aggressive behavior include size >2 cm, spread beyond submucosa (except in the appendix), mitoses, ulceration, necrosis

5 yr survival drops markedly once tumor invades into serosa or beyond (85% down to 5%)

When >2 cm, two thirds will have already metastasized; when <1 cm, <5% will have metastasized

CLASSIC CARCINOID

Solid nests of small monotonous cells

Often invade nerves, muscle, lymphatics, even serosa

ADENOCARCINOID (TUBULAR ADENOCARCINOID)

Glandular formation without solid nests; abundant stroma

Often misdiagnosed as adenocarcinoma

Usually lack seratonin; often positive for glucagon

Seen in small intestine and appendix (tip)

Prognosis same as classic type and depends on location

ATYPICAL CARCINOID

Obvious endocrine features but with invasion, necrosis, mitoses

Better prognosis than adenocarcinoma, but worse than classic carcinoid

MUCINOUS CARCINOID/CLEAR CELL CARCINOID

Essentially unique to the appendix (see later)

Carcinoid Syndrome

Paroxysmal flushing, asthma-like wheezing, right-sided heart failure, attacks of explosive watery diarrhea, abdominal pain, edema

Seen in 1% patients with carcinoid tumors, 10% of those with gastrointestinal carcinoids

Principal agent responsible for symptoms appears to be serotonin

Serotonin (5-hydroxytryptamine, 5-HT) formed by hydroxylating tryptophan to 5-hydroxytryptophan (5-HTP) and then decarboxylating to 5-HT

Foregut carcinoids lack the decarboxylase, and therefore produce mostly 5-HTP rather than 5-HT

Liver usually metabolizes 5-HT and 5-HTP to 5-hydroxyindoleacetic acid (5-HIAA); for distal gastrointestinal carcinoids to produce the carcinoid syndrome, generally need liver metastases

SMOOTH MUSCLE TUMORS

Gastric, esophageal, and rectal tumors are more likely to be benign; small intestinal and proximal colonic tumors are usually malignant

LEIOMYOMA

Small, well defined, <4 cm

Common, often multiple

May ulcerate overlying mucosa—still benign

Smooth muscle tumors in the stomach often have unusual features: extreme cellularity, occasional large cells with bizarre hyperchromatic nuclei, marked diffuse vascularity, palisading of nuclei, clear cytoplasm

≤1 mitosis/10 high power fields (HPF)

Myofibrils may be sparse or even absent; some prefer to refer to these as *stromal tumors*

SMOOTH MUSCLE TUMORS OF UNDETERMINED MALIGNANT POTENTIAL
AKA: STUMP
Generally high cellularity, necrosis, hemorrhage
Fewer than 5 mitoses/10 HPF
Some will behave in a malignant fashion, others benign

LEIOMYOSARCOMA
5 or more mitoses/10 HPF
Usually >5 cm with areas of necrosis, hemorrhage, extreme cellularity, and marked atypia
Often sufficiently poorly differentiated to be diagnosable as a smooth muscle tumor only by immunostain; may even be negative for smooth muscle actin: "malignant stromal tumor"; many of these are CD34+
Most commonly metastasizes to liver and lung
Metastases can develop ≥10 yr after removal of primary

LEIOMYOBLASTOMA
AKA: clear cell or epithelioid leiomyoma/leiomyosarcoma
Round cells with a central nucleus and abundant clear cytoplasm (probably fixation artifact)
Majority are benign, some are malignant
Almost all of these occur in the stomach; malignant ones tend to be on the posterior (vs. anterior) wall, have smaller cells, anaplasia, alveolar arrangement, less reticulin, and *higher mitotic rate*

LYMPHOPROLIFERATIVE DISORDERS
90% of GI tract lymphomas are diffuse, 10% are follicular
Most are large B-cell lymphomas; second most common type is small cleaved
Lymphomas in the GI tract tend to remain localized for prolonged periods before progressing
Overall survival good compared with carcinomas (5 yr = 45%); however, once becomes disseminated, essentially always fatal within 2 yr
Lymphomas used to be classified as "Western type (sporadic)" or "Mediterranean"; the former included large cell lymphomas, Burkitt's, and others; the latter most closely approximated what are now called MALT lymphomas (see later)
Currently, it seems more reasonable to use the conventional (although constantly evolving) classification for nodal lymphomas to subdivide GI tract lymphomas, with some special considerations

LOCALIZED LYMPHOID HYPERPLASIA
AKA: "pseudolymphoma" in the stomach, "rectal tonsil" in the rectum
Lymphoid proliferation usually is diffuse (stomach, proximal small intestine, rectum), although can be follicular (nodular) in the terminal ileum and appendix
Distinguish from "true lymphomas" by polymorphous infiltrate, presence of well-formed reactive lymphoid follicles, proliferation of vessels, associated dense collagenous fibrosis, or ulceration (more common when benign)
Many of these may actually be low-grade MALT lymphomas while still in their reversible state (see later)

DIFFUSE LARGE CELL LYMPHOMA
Most common type; almost all are B-cell; may show immunoblastic cytology
Men affected more commonly than women
Usually found in the stomach (50–60%); 20–30% in the small intestine (usually ileum); 10–20% in the colon
Often are Ki-1 (CD30) positive
Most of these may represent the high-grade form of MALT lymphoma

MUCOSAL ASSOCIATED LYMPHOID TISSUE (MALT) LYMPHOMAS
Men and women affected equally
Cell morphology varies from diffuse small cleaved to intermediate "centrocytic" type
These lesions appear to initially represent an over-reaction to persistent or recurrent antigenic stimulation (e.g., *Helicobacter pylori* in the stomach); at this stage, the "lymphoma" (because often monoclonal) is treatable and reversible by elimination of the antigen (e.g., antibiotics); later, with dissemination, disease becomes antigen independent and, although usually indolent, is no longer reversible
Lymphoepithelial lesions common (distinguishing feature), as are reactive follicles with germinal centers and plasma cells
Low- and high-grade types exist, the latter often arising in the setting of a lower grade lesion

IMMUNOPROLIFERATIVE SMALL INTESTINE DISEASE (IPSID)
AKA: Mediterranean lymphoma
Probably a subtype of the MALT lymphomas, in that this disease appears to be reversible with antibiotics or antihelminthics in early stages, but not later
Presents at 40–45 yr, usually with malabsorption
Usually involves the proximal small bowel
Diffuse proliferation in the lamina propria of initially mature plasma cells and lymphocytes associated with increased serum IgA levels
When undergoes transition to a lymphoma, often a large cell histology with immunoblastic and plasmacytic features and a rapid downhill course

MULTIPLE LYMPHOMATOUS POLYPOSIS
Extranodal mantle zone lymphoma involving the GI tract
Accounts for <5% of all GI lymphomas; most common in stomach and small intestine
Proliferation of intermediate size lymphocytes, usually straddling the muscularis mucosae
Distinguish from MALT lymphomas by lack of lymphoepithelial lesions and absence of germinal centers

BURKITT'S LYMPHOMA
Non-endemic form usually affects older individuals and involves the ileum
(See Hematolymphoid outline)

ENTEROPATHY ASSOCIATED T-CELL LYMPHOMA
Wide age range (30–70 yr)
Usually preceded by a 20–30 yr history of malabsorption, most commonly celiac sprue
Seen in association with the 10% of celiac sprue patients who do *not* have antibodies to alpha-gliatin
Most commonly proximal small bowel
Often CD30+ (large, bizarre multinucleated cells; mimics Hodgkin's disease)

ESOPHAGUS

Normal Anatomy
Extends from C6 to T11 or T12
10–11 cm long in newborn, 25 cm in adult (on average)
Endoscopists measure distances in the esophagus from the incisors (the gastroesophageal junction is therefore usually located at 38–41 cm)

Three points of luminal narrowing:
- Cricoid cartilage
- Where left mainstem bronchus crosses anterior to the esophagus (midway down)
- Diaphragm

Upper and lower sphincters defined manometrically; no morphological landmarks

Outer longitudinal muscle layer is striated for the first 6–8 cm

No serosa; lesions can easily spread into mediastinum

Malformations (Congenital and Acquired)

TRACHEOESOPHAGEAL FISTULAS
(See Lung outline)

HETEROTOPIC TISSUE
GASTRIC MUCOSA
Seen in both children and adults, most commonly just distal to cricoid cartilage

May be detected as a filling defect

Resembles gastric mucosa grossly—may ulcerate

Mostly mucin-secreting cells; chief and parietal cells rare

May give rise to adenocarcinoma
SALIVARY GLAND
Rare; middle or distal esophagus

ESOPHAGEAL RINGS/WEBS
Either fold of mucosa (most commonly) or localized annular thickening of muscle

Generally designated *webs* when above the aortic arch and *rings* when below

Often asymptomatic or episodic dysphagia
WEBS
Usually women, usually >40 yr old, usually upper esophagus

Can be seen in association with iron deficiency anemia (Plummer-Vinson syndrome)
RINGS
AKA: Schatzki's rings

Found in distal 5 cm of esophagus, usually at squamo-columnar junction (squamous mucosa on upper surface, gastric on lower)

2–4 mm thick, protrude <5 mm

DIVERTICULA
ZENKER'S (PULSION)
Upper esophagus at junction with pharynx
TRACTION
Usually lower third of esophagus near hilum of lungs

HIATAL HERNIA
Saclike dilatation of stomach present above the diaphragm
SLIDING HERNIA (90%)
Congenitally short esophagus or acquired from esophageal scarring with traction on the stomach

Extent of herniation and degree of symptoms accentuated by swallowing

Predisposes to reflux
ROLLING (PARAESOPHAGEAL) HERNIA (10%)
Portion of cardia protrudes through the diaphragm into the thorax alongside the esophagus

Vulnerable to strangulation and infarction

LACERATIONS
AKA: Mallory-Weiss tears

Linear irregular lacerations oriented longitudinally usually at the gastroesophageal junction (GEJ)

Occur following fits of vomiting; most commonly in alcoholics

May involve only mucosa or even the full wall

Usually not massive, but do account for 5–10% of cases of massive hematemesis

VARICES
Dilatation of vascular channels (coronary veins) in lower esophagus to divert flow out of the portal system in patient with portal hypertension, usually secondary to cirrhosis

Difficult to visualize postmortem because varices collapse

Massive hematemesis

40% fatality rate; of those who survive, half will rebleed, and 40% of those will die

ESOPHAGEAL DYSMOTILITY
ACHALASIA
Motor dysfunction resulting in: decreased peristalsis, incomplete relaxation of lower esophageal sphincter (LES), increased basal LES tone

Progressive dilatation of the esophagus above the LES

In sporadic form, myenteric plexus may be absent from upper portion of esophagus but is present in region of LES

Cause is usually unknown

2–7% of patients will develop esophageal carcinoma

Can occur in Chagas' disease, in which the trypanosome infection causes destruction of the myenteric plexus of the esophagus, duodenum, colon, and ureter
PLUMMER-VINSON SYNDROME
Anemia, atrophic gastritis, dysphagia; usually affects women

Increased risk of squamous cell carcinoma of the upper esophagus, oropharynx, or tongue

Associated with upper esophageal webs
PROGRESSIVE SYSTEMIC SCLEROSIS
Part of CREST syndrome (calcinosis, Reynaud's, esophageal dysmotility, sclerodactyly, telangiectasias)

Vasculitis with muscle wall degeneration
IDIOPATHIC MUSCULAR HYPERTROPHY
Primary abnormality of neural control of the distal esophageal musculature, resulting in esophageal spasm

Affects predominantly inner circular muscle layer
LEIOMYOMATOSIS

Inflammatory Lesions

REFLUX ESOPHAGITIS
Produced by recurrent or prolonged reflux; promoted by elevated acidity and disordered esophageal motility

Often associated with sliding hiatal hernia, Zollinger-Ellison syndrome, scleroderma

Histologic changes include basal hyperplasia (>15–20% of the epithelial thickness), elongation of the vascular papillae to greater than one half to two thirds of mucosal height, intraepithelial eosinophils, numerous intraepithelial neutrophils

INFECTIOUS ESOPHAGITIS
BACTERIAL
VIRAL
Cytomegalovirus (CMV): submucosal cells with inclusions

Herpes: epithelial cells with ground-glass nuclei; often form multinucleated giant cells
FUNGAL
Candida: white plaques, usually in middle to distal esophagus; budding blastospores and pseudohyphae
Mucormycosis
Aspergillosis

OTHER CAUSES OF ESOPHAGITIS
Ingestion of irritants
Prolonged gastric intubation
Radiation/Anticancer therapy
Crohn's disease
Pemphigus vulgaris
Uremia
Graft-vs.-host disease

BARRETT'S METAPLASIA
Conversion of stratified squamous epithelium to columnar epithelium in the lower portion of the esophagus
Complications: ulceration, stricture, adenocarcinoma (~10%)
Classification:
• Barrett's type I: no residual squamous islands are present
• Barrett's type II: squamous islands persist among the columnar mucosa

Types
SPECIALIZED TYPE (INTESTINAL OR COLONIC)
Goblet cells and columnar cells (goblet cells contain sialomucin [acid mucin] and stain positively with Alcian blue at pH 2.5)
Most common type seen in adults
Incomplete: gastric foveolar cells intermixed with intestinal goblet, absorptive, Paneth, and endocrine cells
Complete: only intestinal-type cells present
CARDIAC OR JUNCTIONAL TYPE
Almost entirely mucin cells
Generally need to see ≤3 cm above the GEJ (i.e., <35 cm) to be comfortable calling this more than an irregular Z-line
Some pathologists do not consider this Barrett's at all, but rather simply a very irregular Z-line
ATROPHIC FUNDAL TYPE
Contains few parietal and chief cells
Rare; usually the type seen in children

Dysplasia
• Hyperchromatic and crowding nuclei = low-grade dysplasia
• Glandular distortion and nuclear hyperchromasia extending to upper portions of epithelium = high-grade dysplasia
In general, when high-grade dysplasia is present in a biopsy, there is a 70% chance that carcinoma is already present

Neoplasms

BENIGN LESIONS
Uncommon; usually small and asymptomatic
INFLAMMATORY FIBROUS POLYP
AKA: fibrovascular polyps, inflammatory pseudotumors
Usually pedunculated and solitary

85% located in upper third of esophagus
Submucosal proliferation of vascularized, inflamed fibrous stroma with eosinophils frequently present
Similar to lesion in stomach
SQUAMOUS PAPILLOMA
Usually lower esophagus; men over 40 yr; may be multiple
ADENOMA
Arises in Barrett's mucosa
LEIOMYOMA
GRANULAR CELL TUMOR
LOCALIZED AMYLOIDOSIS

SQUAMOUS CELL CARCINOMA
80–85% of esophageal carcinomas
10% of all cancers of the GI tract
More common among blacks and males
Risk factors: lye strictures (1000× risk), chronic *alcohol* (20–30× risk, esp. hard liquor), and *tobacco* (10–20× risk) use, consumption of foods rich in *Aspergillus,* nitrites, or nitrosamines; chronic vitamin deficiency, achalasia, esophagitis, Plummer-Vinson syndrome
20% upper third, 50% middle third, 30% lower third
May present as hemorrhage, sepsis, tracheoesophageal fistula
Most commonly fungating polypoid lesion (60%), less commonly necrotic deeply ulcerating lesion (35%), rarely diffusely infiltrating wall with thickening, rigidity, luminal narrowing
Extensive circumferential and/or longitudinal spread common because of rich lymphatic supply
Usually well into wall or beyond by time of diagnosis; only about half of cases resectable
30% 1 yr survival; 5–10% 5 yr survival
SUPERFICIAL (EARLY) SQUAMOUS CARCINOMA
Limited to mucosa or submucosa (stage I)
May be inapparent grossly
5 yr survival good: 65–90%
VERRUCOUS CARCINOMA
Rare
Predominantly exophytic growth with pushing margins
Slow growing; rarely if ever metastasizes
EPIDERMOID CARCINOMA WITH SPINDLE-CELL STROMA
AKA: pseudosarcoma, carcinosarcoma, spindle cell carcinoma
Usually large (~6 cm) polypoid lesion of the middle to lower esophagus, often with very inconspicuous epithelial component, which is usually squamous
Spindle component resembles malignant fibrous histiocytoma; may have focal cartilage or bone or skeletal muscle differentiation
Prognosis actually better than traditional squamous cell carcinoma: 3 yr survival ~40%

Staging
T1   Lamina propria or submucosal invasion
T2   Muscularis propria invasion
T3   Adventitial invasion
T4   Adjacent structures
N1   Regional nodes involved

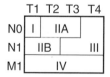

ADENOCARCINOMA

5–10% of esophageal carcinomas

Almost always white; male : female = 5 : 1; median age 50

Usually middle or lower third, often GEJ

Vast majority probably arise in setting of Barrett's mucosa

Gross: mass or nodular elevation in otherwise intact mucosa

Histologic types:

- Intestinal: as seen in stomach or intestines
- Diffuse: diffuse infiltration of mucin-producing cells
- Adenosquamous: mixture of squamous cell and adeno-carcinoma

Same staging as for squamous cell carcinoma (SCC)

As with SCC, most are high stage at diagnosis

OTHER TUMORS OF THE ESOPHAGUS

BASALOID TYPE CARCINOMA

Thought by many to be a type of adenoid cystic carcinoma

Small, blue cells with peripheral palisading, round glandular lumina, abundant basal lamina material

Extremely aggressive behavior

SMALL CELL CARCINOMA

Highly malignant; neuroendocrine carcinoma

Usually fungating grossly

Distinguish from better differentiated carcinoid tumor

OTHER MALIGNANT TUMORS

Mucoepidermoid carcinoma

Leiomyosarcoma

Malignant melanoma

Malignant lymphoma

Plasmacytoma

STOMACH

Normal Anatomy

Mucosal surface and gastric pits lined by surface mucous cells

Neck mucous cells are the progenitor cells for the glandular epithelium and the pit and surface epithelium

Glands of cardia and antrum are similar to neck mucous cells

Fundic glands contain the parietal (HCl and intrinsic factor) and chief (pepsinogen) cells

Antrum contains endocrine cells, variably designated as enteroendocrine, enterochromaffin, Kulchitsky's, or APUD (amine precursor uptake and decarboxylase) cells

Malformations (Congenital and Acquired)

HIATAL HERNIAS

(See earlier under Esophagus)

HETEROTOPIC PANCREAS

Relatively common: 1–2% of the general population

Dome-shaped mass (1–2 cm), nipple-like projection, or symmetric cone

75–85% occur in submucosa, rest in muscularis

61% are in the antrum, 24% in the pylorus

Endocrine pancreas (islets) present in only one third

PYLORIC STENOSIS

CONGENITAL HYPERTROPHIC PYLORIC STENOSIS

Familial malformation; seen in 1/300–900 births; male : female = 4 : 1; most common in first born

Hypertrophy and perhaps hyperplasia of the circular muscle of the muscularis propria of the pylorus

Present with regurgitation and vomiting in 2nd or 3rd wk

ACQUIRED PYLORIC STENOSIS

Long-term complication of chronic antral gastritis and/or peptic ulcer disease

Can also be seen in carcinomas of the pylorus, head of pancreas, or lymphomas

GASTRIC ANTRAL VASCULAR ECTASIA

AKA: watermelon stomach

Persistent blood loss; may be severe

Prominent radiating mucosal stripes arising in the pylorus

Unknown etiology

Inflammatory/Non-Neoplastic

ACUTE GASTRITIS

Acute mucosal inflammation, usually transient

Continuum including acute gastritis, acute hemorrhagic gastritis, acute erosive gastritis, and acute stress erosions

Usually only partial erosion of the mucosa, not penetrating the muscularis mucosa

Often accompanied by focal hemorrhage into mucosa

In severe forms can have sloughing of the mucosa and extensive lamina propria hemorrhages

Can be caused by excessive ethyl alcohol consumption, chronic aspirin (or other nonsteroidal antiinflammatory drug) use, heavy smoking, shock, severe stress (see later)

When severe (acute hemorrhagic erosive gastritis), mortality can exceed 50%

CHRONIC GASTRITIS

Infiltration of lamina propria by lymphocytes and plasma cells combined with varying degrees of gastric atrophy

Many classification schemes used

IMMUNE GASTRITIS (TYPE A; FUNDAL)

Involves fundic mucosa preferentially; antrum usually spared

Patients have circulating antibodies to parietal cells and/or intrinsic factor

Hypochlorhydria, loss of parietal cells, hypergastrinemia

Significant gastric atrophy and intestinal metaplasia

10% will develop pernicious anemia after several years

Associated with other autoimmune disorders (Hashimoto's thyroiditis, Addison's disease)

NON-IMMUNE GASTRITIS (TYPE B; ANTRAL)

No associated parietal cell antibodies or pernicious anemia

Four times more common than type A

Helicobacter pylori implicated in many cases as causal agent; it is present on the surface of the epithelium and is *not* seen in areas of intestinal metaplasia

- Hypersecretory subtype:

    Restricted to the antrum; usually minimal fundic atrophy

    Hyperacidity, often leading to duodenal ulcers

    Normal gastrin levels

- Environmental subtype:
    Most common form of chronic gastritis
    Involves both fundus and antrum
    Initially patchy in antrum, later diffuse in antrum and fundus
    Strong association with atrophy, metaplasia, carcinoma
    Begins as superficial gastritis, progresses to atrophic
    Etiologically related to ethyl alcohol use, but not to smoking

Histologic Classification

CHRONIC SUPERFICIAL GASTRITIS
Inflammation confined to superficial mucosa (upper one third)
Mild flattening of mucosa

CHRONIC ATROPHIC GASTRITIS
More obvious thinning of mucosa—may appear red grossly since submucosal vessels more visible
Full-thickness inflammation involving the glandular portion of mucosa as well as more superficial areas
Graded mild, moderate, and severe based on thickness of glandular portion in relation to mucosa
With atrophy, glands become cystically dilated, commonly metaplastic (see later); in type A, there is an absence of parietal cells

GASTRIC ATROPHY
Thinning of gastric mucosa in absence of inflammation, usually seen as an end stage of chronic gastritis

Sydney System
Need at least two biopsies each from the fundus and antrum
Diagnosis is given a multipart name including the following:
- Etiology: (if known) for example, autoimmune
- Type: acute, chronic, special (granulomatous, eosinophilic)
- Distribution: antral, fundic, or pangastritis
- Graded variables: inflammation, activity (mild = one-third pits, moderate = one- to two-thirds pits, severe = greater than two-thirds pits), metaplasia, atrophy, *Helicobacter pylori* density

SPECIFIC GASTRIDITIES

GRANULOMATOUS GASTRITIS
Seen in sarcoidosis but also as an isolated disorder
Generally 40 yr or older
?TB, mycosis, Crohn's

LYMPHOCYTIC GASTRITIS
T-cell infiltration of foveolae and surface epithelium
Frequently seen in patients with Celiac sprue

EOSINOPHILIC GASTRITIS
Infiltration of the mucosa and sometimes submucosa by eosinophils
Usually involves the distal stomach and the proximal duodenum
Necrotizing vasculitis may be present
Probably allergic reaction to ingested material

GASTRITIS IN IMMUNOSUPPRESSED
CMV, herpes simplex virus (HSV), cryptosporidiosis, mycobacteria

GASTRIC ULCERS

STRESS ULCERS
Multiple small lesions, mainly gastric, sometimes duodenum

Shedding of superficial epithelium to full-thickness ulceration
Occurs in setting of "severe stress," for example, shock, sepsis, severe trauma, etc.
Pathogenesis usually unclear
- Cushing's ulcers: in setting of elevated intracranial pressure; increased acid secretion caused by increased vagal tone
- Steroid ulcer: following steroid use
- Curling's ulcers: associated with extensive burns

PEPTIC ULCERS
Chronic, usually solitary lesion (80%) occurring at any level of GI tract exposed to acid-peptic juices
Most commonly 1st portion duodenum (~80%), antrum of stomach (~20%), Barrett's esophagus, Meckel's
Remitting and relapsing course; male : female = 3 : 1 (duodenal); 1.5–2 : 1 (gastric); pain after eating
50% <2 cm, 75% <3 cm, 10% >4 cm
Oval, sharply delimited defect with tendency for overhanging mucosal margins, especially proximally
Minimal if any heaping up of margins (common in carcinoma)
Gastric folds radiate out from ulcer
Nearly all patients have concurrent chronic antral gastritis (e.g., *Helicobacter pylori*); those who don't are usually habitual aspirin users
Fatal in ~5%: 70% caused by perforation, 10% due to bleeding
- Duodenal:
    Genetic influences appear to be involved
    Increased incidence in alcoholic cirrhosis, chronic renal failure, chronic obstructive pulmonary disease (COPD), hyperparathyroidism
    Increase in both the basal and stimulated level of acid secretion, and more rapid gastric emptying are common
    Anterior wall more commonly than posterior
- Gastric:
    Genetic influences do not appear to be involved
    Low to normal acidity; probably abnormal mucosal resistance
    Usually lesser curve
    1–3% will develop gastric carcinoma

GASTRIC HYPERPLASIAS
AKA: hypertrophic gastritis
Neither hypertrophic nor inflammatory—hyperplastic
Giant, cerebriform enlargement of the rugal folds
Radiologically, can be confused with lymphoma

MÉNÉTRIER'S DISEASE
Hyperplasia of the surface mucous (foveolar) cells with tortuous, corkscrew cystic dilatation extending to the base of the glands
Hypochlorhydria, often hypoproteinemia
Usually chronic and severe; progressive
Antrum usually uninvolved
May show slightly increased risk of carcinoma

ZOLLINGER-ELLISON SYNDROME
Hyperplasia, predominantly of the glandular cells (mainly parietal cells, which tend to crowd out the chief cells; sometimes enterochromaffin-like cells also proliferate) secondary to gastrin-secreting tumor (20% are associated with multiple endocrine neoplasia I)
Gland lumen size is normal; no cyst formation
Hyperchlorhydria

HYPERPLASIA OF PARIETAL AND CHIEF CELLS

AKA: hypertrophic hypersecretory gastropathy
Two variants of unknown etiology:
- Protein losing:
    Patients are often hypergastrinemic
    Histology mimics that of Ménétrier's disease
- Non–protein losing:
    Patients are hyperchlorhydric but *not* hypergastrinemic
    Histology mimics Zollinger-Ellison syndrome

METAPLASIA

Most commonly, but not exclusively, seen in the setting of atrophic gastritis
PYLORIC METAPLASIA
With age, fundic gland mass decreases and is replaced by pyloric glands
CILIATED CELL METAPLASIA
INTESTINAL METAPLASIA
Replacement by mucosa with goblet cells, absorptive cells, Paneth cells, etc.
Small bowel (intestinal) and large bowel (colonic) types
Both may be either complete or incomplete:
- Complete (type I): sialomucin predominates (goblet cells)
- Incomplete (type II): absorptive cells absent; gastric foveolar cells retained
    Type IIA: foveolar cells contain neutral mucins
    Type IIB: foveolar cells contain sulphomucins
When incomplete, special stains needed to detect the different staining properties of the mucins

POLYPS
HYPERPLASTIC (85%)
AKA: inflammatory, regenerative
Exaggerated regenerative response to injury
Usually multiple, most sessile, <1 cm, randomly distributed
Elongated and distorted glands, tubules, microcysts with a single layer of regular cells, predominantly foveolar
Stroma often inflamed, edematous, with patchy fibrosis
Often seen coexisting with gastric carcinoma elsewhere
ADENOMATOUS (10%)
Neoplastic lesion
Usually single, antral, up to 3–4 cm; larger are pedunculated
Closely packed glandlike tubular structures or villi with dysplastic cells; probably arise in intestinal metaplasia
Tubular, villous, and tubulovillous varieties; 10% are flat or depressed (higher rate of malignant transformation)
Estimated risks of synchronous and metachronous gastric adenocarcinomas has varied widely among different studies: 4–50% and 3–75%, respectively
FUNDIC GLAND POLYPS
Multiple small polyps with cystically dilated fundic glands forming microcysts lined by fundic epithelium
Can arise secondary to omeprazole therapy
INFLAMMATORY FIBROID POLYP
Can occur anywhere in GI tract, but ~75% occur in stomach, usually the antrum
Mean age 53; presents with pain and/or obstruction
Can become quite large
Proliferation of loose connective tissue in the submucosa with small-caliber, thin-walled vessels surrounded by hypocellular stroma; inflammatory cells
Overlying mucosa is stretched and eventually ulcerates
HAMARTOMATOUS
Peutz-Jeghers syndrome
Juvenile (retention) polyps

POLYPOID MUCOSAL PROLAPSE
AKA: polypoid cystic gastritis, polypoid hypertrophic gastritis
Occurs on the gastric side of a gastroenterostomy stoma
Same histology as hyperplastic polyps

Neoplasms

Staging
T1 Lamina propria or submucosal invasion
T2 Muscularis propria or subserosal invasion
T3 Penetration of serosa
T4 Adjacent structures
N1 Perigastric nodes within 3 cm of primary involved
N2 Perigastric nodes >3 cm from primary or other local lymph nodes (LNs)

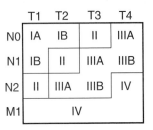

	T1	T2	T3	T4
N0	IA	IB	II	IIIA
N1	IB	II	IIIA	IIIB
N2	II	IIIA	IIIB	IV
M1	IV			

ADENOCARCINOMA
85–90% of gastric malignancies
Incidence particularly high in Japan, Chile, Scotland, Finland; lower in U.S., U.K., Canada, Greece; more common in blacks
Overall incidence in U.S. has been steadily dropping over past several years, but the incidence of carcinoma in the cardia is increasing; currently, 50% of gastric cancers in white men are in the cardia; (Male : female = 8 : 1)
Risk factors: dietary/environmental (still unidentified)—salt, low intake of animal fat/protein, complex carbohydrates, nitrates; chronic gastritis and pernicious anemia; gastric adenomatous polyps
Accompanied by hypochlorhydria in 85–90% cases, and chronic atrophic gastritis is usually present
Lesser curvature involved 3× more frequently than greater
Cells generally positive for keratin, EMA, CEA
Often present in advanced stage; may present with metastases; only about 50% resectable at diagnosis; 80–90% have local LN metastases
Virchow's node: isolated metastasis to left supraclavicular LN (also called Trousseau's sign)
Overall 5 yr survival still 5–15%
SUPERFICIAL SPREADING (EARLY) CARCINOMA
10–35% of gastric carcinomas
Limited to mucosa and submucosa
Less than 20% have LN metastases; 5 yr survival 80–95%

Histologic Types
INTESTINAL TYPE
AKA: expanding carcinoma
Relatively cohesive mass of tumor cells; pushing margins
May be nodular, polypoid, or ulcerated
Usually well demarcated grossly
Can be composed of foveolar cells, intestinal columnar, and/or goblet cells
Arise from metaplastic epithelium

Used to be the more common type, but incidence has been decreasing relative to the diffuse type

DIFFUSE TYPE
AKA: infiltrative carcinoma; linitis plastica

Individually invading tumor cells with intracellular mucin vacuoles, often forming signet ring cells

Extent of tumor cannot be appreciated grossly

Does not appear to be related to environmental factors; occurs at a younger age than the intestinal type; incidence has been steady for many years

Marked degree of inflammation and desmoplasia, and the inconspicuous tumor cells may lead to missed diagnosis

Prognostic Factors
Good: distal gastric involvement (vs. proximal), pushing margin, small size, intestinal type, inflammatory infiltrate

Poor: young age, deep invasion, infiltrative margin, diffuse type, positive margins, LN involvement

Metastases
Liver metastases most common with intestinal type

Diffuse type: peritoneum, lung, adrenal gland, ovary

Krukenberg's tumor: bilateral ovarian involvement

CARCINOID TUMORS
(See also beginning of this outline)

5% of GI carcinoids occur in stomach

Slow growing, but always malignant

When metastasize (30%), usually regional LNs only

Much better prognosis than adenocarcinoma, but clearly more aggressive than carcinoid tumors of the appendix

Two subtypes:
- G-cell tumor (gastrinoma): antral, immunoreactive for gastrin, sometimes associated with peptic ulcer
- Enterochromaffin-like cells (ECL tumor): multiple, often polypoid, fundic; believed to result from gastrin stimulation

OTHER CARCINOMAS
SMALL CELL CARCINOMA
Highly malignant; neuroendocrine carcinoma

ADENOSQUAMOUS AND SQUAMOUS CELL CARCINOMA
Less than 1% gastric carcinomas

MUCINOUS CARCINOMA
Relatively good prognosis

HEPATOID ADENOCARCINOMA
PARIETAL GLAND CARCINOMA

LYMPHOMA
(See also beginning of this outline)

3–5% of all gastric malignancies

Most common site for primary lymphomas in GI tract

Some of the MALT-type lymphomas are associated with *Helicobacter pylori*

Much better prognosis than gastric adenocarcinomas

Can be treated with radiation alone; if transmural, risk gastric perforation

SMOOTH MUSCLE TUMORS
(See also beginning of this outline)

Most smooth muscle tumors in the stomach are benign

Smooth muscle tumors in this location often have bizarre features (extreme cellularity, occasional large cells with bizarre hyperchromatic nuclei, marked diffuse vascularity, palisading of nuclei, clear cytoplasm) and still be benign; base determination on mitotic rate

OTHER TUMORS
GLOMUS TUMOR
Clear epithelioid cells arranged around dilated vessels

Morphologically similar, perhaps histogenetically, to leiomyoblastoma

LIPOMA
GRANULAR CELL TUMORS
NEUROFIBROMA, SCHWANNOMA
Usually well demarcated, firm, <4 cm; arise in muscularis

May be leiomyomata with minimal to no myofibers

Many prefer to refer to all such tumors as *stromal tumors*

SMALL INTESTINE

Normal
Length: in an adult, averages 6–7 m (20 ft)

Epithelium regenerates every 72–96 hr (3–4 days)

Cell types: undifferentiated, Paneth, goblet, endocrine

Malformations (Congenital and Acquired)

ATRESIA/STENOSIS
Atresia: failure to canalize; blind pouch or fibrous cord

85–90% are solitary

Radiographically: "string of pearls"

May be related to in utero mechanical injury

Types of atresia:
- Type I: 20%; continuous bowel lumen interrupted by a mucosal septum and an intact mesentery
- Type II: 35–40%; blind proximal and distal ends connected by a fibrous cord; mesentery intact
- Type III: 40–45%, blind proximal and distal ends; unattached
- (Type IV: subset of Type III (~one third) with V-shaped mesenteric defect)

"Apple peel" atresia: interruption in distal duodenum or proximal jejunum with absence of the dorsal mesentery and obliteration of the superior mesenteric artery; the distal small intestine is shortened and has a spiral configuration

Stenosis: narrowing of canalized lumen (by fibrosis, stricture)

ABDOMINAL WALL DEFECTS
OMPHALOCELE
1/5000 live births

Amnion-enclosed extra-abdominal sac contains intestines and sometimes the liver

Arises in midline and involves the umbilical stump

Failure of intestines to return to abdomen at 10–11 wk

50% mortality

GASTROSCHISIS
1/12,000 live births

Non-enclosed paraumbilical abdominal wall defect
Abdominal contents (usually just bowel) externalized

DIVERTICULA
MESENTERIC
Congenital defects in the muscular wall (thinned)
Pseudodiverticula (muscle wall not present in outpouching)
Rare; most common in duodenum
MECKEL'S
Persistence of omphalomesenteric (vitelline) duct (connection between GI tract and umbilicus present at 4 wk; normally becomes obliterated to form a fibrous band, which is subsequently absorbed)
Solitary; antimesenteric; usually ileal (~30 cm from cecum)
Present in 2% of population, more commonly males
50% have some gastric mucosa; peptic ulceration may occur, usually in adjacent intestinal mucosa
Ectopic pancreas may also be seen in wall
Complications: perforate, ulcerate, bleed, intussusception

HETEROTOPIC TISSUE
PANCREAS
1–2 cm mucosal elevation
Ducts and acini, usually without islets
Can occur anywhere in small bowel; most common in duodenum (periampullary); least common in jejunum
May serve as a lead point for intussusception
GASTRIC MUCOSA
Discrete small nodules or sessile polyps in the duodenum
Fundic type mucosa with chief and parietal cells
ENDOMETRIOSIS

INTUSSUSCEPTION
Usually in infants or children; one segment of small bowel (the intussusceptum) becomes telescoped into the immediately distal segment of bowel (the intussuscipiens) and is propelled further inward by peristalsis, taking the mesentery with it; can lead to infarction
When occurs in adults, usually caused by a mass lesion, which forms the leading point of traction
In children, lymphoid hyperplasia often serves as the mass that forms the leading edge
Barium enema may reduce the lesion

Inflammatory Disorders

ISCHEMIC BOWEL DISEASE
Mesenteric artery successively branches; intermediate branches have numerous anastomoses with each other
May mimic Crohn's disease
• Obstruction of a main branch: extensive infarction
• Obstruction of a secondary branch: no effect (collaterals)
• Obstruction of a terminal branch: localized infarction

Transmural Infarction (Gangrene)
Short segment or more commonly substantial length
Grossly hemorrhagic, whether arterial or venous in origin
Arterial occlusions tend to have sharper margins; venous occlusions tend to fade gradually into normal bowel
Intense congestion, subserosal and submucosal hemorrhages, edema, later blood in lumen
Perforation likely within 3–4 days

ARTERIAL THROMBOSIS
Usually associated with/triggered by atherosclerosis
Other etiologies: vasospasm, dissecting aneurysm, tumor, fibromuscular hyperplasia of the intestinal arteries (seen in some patients on digoxin), acute arteritis (polyarteritis nodosa)
EMBOLIC OCCLUSIONS
Usually superior mesenteric because inferior has a more oblique take–off from aorta
Intracardiac or intra-aortic mural thrombi most commonly
VENOUS THROMBOSIS
25% of cases of transmural infarction
Following surgery, cardiac failure, polycythemia, mass

Hemorrhagic Gastroenteropathy
Usually related to hypoperfusion (e.g., shock)
Superficial layers affected first; extends deeper with increasing severity
Similar histology to transmural, but less severe

Chronic Ischemia
Fibrosis most pronounced in mucosa
Fibrotic narrowing can occur

MALABSORPTION SYNDROMES
Abnormal absorption of fat, fat-soluble vitamins, other vitamins, proteins, carbohydrates, minerals, usually with abnormal fecal excretion of fat (steatorrhea: >6 g/day)
Can be caused by defective intraluminal hydrolysis, mucosal abnormality, lymphatic obstruction, infection, etc.
Appearance of mucosa under dissecting scope can be correlated, roughly, with histology; patterns:

Appearance	Histology
Villous, finger-like	Normal
Villous, leaflike	Normal
Convoluted (cerebroid)	Partial villous atrophy
Mosaic	Subtotal villous atrophy
Flat	Near total villous atrophy

CELIAC DISEASE
AKA: celiac sprue, nontropical sprue, gluten sensitive enteropathy
Affects predominantly the proximal small bowel
Etiology is almost certainly a hypersensitivity response to gliadin (gluten) in the diet
80–90% are HLA-B8 or DR3
Associated with dermatitis herpetiformis (DH): 60–80% of patients with DH have abnormal intestinal villi; 75% show improvement of the skin lesions when placed on a gluten-free diet
Absence of villi (or marked flattening [should be 3× depth of crypts]), resulting in a flat mucosa, with plasma cells, absence of alpha₁-antitrypsin from crypt cells, and accumulation of large fat globules
Not diagnostic: same changes can be seen in kwashiorkor, dermatitis herpetiformis, and severe tropical sprue
90% of patients contain circulating antibodies to alpha-gliadin; antibody level does not correspond well to the severity of disease
Course of disease can be followed by monitoring serum IgA anti–smooth muscle endomesium levels
When increased lamina proprial accumulation of hyaline material occurs, some refer to as *collagenous sprue*

Complications:
- Intestinal malignant lymphoma (see also beginning of this outline) following longstanding disease in the 10% of patients who do *not* have antibodies to alpha-gliadin
- Chronic nonspecific ulcerative duodenojejunoileitis: may be an initial stage of the lymphoma described earlier
- Gastrointestinal carcinoma: rare; usually in jejunum; usually adenocarcinoma

TROPICAL SPRUE
Unrelated to gluten ingestion
Almost exclusively limited to tropics (living in or visiting)
May be related to enterotoxigenic *E. coli*
Responds to folic acid, Vitamin B_{12}, and tetracycline
Partial villous atrophy seen in most cases, more prominent in the distal small bowel
Inflammatory infiltrate has large numbers of lymphocytes and occasional eosinophils

WHIPPLE'S DISEASE (INTESTINAL LIPODYSTROPHY)
Large macrophages (stuffed with diastase-resistant PAS+ "bacilliform bodies") packing the lamina propria and distorting the villi, alternating with dilated lymphatic channels and empty spaces containing neutral lipids (occasionally with giant cells: lipogranulomas)
No significant inflammatory response
Organism not consistently identified on culture
Usually whites, male : female = 10 : 1, 30s–40s
Not restricted to bowel; similar macrophages can be seen in other parts of GI tract, LNs, heart, lung, liver, spleen, adrenals, nervous system

OTHER CAUSES OF MALABSORPTION
Biliary obstruction with bile acid deficiency
Chronic pancreatitis
Amyloidosis
Reduced small bowel length after surgical resection
Infections
Lymphatic obstruction

PEPTIC ULCER DISEASE
(See earlier under Stomach)

INFECTIOUS ENTEROCOLITIS
(See also Infectious Agents outline)

ORGANISMS ASSOCIATED WITH ENTEROINVASION
Usually ulceroinflammatory
- *Shigella* (see later under Colon)
- *Salmonella:*
    Invades and produces endotoxin (like *Shigella*) but generally does not ulcerate
    Immune response produces massive lymphoid hypertrophy (e.g., typhoid fever)
    May have secondary necrosis of mucosa overlying the lymphoid follicles
    Involves both the small and large intestine
- Others:
    Campylobacter jejuni, some strains of *E. coli,* TB, *Yersinia*
    Also viral, fungal, protozoal

ORGANISMS THAT ADHERE BUT DO NOT INVADE (TOXIN PRODUCING)
Vibrio cholerae and toxigenic *E. coli* produce toxin that activates adenylate cyclase; no histopathologic changes
Preformed *Clostridium* toxins or staphylococcal toxins can produce pathology without the organism

RADIATION ENTERITIS
Grossly, thickening of bowel wall caused by fibrosis, particularly in the submucosa

Mucosal ulceration
Early changes: increased mucus production, nuclear changes in the lining epithelium
Later: submucosal edema, then fibrosis and ulceration
Subendothelial accumulation of lipid-laden macrophages in vessels, with thrombosis and calcification

NONSTEROIDAL ANTI–INFLAMMATORY DRUG–INDUCED GUT LESIONS
Can see erosions or ulcers
Most characteristically, see strictures of the small intestine with diaphragm formation

CROHN'S DISEASE (REGIONAL ILEITIS)
Idiopathic, chronic, and recurrent inflammatory bowel disease with variably distributed but usually sharply delimited, typically transmural involvement of bowel at any level by noncaseating granulomatous inflammation, ulceration, and fibrous constriction
Onset usually in 20s and 30s; higher incidence in U.S., U.K., and Scandinavia than in U.S.S.R., South America
White > black; female ≥ male
Often intermittent attacks of diarrhea, fever, abdominal pain; attacks can be triggered by physical or emotional stress
Most commonly affects terminal ileum (65–75%) and/or colon (50–70%); colonic involvement alone in only 20–30%
Frequently "skip lesions" in GI tract, with intervening unaffected segments
Related lesions may be seen in skin, bone, muscle, lung
Pathogenesis unknown: theories include infectious, immunologic, vasculitis, etc.
Inflammation in wall initially edematous, but then becomes fibrous with longitudinal mucosal ulcerations, creeping fat, luminal narrowing, fissure formation (25–30%), and fistulous tracts
Histologically, transmural inflammation, relatively poorly formed noncaseating granulomas (present in only 65%), lymphoid aggregates and germinal centers, dilation or sclerosis of lymphatic channels
Complications: strictures, fistulae, abscesses, protein-losing enteropathy, Vitamin B_{12} malabsorption, ankylosing spondylitis
Increased risk of carcinoma (3%)

Neoplastic Diseases

Account for less than 5% of the tumors of the GI tract
Malignant tumors are about 50% more common than benign
Most of the malignant tumors are in the ileum

ADENOMA
Most often in duodenum and ileum
Similar to those of the colon
Larger ones, particularly villous adenomas, frequently undergo malignant transformation

BRUNNER'S GLAND ADENOMA
AKA: polypoid hamartoma, brunneroma
Nodular proliferation of all elements of normal Brunner's glands (ducts, stroma)
Probably not true neoplasm; hyperplasia

PEUTZ-JEGHERS SYNDROME
Hamartomatous polyps
Glands supported by broad bands of smooth muscle
Columnar and goblet cells on surface, Paneth and endocrine cells near base

ADENOCARCINOMA
Can grow in napkin-ring or polypoid fashion
Most arise in the duodenum
40–60× less common than in the colon
Staging is similar to that in the colon EXCEPT:
• Only N0 and N1 for regional nodes uninvolved/involved
• Tis is intraepithelial only; intramucosal is T1
AMPULLARY CARCINOMA
Often arises from pre-existing villous adenoma, often with "benign" glands in villi but malignant cells in base
Intraampullary, periampullary, and mixed forms
Usually poorly differentiated adenocarcinoma
Metastatic at diagnosis (regional LNs) in 35–50%
Distinction from bile duct carcinoma or pancreatic carcinoma important because prognosis better: 25% 5 yr, 50% if node negative
Prognosis relates to size

OTHER CARCINOMAS
Small cell carcinoma
Adenosquamous carcinoma
Anaplastic (sarcomatoid) carcinoma

CARCINOID TUMOR
(See also beginning of this outline)
Most common malignant tumor of the small bowel
~30% of patients with small intestine carcinoids will have either concurrent malignancies (intestinal or extraintestinal) elsewhere, most commonly GI adenocarcinoma

GANGLIOCYTIC PARAGANGLIOMA
AKA: nonchromaffin paraganglioma, paraganglioneuroma
Benign tumor; almost exclusively 2nd portion of duodenum, especially near ampulla of Vater
Most are small, submucosal, pedunculated; frequently ulcerate and bleed
Composed of a mixture of three cell types: endocrine cells (carcinoid-like, usually positive for pancreatic polypeptide), ganglion cells, and spindle-shaped S-100 positive Schwann-like cells

SMOOTH MUSCLE TUMORS
(See also beginning of this outline)
Much more likely to be malignant than esophageal or gastric
10% duodenal, 37% jejunal, 53% ileal
Leiomyoblastoma type very uncommon

MALIGNANT LYMPHOMA
(See also beginning of this outline)
ENTEROPATHY ASSOCIATED T-CELL LYMPHOMA
IMMUNOPROLIFERATIVE SMALL INTESTINE DISEASE
DE NOVO LYMPHOMAS
80–90% solitary, usually ileum
Diffusely infiltrating, often bulky
Most are large B cell, followed by small lymphocytic

OTHER TUMORS
Lipomas
Hemangioma
Neurofibroma
Granulocytic sarcoma

METASTATIC TUMORS
By far the most common tumor in the small intestine
Can often involve multiple polypoid lesions
Most common primaries: malignant melanoma, lung carcinoma, breast carcinoma, choriocarcinoma

COLON

Normal
Colon retroperitoneal along most of its length
Rectum ~6 inches long; proximal portion in peritoneal cavity; distal portion is extraperitoneal, with the peritoneal reflection forming the pouch of Douglas (common site for tumor implantation)
VASCULAR SUPPLY
• Superior mesenteric: cecum, right colon, transverse colon
• Inferior mesenteric: descending (left) colon, sigmoid colon, proximal rectum
• Hemorrhoidal branches of internal iliac: distal rectum
Watershed areas:
• Splenic flexure: between superior and inferior mesenteric arteries
• Rectum: between inferior mesenteric and hemorrhoidal arteries
Collateral blood supply from posterior abdominal wall makes transmural infarction uncommon
Superior hemorrhoidal veins (drain to portal system) anastomose with the inferior hemorrhoidal veins (drain to inferior vena cava)—become dilated in portal hypertension
NERVOUS SUPPLY
Auerbach's plexus (within muscularis) and Meissner's plexus (submucosal) form from neuroblasts, which migrate in a cephalocaudal direction during development; usually reach rectum by 12 wk gestational age

Malformations (Congenital and Acquired)

MISCELLANEOUS MALFORMATIONS
Malrotation
Duplication
Imperforate anus

HIRSCHSPRUNG'S DISEASE
AKA: congenital megacolon
Failure of neuroblasts to migrate to the end of the bowel, resulting in an aganglionic segment, which always involves the rectum and extends varying distances proximally
80% patients are male; 10% have Down syndrome
4% risk in sibling of an affected patient
Usually manifests early in neonatal period

Absence of ganglion cells accompanied by erratic hyperplasia of nerves within the submucosa and increased acetylcholinesterase activity in the lamina propria and muscularis mucosa

Restricted to the rectum in 90%

Lack of peristalsis results in a functional obstruction and dilatation to form "megacolon"

Surgical correction required; 5–10% mortality from electrolyte disturbances and infections

DIVERTICULAR DISEASE

AKA: diverticulosis

Outpouchings of mucosa and submucosa through a weakened area in the muscularis, often with hypertrophy of adjacent muscularis

Symptomatic in only ~20% of affected patients

Symptoms of lower abdominal discomfort and/or cramping pains may or may not be present, independent of whether or not inflammatory changes (diverticulitis) are present

>95% diverticula are located in the sigmoid colon

Pathogenesis involves both focal weakness in the muscularis and increased intraluminal pressure

When inflamed, peridiverticular acute and chronic inflammation is seen with fibrosis and sometimes abscess or fistula tract formation

HEMORRHOIDS

Variceal dilations of the anal and perianal venous plexi

Affects ~5% of population; unusual before 30 yr of age, except in pregnant women

Predisposing factors: constipation with straining at stool, venous stasis of pregnancy, increased portal hypertension

Types:
• External: inferior hemorrhoidal plexus; below anorectal line
• Internal: superior hemorrhoidal plexus; above anorectal line

ANGIODYSPLASIA

Dilatation and increased tortuosity of the submucosal veins in the cecum and occasionally ascending colon

Can cause lower GI bleeding in elderly

Probably acquired

May develop in the cecum because of its largest diameter, causing its wall tension to be the greatest, compressing the veins in the muscularis and thereby shunting more blood through the submucosal veins

Inflammatory Disorders

NECROTIZING ENTEROCOLITIS

Acute necrotizing inflammation of small and large intestine

Affects 10% of full-term infants; more common in prematurity

Peak incidence is 2–3 days of age following initiation of oral feeding

More common among formula-fed vs. breast-fed infants

Symptoms vary from mild abdominal tenderness to frank bleeding, perforation, and sepsis

Radiography may reveal air in bowel wall (pneumatosis intestinalis)

Most common sites: terminal ileum, cecum, ascending colon

Mucosal necrosis with fibrinous exudate, sometimes pseudo-membrane formation, neutrophils, lymphocytes

ULCERATIVE COLITIS (UC)

Idiopathic; inflammatory bowel disease

Recurrent acute and chronic inflammatory disorder affecting principally the rectum and left colon, but often extending more proximally; never beyond the cecum

Patients often present with attacks of bloody mucoid diarrhea, which may persist for days, weeks, or months

4–6/100,000 in U.S.; whites > black; female > male; peak onset 20–25 yr

Like Crohn's, patients may also have migratory polyarthritis, ankylosing spondylitis, uveitis, skin lesions

Continuous involvement from rectum (in untreated cases); no skip lesions, although different segments may be in different stages of healing/activity; with treatment, can have patchy involvement, even in the rectum

Active lesions marked by mucin depletion, crypt abscesses, ulcerations which tend to be broad based and may extend deep into submucosa but usually not far into muscularis, extensive mucosal destruction, islands of residual mucosa (pseudopolyps), undermining and mucosal bridging

Chronic changes include distortion of crypt architecture (branching and irregular glands), basal lymphoplasmacytic infiltrate, Paneth cell metaplasia, adipose islands in lamina propria

Dysplasia should be graded on every biopsy as absent, indefinite, low grade, or high grade

2–5% will develop primary sclerosing cholangitis

25% are anti-neutrophil cytoplasm antibody positive (P-ANCA): more likely to develop primary sclerosing cholangitis (PSC)

Fulminant UC: 25% of cases; sudden onset of intractable, bloody diarrhea, fever, electrolyte imbalances; can be fatal

COMPLICATIONS

Toxic megacolon: sudden cessation of bowel function with dilatation and potentially rupture

Carcinoma: incidence of carcinoma is 1% at 10 yr, 3.5% at 15 yr, 10–15% at 20 yr, 30% at 30 yr duration (when most of colon involved; lower for limited disease); tumors may be multiple; usually preceded by dysplasia; tumors tend to be higher grade/stage than those arising in uninflamed mucosa

CROHN'S DISEASE

(See earlier under Small Intestine)

ISCHEMIC COLITIS

Most commonly splenic flexure, descending, sigmoid; occurs in elderly

Edema, hemorrhage, later ulcerations, fibrosis, pseudo-membranes, pseudopolyps; not uncommonly with adjacent normal mucosa

Hemosiderin usually abundant

Lymphoid follicles and granulomas are absent

Differential diagnosis includes Crohn's disease, ulcerative colitis, and pseudomembranous colitis

INFECTIOUS COLITIDES

ACUTE SELF-LIMITED COLITIS

AKA: nonspecific bacterial colitis

Edema, inflammation, hyperemia, hemorrhage

Most commonly *Campylobacter*, *Salmonella*, *Shigella*

Salmonella and *Shigella* can simulate ulcerative colitis
E. coli can cause an acute hemorrhagic colitis
- *Shigella*
  Bacillary dysentery
  Penetrates mucosa; replicates within lamina propria; elaborates cytotoxic endotoxin
  Shallow ulcerations
  Preferentially involves large bowel
- *Salmonella* (see earlier under Small Intestine)

PSEUDOMEMBRANOUS COLITIS
Acute colitis in which the inflamed, focally necrotic mucosa is covered by pseudomembranes composed of fibrin and inflammatory cells spewing out from the crypts
Caused by toxin of *Clostridium difficile,* which overgrows normal flora, usually following treatment with a broad-spectrum antibiotic, particularly clindamycin or lincomycin
More often involves the right colon; may occasionally involve the distal small bowel
Membranes gray-yellow; may coalesce and become greenish
Differential diagnosis: ischemic colitis

OTHER INFECTIOUS COLITIDES
- Amebic: predilection for cecum and ascending colon, flask-shaped ulceration with minimal inflammation
- TB: most commonly ileocecal; mass (tuberculoma) present in 50% of cases; currently, most commonly acquired from swallowing infected pulmonary secretions
- CMV: most commonly ileocecal; extensive ulceration, inclusion bodies most prominent in vascular endothelial cells
- Cryptosporidiosis: most common cause of severe watery diarrhea in AIDS; organism present in large numbers; difficult to treat

"MICROSCOPIC COLITIS"
Chronic or episodic watery diarrhea with radiographically and endoscopically normal bowel
Patients almost always >30 yr old (mean age 55); male:female = 1:6; may have autoimmune disease
Histologic features vary from field to field—patchy

LYMPHOCYTIC COLITIS
Surface epithelium is somewhat flattened, with loss of mucin and cytoplasmic vacuolization, and is infiltrated by lymphocytes, neutrophils, eosinophils
Occasional crypt abscesses may be present

COLLAGENOUS COLITIS
Lymphocytic colitis with deposition of ≥10 μm thick hypocellular collagenous band beneath surface mucosa, occasionally with trapped congested capillaries

OTHER COLITIDES
DIVERSION COLITIS
Occurs in distal bowel isolated from fecal stream by diversion colostomy
Marked lymphoid follicular hyperplasia with germinal centers, acute cryptitis, and crypt abscesses

RADIATION COLITIS
Acute: within 2 wk; epithelial injury with inflammation
Chronic: 2 months to 20 yr; proliferative endarteritis, fibrosis

OTHER NON-NEOPLASTIC LESIONS
COLITIS CYSTICA PROFUNDA
Intramural mucus-containing cysts in colon and rectum

Localized form typically occurs in rectum; AKA hamartomatous inverted polyp
Diffuse form results from inflammation and ulceration

MELANOSIS COLI
Brown-black discoloration of the colonic mucosa caused by accumulation within the lamina propria of macrophages filled with pigmented material composed of melanin and lipofuscin; usually PAS and Fontana-Masson positive
Attributed to use of anthracene-type laxatives, which damage the mucosal cells; macrophages phagocytose debris
No clinical or physiologic significance

Neoplasms

POLYPS

Non-Neoplastic Polyps
HYPERPLASTIC POLYPS
Most common non-neoplastic polyp in the GI tract
Generally sessile, <5 mm; single or multiple
Found in 25–50% of individuals at autopsy; account for 90% of epithelial polyps at autopsy, but only 20% of biopsied polyps
60–80% in rectosigmoid
Epithelium has normal mucinous component with a scalloped sawtooth pattern, esp. on the surface

JUVENILE (RETENTION) POLYPS
Most frequent polyp in children; one third of cases seen in adults
Most common in rectosigmoid; autoamputation is common
Granular, red grossly; mucus-filled cystic glands
Stroma is inflamed and edematous (crypt rupture)

HAMARTOMATOUS (PEUTZ-JEGHERS TYPE) POLYPS
May be single or multiple (in the Peutz-Jeghers syndrome)
Glands supported by broad branching bands of smooth muscle, which extend upward from the muscularis mucosae into the lamina propria
Columnar and goblet cells on surface, Paneth and endocrine cells near base
Minimal to no atypia

PSEUDOPOLYPS
Islands of residual mucosa surrounded by ulceration, seen in ulcerative colitis

INFLAMMATORY FIBROID POLYPS
Mainly occur in the small intestine and stomach (see earlier)
Broad based, 1–15 cm, ulcerated surface
Fibroblasts, inflammatory cells (often eosinophils) in collagenous or myxoid stroma
May present as intussusception

SOLITARY RECTAL ULCER
AKA: benign idiopathic recurrent rectal ulceration
Solitary (may be multiple), ulcerated (may have intact overlying mucosa), polypoid lesion 4–18 cm from anal margin (may be anal or in sigmoid colon), often associated with mucosal prolapse
Obliteration of lamina propria by fibrosis, smooth muscle proliferation within and extending up from the muscularis mucosa, decreased numbers of lymphocytes
Inflammatory cloacogenic polyp and *mucosal prolapse syndrome* are probably variations on this

LYMPHOID POLYPS
Mucosal protrusion secondary to lymphoid hyperplasia, most commonly seen in the rectum

Neoplastic Polyps
ADENOMATOUS POLYPS (TUBULAR ADENOMAS)
May be pedunculated; stalk usually has normal epithelium; stalks longer in left colon

75% of all neoplastic polyps; male : female = 2 : 1

0.3–3.5 cm; most are located in the sigmoid colon and rectum, but 25–40% are found in the right colon

Thicker mucosa with goblet cell depletion, multiple cell layers, mitoses off basal layer

Superficial areas affected first

Dysplasia can be graded as mild, moderate, and severe

Although "premalignant," few adenomatous polyps progress to cancer; risk of malignancy only 1–3%; increases with number and size (esp. if >2 cm) of polyps

Larger lesions usually have some villous component: "villoglandular polyps" or "tubulovillous polyps"; increased risk of malignant progression

Pseudoinvasion of the stalk distinguished from carcinoma by similarity to surface glands, presence of lamina propria between glands, lack of a desmoplastic response, hemosiderin granules, or hemorrhage

VILLOUS ADENOMA

Account for <10% of all neoplastic polyps

>50% villous in architecture

Tend to occur in elderly patients, usually single, rectosigmoid, sessile, large

Associated with hypoproteinemia and hypokalemia

Much more prone to undergo progression to malignancy than tubular adenomas (30–70%)

SERRATED ADENOMA

Uncommon (<1% of all polyps)

Mixed hyperplastic and adenomatous polyp

On low power, contains the serrated surface and glands of a hyperplastic polyp, but has the cellular immaturity of an adenoma

Probably represents a transitional state

Polyposis Syndromes

COWDEN SYNDROME

Multiple hamartomatous polyps, but not Peutz-Jeghers type (disorganization and proliferation of muscularis mucosa)

Autosomal dominant

Facial trichilemmomas, acral keratoses, oral mucosal papillomas

Increased incidence of malignancy in various sites (esp. breast, thyroid)

CRONKHITE-CANADA SYNDROME

Nonhereditary

Multiple juvenile polyps associated with alopecia, nail atrophy, and hyperpigmentation

FAMILIAL POLYPOSIS

Autosomal dominant, gene on chromosome 5q21 (APC gene)

Polyps not present at birth

Early development (teens–20s) of numerous tubular adenomas throughout GI tract (including small intestine and stomach); usually need 100 polyps to make diagnosis

High incidence of malignant transformation; almost 100% will develop carcinoma by early 30s

GARDNER'S SYNDROME

Autosomal dominant

Colonic polyposis in association with multiple osteomas of the skull and mandible, keratinous cysts of the skin, soft tissue tumors (esp. fibromatosis)

Risk of colonic carcinoma as high as for familial polyposis

MULTIPLE JUVENILE POLYPOSIS SYNDROME

Autosomal dominant

Associated with development of adenomatous polyps and adenocarcinoma

PEUTZ-JEGHERS SYNDROME

Autosomal dominant

Multiple hamartomatous (juvenile) polyps in colon (30%), small bowel (100%), and stomach (25%); melanotic mucosal and cutaneous pigmentation around the lips, mouth, face, genitalia, palmar surfaces of hands

Increased risk of developing carcinomas of the pancreas, breast, lung, ovary, and uterus

TURCOT'S SYNDROME

Autosomal recessive

Colonic adenomatous polyps seen in association with brain tumors, usually glioblastomas

ADENOCARCINOMA

Second leading cancer killer in the U.S.; 15% of all cancer deaths

Accounts for 98% of all cancers of the large intestine

50–70% are rectosigmoid

Incidence appears to parallel socioeconomic status

Cecum and ascending colon in low incidence areas, more frequently rectum and sigmoid in higher incidence areas

Increasing use of sigmoidoscopy has led to decreased frequency in rectosigmoid recently

Dietary factors predisposing to carcinoma include low content of unabsorbable vegetable fiber, high content of refined carbohydrates, high fat content

Peak incidence in 60s; <20% in patients <50 yr

On the left side, tend to grow as annular encircling lesions with early obstruction; on the right: polypoid, fungating masses, generally don't obstruct, diagnosed later

Usually well to moderately differentiated adenocarcinoma, often with T-cell inflammatory response at leading edge

Tumor is keratin and CEA positive (latter equally distributed vs. apical distribution in normal mucosa)

ras, p53 (17p13), DCC (18q21) mutations common

Staging

(Lamina propria of colon lacks lymphatics; therefore, even if tumor invades lamina propria, it is still considered in situ)

Tis	Intraepithelial carcinoma or lamina propria invasion
T1	Submucosal invasion
T2	Muscularis propria or subserosal invasion
T3	Subserosal or other pericolic invasion
T4	Adjacent structures or through peritoneum
N1	1–3 pericolic or perirectal nodes
N2	≥4 pericolic or perirectal LNs
N3	LNs along vascular trunk or apical node involvement

	AJCC		Dukes			5 yr survival (%)			
	T1, T2	T3, T4	T1	T2	T3, T4	T1	T2	T3	T4
N0	I	II	A	B1	B2	99	85	70	30
N1						60			
N2	III		C1		C2	30			
N3									
M1	IV			D		3			

Prognostic Factors
Metastases most commonly to liver, often as a single or small number of large, well-defined lesions, often central necrosis

Good prognostic factors: females, low stage, pushing margins and inflammatory infiltrate, eosinophil infiltration

Bad prognostic factors: very young or very old, males, obstruction, perforation; mucinous, small cell or signet ring cell; vascular or perineural invasion

Special Histologic Types
MUCINOUS
Collections of tumor cells suspended in lakes of extracellular mucin

15% of colorectal carcinomas, most commonly rectum, commonly associated with villous adenomas

Slightly worse prognosis, independent of histologic grade

SIGNET RING
Rare, usually younger patients

Signet ring cells with diffuse infiltration and thickening of wall

Metastases more likely to LNs, peritoneal surface, and ovary, rather than liver

Extremely poor prognosis

SQUAMOUS
More common in cecal neoplasms

Usually adenosquamous; rarely purely squamous

NEUROENDOCRINE FEATURES
If scattered cells in otherwise typical adenocarcinoma, usually mucinous type, does not influence prognosis

Small cell pattern caries a poor prognosis

OTHERS
Clear cell change

Basaloid (cloacogenic)

Choriocarcinomatous

CARCINOID TUMOR
(See also beginning of this outline)

Most commonly in rectum, sometimes in distal sigmoid

Generally are well behaved

In the rectum, >70% are positive for prostatic acid phosphatase (in both men and women) but are negative for prostate specific antigen

CARCINOMA OF THE ANAL CANAL
Present with bleeding (50%), pain (40%)

More common in women, but increasing frequency among homosexual men

Most are epidermoid (squamous cell) carcinomas

~20% will show a basaloid appearance with areas of palisading; this has been variably termed *basaloid, transitional,* or *cloacogenic,* but is probably a variant of squamous cell carcinoma

May be massively infiltrated by eosinophils

Human papilloma virus (HPV) is strongly suspected in pathogenesis

OTHER VARIANTS/CARCINOMAS INCLUDE
Sarcomatoid carcinoma

Verrucous carcinoma

Mucinous adenocarcinoma

Basal cell carcinoma

Bowen's disease

Paget's disease

OTHER TUMORS OF THE ANAL CANAL
Malignant melanoma

Embryonal rhabdomyosarcoma

Malignant lymphoma

OTHER NEOPLASMS
LIPOMA
LIPOMATOSIS OF THE ILEOCECAL VALVE
SMOOTH MUSCLE TUMORS
Most are in the rectum, are small, and are benign

Proximal tumors tend to be larger; more likely to be malignant

KAPOSI'S SARCOMA

APPENDIX

Normal
Extremely rich in lymphoid tissue in young individuals

Lymphoid tissue and epithelium undergoes atrophy during life; may result in complete fibrous obliteration of the lumen (may be a schwannoma-related lesion, since often there is associated hypertrophy of the nerves)

ACUTE APPENDICITIS
Mainly a disease of adolescents; may affect any age

Classically, pain is initially periumbilical, then migrates to right lower quadrant; fever, nausea/vomiting, abdominal tenderness, leukocytosis; rarely are all elements present

Most commonly arises in setting of obstruction by fecalith, vermicularis, foreign body, cecal tumor

Obstruction and continued mucin secretion lead to increased luminal pressure, collapse of drainage veins, ischemic injury, bacterial invasion, further ischemia, etc.

Most surgeons accept a 20% false-positive rate of operating for acute appendicitis because rupture carries a 2% mortality

Usually require neutrophils in muscularis to make diagnosis, because neutrophils in mucosa or submucosa can result from drainage from an infection higher in bowel

Some divide degree of inflammation into early (focal), suppurative, gangrenous, and perforative

EOSINOPHILIC APPENDICITIS
Diffuse eosinophilic infiltration, often with granulomas

Correlated with present of *Strongyloides stercoralis* in stool

APPENDICEAL "INFECTIONS"
OXYURIS VERMICULARIS
Seen in about 3% of appendices removed surgically

Most common in children between 7 and 11 yr

May induce granulomatous inflammation

CAMPYLOBACTER
MEASLES
INFECTIOUS MONONUCLEOSIS
ADENOVIRUS

Neoplasms

MUCINOUS CYSTADENOMA
AKA: mucocele

Diffuse globular enlargement of appendix by large amount of tenacious mucus; lumen lined by atypical mucinous epithelium with at least focal papillary growths

Four times more common than malignant counterpart

20% will be associated with appendiceal perforation and implantation of mucin within the peritoneum; malignant cells will *not* be found in the mucin

May have coexisting mucinous cystadenoma of the ovary with identical histology

Some pathologists reserve the term *mucocele* for mucinous distention secondary to non-neoplastic obstruction

MUCINOUS CYSTADENOCARCINOMA

Similar to benign counterpart except cells are more atypical, often invade bowel wall, and viable tumor cells can be found in the mucin lakes

When mucin is present in the peritoneal cavity associated with malignant cells, called *pseudomyxoma peritonei*

ADENOCARCINOMA

May be secondarily involved by a cecal carcinoma

Histology same as for colonic tumor

Signet ring variant exists

CARCINOID TUMOR

(See also beginning of this outline)

Most common site for carcinoid tumor in the body

Found in 1/300 routine appendectomies

Tip of appendix most common site (70%); when more proximal, may cause obstruction and appendicitis

Large majority are benign

Rarely cause carcinoid syndrome

Immunoreactive for seratonin and S-100

CLASSIC TYPE

Solid nests of small monotonous cells; insular growth pattern

Often invades nerves, muscle, lymphatics, even serosa

TUBULAR ADENOCARCINOID

Glandular formation without solid nests

Usually tip of appendix

Usually lacks serotonin; often positive for glucagon

Often misdiagnosed as adenocarcinoma; important distinction because behavior is benign

CLEAR CELL CARCINOID

Cells have clear cytoplasm but lack mucin and glycogen

Behaves like classic type

MUCINOUS CARCINOID

AKA: Goblet cell carcinoid, microglandular carcinoma, crypt cell carcinoma

Unique to the appendix

Cells may have signet ring configuration

Grows in a concentric pattern within the submucosa

More aggressive than other two types with 10–20% metastasizing, often to bilateral ovaries

PERITONEAL CAVITY

Peritoneum

Normal

Lined by mesodermally derived keratin positive mesothelium

Subserosal cells are vimentin positive, fibroblast-like, and believed to be pluripotent

PERITONITIS

May completely resolve, become walled off (abscess), or heal as fibrous adhesions

- Chemical: bile, pancreatic juices, gastric juice, barium
- Meconium: intrauterine perforation of small bowel
- Bacterial:
  Primary infections: streptococci, usually children
  Secondary infections: perforation of viscus, TB
- Foreign body: granulomatous inflammation

CYSTS

PSEUDOCYST

No lining; results from inflammatory processes

SOLITARY CYST

1–6 cm

Attached to wall or lying loose

Usually watery fluid in lumen, single layer of cuboidal to flat mesothelial cells

MULTICYSTIC BENIGN MESOTHELIOMA

Usually adult females

Cysts are microscopic to >15 cm in diameter

Flattened cuboidal mesothelium, clear fluid, mild chronic inflammation in walls

Probably reactive process; frequently recur

MÜLLERIAN CYSTS

Usually fallopian tube type epithelium

Seen in males: residual Müllerian structures

HYPERPLASIA/METAPLASIA

MESOTHELIAL HYPERPLASIA

Reaction to irritation

Nodular or papillary; psammoma bodies may be present

METAPLASIA

Squamous

Müllerian (endometriosis, endosalpingiosis, ectopic decidual reaction)

Cartilaginous

MESOTHELIOMA

(See also Pleura in Lung outline)

FIBROUS

<25% of peritoneal tumors (much less common than in pleura)

May arise from submesothelial connective tissue

May be associated with hypoglycemia

Generally benign

BENIGN EPITHELIAL MESOTHELIOMA

Small, solitary, papillary structure

Resembles choroid plexus

May be extension of mesothelial hyperplasia

MALIGNANT EPITHELIAL MESOTHELIOMA

Most are in males over 40 yr

~50% associated with (heavy) asbestos exposure

Multiple plaques/nodules on visceral and parietal peritoneum

Ascites almost always present

Advanced lesions may obliterate peritoneal cavity

Histology is variable: papillary, tubular, solid; psammoma bodies; may have sarcomatoid component

Generally keratin positive; CEA and LeuM1 negative

Electron microscopy: long microvilli

Omentum

Hemorrhagic infarct (torsion, strangulation)
Cystic lymphangioma
Most tumors are metastatic implants

Mesentery

Panniculitis
Mesenteric cysts (same as peritoneal "solitary cysts")
Giant lymph node hyperplasia (Castleman's disease)

14

LIVER AND GALLBLADDER

NORMAL ANATOMY

Liver averages 1400–1600 g in adult

Covered by Glisson's capsule

Receives 70% of blood flow from portal vein, 30% from hepatic artery

Grossly divided into left, right lobes; right is 6× larger and contains quadrate (inferior) and caudate (posterior) lobes

Enormous reserve and regenerative capacity; regenerated liver often has abnormal biliary connections

Microscopically divided into "lobules," 1–2 mm in diameter

- Classical: hexagonal—central vein in middle
- Portal: triangular—portal tract in middle and three central veins
- Acinar: diamond—two central veins + two portal tracts
    Zone 1: periportal; most sensitive to toxins
    Zone 2: intermediate
    Zone 3: pericentral vein; stellate, not circular; most active P-450 oxidase system; most sensitive to ischemic injury

Portal tracts contain portal vein, hepatic artery, bile duct (one per artery), lymphatics, nerves, connective tissue

Limiting plate: lineup of hepatocytes surrounding portal tract

Cords are one cell thick in adult, two cells thick in newborns (and in regenerating liver)

Nuclear size in hepatocytes varies significantly; ploidy ranges up to octaploid

Sinusoids lined by discontinuous, fenestrated endothelium

Lymphatic flow: perisinusoidal space of Disse, periportal space of Mall, portal tract lymphatics, etc.

Bile flow: canaliculi, canals of Hering (cells intermediate between hepatocytes and duct cells), portal bile ducts, left and right hepatic ducts, common hepatic bile duct, etc.

Bile flow is energy dependent (probably active transport of ions is required)

Little variation in hepatocyte size; significant anisonucleosis

Kupffer cells: monocyte/phagocyte system—in sinusoids; can be visualized by staining with Cam56

Perisinusoidal "Ito" cells: fat-containing mesenchymal cells in space of Disse; important for Vitamin A storage (become swollen in hypervitaminosis A)

Iron accumulation is predominantly periportal, vs. lipofuscin accumulation, which is predominantly pericentral vein

IMMUNOHISTOCHEMISTRY

KP-1 (CD68) stains Kupffer's cells

Low molecular weight (MW) keratin stains bile ducts

EMA/CEA stains canaliculi

BIOPSY

Blind percutaneous liver biopsy: mortality rate 1/5000–7000 biopsies

For patients with clotting abnormalities, use transjugular approach

Indications: mass lesion, abnormal/unexplained chemistries, failure of unknown cause, staging of known disease

EMBRYOLOGY

Arises as ventral bud from the caudal foregut early in the 4th wk

Hepatic diverticulum separates from primitive gallbladder

Hepatocytes and intrahepatic bile ducts endodermally derived

Initially, right and left lobes same size; then right lobe enlarges, develops caudate and quadrate lobes

Hematopoiesis begins during the 6th wk; continues to term

9th wk: liver represents 10% fetal weight (5% at term)

12th wk: bile formation begins

Extrahepatic biliary tree initially occluded with endodermal cells, later recanalized

HETEROTOPIA

Has rarely been seen in gallbladder, spleen, pancreas, umbilicus, adrenal glands, omentum

JAUNDICE (ICTERUS)

Yellow-green discoloration of skin or sclerae by bilirubin; pruritus common (because of bile acids in serum, not bilirubin)

Kernicterus: deposition of bilirubin in brain (disappears within 24 hr of death; to diagnose, need to cut brain fresh)

Not clinically evident until serum bilirubin exceeds 2 mg/dl

70% bilirubin derived from catabolism of hemoglobin

Heme (red) → biliverdin (green) → bilirubin (yellow) → conjugated (glucuronidated) in liver, secreted in bile → converted to urobilinogen by bacteria → most oxidized to urobilin (stercobilin) and excreted; 10% reabsorbed, returns to liver, some excreted by kidneys

Unconjugated bilirubin not water soluble (binds albumin in serum, cannot be excreted by kidneys); toxic to tissues

Unconjugated (Indirect) Hyperbilirubinemia

INCREASED PRODUCTION

AKA: hemolytic jaundice

Pernicious anemia, thalassemia

DECREASED UPTAKE BY LIVER

Constitutional hepatic dysfunction = Gilbert's syndrome; affects 7% of population

IMPAIRED CONJUGATION

Physiologic jaundice of the newborn

Crigler-Najjar syndrome

- Type I: autosomal recessive deficiency of glucuronyltransferase; progressive kernicterus; invariably fatal
- Type II: autosomal dominant with variable penetrance, moderate decrease in glucuronyltransferase; normal liver histology

Conjugated (Direct) Hyperbilirubinemia

LIVER DAMAGE (INTRAHEPATIC CHOLESTASIS)

Secretion of bilirubin into canaliculus is compromised before ability to conjugate is lost

DUBIN-JOHNSON SYNDROME
Autosomal recessive defect in canalicular transport of organic anions, including conjugated bilirubin
Liver becomes black because of accumulation of an unknown pigment (not related to bilirubin)

EXTRAHEPATIC DUCT OBSTRUCTION
(See later)

INFLAMMATORY/NON-NEOPLASTIC DISORDERS OF THE LIVER

GENETIC/CHILDHOOD DISORDERS

NEONATAL HEPATITIS SYNDROME
Onset of jaundice between 1 wk and 2 months
Usually idiopathic (may be caused by sepsis, *Listeria, Toxoplasma,* hepatitis B (HepB), cytomegalovirus (CMV), herpes simplex virus (HSV), alpha₁-antitrypsin, galactosemia, cystic fibrosis, tyrosinemia . . .)
Lobular disarray, focal liver cell necrosis, prominent giant cell transformation, mononuclear infiltrate into portal areas, cholestasis, reactive changes in Kupffer cells
Long-term prognosis generally not good; surgery to rule out biliary atresia can further increase morbidity/mortality
Usually don't see bile duct proliferation (vs. in atresia)

ALPHA₁-ANTITRYPSIN (AAT) DEFICIENCY
May present as liver disease, lung disease, or both
More than 30 variants exist
Abnormal allele is "Z" vs. M for the Pi (protease inhibitor) locus (chromosome 14); mutant protein (single amino acid change: glu342 → lys) is not secreted
ZZ individuals (1 in 2000–4000) have 10–15% normal level of AAT; two thirds develop liver disease; 2.5% die by 4 yr
May present later in adult life with cirrhosis and liver failure; usually shows massive accumulation of AAT
Increased risk for hepatocellular carcinoma in males
PAS+, diastase resistant, round to oval cytoplasmic globules in periportal regions; by electron microscopy (EM), these are in the endoplasmic reticulum; composed of the mutant protein
May also see giant cell formation, cholestasis, portal fibrosis

CYSTIC FIBROSIS
Liver usually unaffected at birth—worsens through life
Steatosis most common lesion, panlobular
Focal biliary cirrhosis with inspissated granular eosinophilic material within portal bile ductules is pathognomonic
10% develop cirrhosis by age 25
(See Congenital Syndromes outline for more details)

REYE'S SYNDROME
Encephalopathy and fatty degeneration of liver, usually lethal
Associated with elevated serum ammonia
Linked in children to the use of aspirin for viral illnesses
Panlobular steatosis, microvesicular, without inflammation
May lead to zonal or massive hepatic necrosis
EM: enlarged, pleomorphic mitochondria with swollen matrix
Microvesicular fat also accumulates in proximal tubules of kidney and in myocardium and skeletal muscle

HEMOCHROMATOSIS
Autosomal recessive (chromosome 6p21.3): incidence 1–2/1000; male : female = 7 : 1
Hepatic iron index: μmoles Fe/g dry weight liver/age
  Homozygotes: >2, may be >20
  Heterozygotes: 0.2–2
  Normal: 0.1–1
Quantitative iron can help distinguish primary hemochromatosis from secondary hemosiderosis (iron overload without associated tissue damage; iron preferentially accumulates in the Kupffer cells)
If cirrhosis (usually micronodular) develops, increased risk of hepatoma, decreased life span
Associated with HLA-A3 and HLA-B14
• Familial (Idiopathic) Hemochromatosis
  Excessive iron absorption
  Iron accumulates in Kupffer cells, periportal hepatocytes
  Some fibrosis may be present—not related to amount of iron
• Neonatal Hemochromatosis
  Not familial: affects premature infants
  Progressive iron deposition in liver and other tissues

WILSON'S DISEASE
AKA: hepatolenticular degeneration
Autosomal recessive inability to excrete copper into the bile
Present late childhood/early adulthood with neurologic dysfunction, hepatic disease, or hemolytic anemia
Variable liver picture: acute hepatitis, chronic active hepatitis (CAH), fulminant, cirrhosis; typically CAH with fibrosis and glycogen nuclei
Histochemical stains for copper inadequate as screening test; need chemical determination of serum or liver biopsy
Patients usually have Kayser-Fleischer rings on cornea

CONGENITAL HEPATIC FIBROSIS
Bands of fibrous septa (with numerous bile ducts) surrounding islands of normal parenchyma
Not cirrhosis: no inflammation, no regenerative nodules
May belong to spectrum of diseases including Caroli's disease and polycystic liver disease

INTRAHEPATIC BILIARY ATRESIA
Absence or loss of intrahepatic ducts with minimal if any regenerative effort
Usually need <0.5 ducts per portal tract (normal = 1) to make diagnosis
Alagille syndrome (arteriohepatic dysplasia): autosomal dominant syndromic form with vertebral arch anomalies, pulmonic stenosis, abnormal facies, hypogonadism; progressive loss of bile ducts with age
Nonsyndromic form: usually congenital absence of the ducts

CIRCULATORY/VASCULAR CHANGES
May be caused by obstruction of blood inflow (hepatic artery or portal vein) or blood outflow (central or hepatic vein)

INFARCTION
Rare—requires sudden obstruction of hepatic artery

PORTAL VEIN THROMBOSIS
Abdominal cancers, peritoneal sepsis, pancreatitis, postsurgery; cirrhosis, metastatic cancer
Abdominal pain and ascites

CHRONIC PASSIVE CONGESTION
Slightly enlarged, blood filled, rounded edges
Nutmeg appearance, with central congested areas and relative pallor of the periportal zones
Distention of central veins and perivenous sinusoids

Erythrocytes may be extruded into the cords, where they become trapped

CENTRILOBULAR NECROSIS
Seen in prolonged congestive heart failure

Grossly, nutmeg appearance with central depressions

Necrosis of liver cells around central veins—may bridge

May also be seen in left heart failure alone—ischemic

Cardiac sclerosis: centrilobular necrosis with delicate central fibrous scarring, extending out into surrounding liver

VENO-OCCLUSIVE DISEASE
Sclerotic occlusion of the central veins with associated sinusoidal congestion; sclerosis may extend into outflow veins, simulating Budd-Chiari

Can be seen with pyrrolozidine alkaloids, azathioprine, thioguanine, hepatic radiation, bone marrow (BM) transplantation with graft vs. host reaction

BUDD-CHIARI SYNDROME
Unexplained partial or complete thrombosis and/or fibrous obliteration of the major hepatic veins or inferior vena cava, usually with membranous webs

Can be seen with polycythemia vera, pregnancy, oral contraceptives, hepatoma, intraabdominal malignancies

Acute form is rapidly lethal; chronic is 50% lethal at 5 yr

PELIOSIS HEPATIS
Caused by rickettsial organism: *Rochalimaea henselae* or *Rochalimaea quintana* (related to agent that causes bacillary angiomatosis in the skin)

Hepatocytes die and drop out; red cells are extruded into the space of Disse, occupying the space where the hepatocytes used to be; eventually walls of the now empty sinusoids break down, producing cystic pools of blood lined by hepatocytes rather than endothelial cells

Can be seen with anabolic steroid use, exposure to vinyl chloride, following renal transplants, hematologic disorders

VIRAL HEPATITIS

Viruses

HEPATITIS A
Non-enveloped ssRNA, icosahedral, 27 nm (picornavirus)

Not cytopathic directly

~1 month incubation period; antibodies (Abs) begin to appear ~2 wk later

Most infections are anicteric; self-limited illness

Inflammation tends to be restricted to portal and periportal areas (in contrast with Hepatitis B,C, which tend to be panlobular)

IgG indicates exposure to HAV at some point in life; IgM is marker for acute infection; IgM may persist for 1 yr

Fatalities in <0.5%; no chronic carrier state exists

HEPATITIS B
Enveloped (42 nm) "Dane particle"; 27 nm hexagonal inner core with circular dsDNA genome

Present in blood near end of incubation period (1–6 months); can be transmitted by blood exposure

Most cases subclinical; 10% symptomatic cases develop acute fulminant hepatitis or chronic disease

Virus is *not* cytopathic (integrates into host DNA); injury caused by inflammation

May cause "ground glass" cytoplasm—distention of smooth endoplasmic reticulum with virions; indication of chronic carrier state

Incubation period ~2 months

Antibody to hepatitis B surface antigen (HBsAg) appears first, followed shortly by hepatitis B e antigen (HBeAg), which peaks early and then disappears with IgM-anti-HBc

and anti-HBe; HBsAg drops after ~2 mo, and there is a 1–4 mo "window period" before anti-HBs appears

Persistence of HBeAg indicates continued active infection and probable progression to chronic hepatitis

Progression to chronic hepatitis more common in immunocompromised patients

Symptoms appear with IgM-anti-HBc

HEPATITIS C (NON-A/NON-B)
Enveloped ssRNA 9.4 kb flavivirus

Causes most (80–90%) cases of transfusion-related hepatitis; also common in IV drug users

Directly cytopathic

Seropositivity occurs late in infection

Tends to produce a greater degree of fat accumulation (macrovesicular and microvesicular) and eosinophilic changes in the hepatocytes

Inflammation may involve the bile ducts

Insidious progression; chronic hepatitis may develop in ~50% of patients

May progress to cirrhosis, even without significant piecemeal necrosis

HEPATITIS DELTA
Defective RNA virus (small, only 1.7 kb, requires concurrent infection with HepB)

Can be directly cytopathic; tends to be more severe than other hepatitis infections (marked intralobular involvement)

Microvesicular fat and many acidophil bodies are seen

IgM anti-D is a reliable marker

HEPATITIS E
RNA virus (calicivirus)

Uncommon—not much known

Commonly produces cholestasis

Causes high mortality in pregnancy

HepE antigen can be detected in hepatocytes

Acute Viral Hepatitis
May be icteric or non-icteric

Panlobular disease with irregular cords, lobular disarray, variation in hepatocyte size, inflammation (predominantly mononuclear, some neutrophils and eosinophils)

Ballooning degeneration: rapid swelling of preterminal hepatocytes with rarefaction of the cytoplasm

Acidophil (Councilman) bodies: eosinophilic apoptotic degeneration of hepatocytes; shrunken cells are extruded into the sinuses

Typically, multiple small foci of hepatocyte dropout

Histologic changes essentially independent of etiologic agent

Bridging necrosis: when present, indicates greater likelihood of atypical outcome—progressive failure and death, cirrhosis

FULMINANT HEPATITIS
Severe form with submassive to massive necrosis

2–3 wk downhill course to death

50–60% of cases caused by virus; drugs (isoniazid, halothane, acetaminophen) and chemicals can also cause

ACUTE CHOLESTATIC VIRAL HEPATITIS
To distinguish from obstructive cause, must identify hepatitis in areas without cholestasis

INFECTIOUS MONONUCLEOSIS
Less hepatocellular injury but marked lymphocytosis and plasmacytosis within the portal tracts, often in an "Indian-file" configuration

AIDS HEPATITIS
Wide variety (any) of histologic patterns, plus often see *Mycobacterium avium-intracellulare* (MAI), CMV, *Crypto-*

sporidium, Microsporida, Kaposi's sarcoma, malignant lymphoma

Chronic Hepatitis (Traditional Classification)

Distinction of chronic from acute hepatitis is made *clinically* (not histologically); usually need persistent elevation of liver aminotransferase levels in the serum for >6 months

CHRONIC PERSISTENT HEPATITIS (CPH)

Inflammatory infiltrate restricted to portal tracts

Most common long-term sequelae of viral hepatitis (B or C)

Can tolerate minimal erosion of the limiting plate but must have no cell necrosis

CHRONIC LOBULAR HEPATITIS (CLH)

Patchy inflammation within the lobules with only minimal portal tract inflammation

May mimic acute hepatitis—need clinical history

Some pathologists consider this a variant of CPH

CHRONIC ACTIVE HEPATITIS

AKA: chronic aggressive hepatitis

Piecemeal necrosis: destruction of the liver cells at the interface between the parenchyma and the portal tracts

Bridging necrosis: collapse of reticulin network caused by coalescence of islands of focal necrosis

Pattern ranges from minimal to widespread necrosis

More likely to progress to end-stage liver disease, esp. if associated with HepBsAg

Autoimmune chronic hepatitis: variant with clinical hypergammaglobulinemia, autoantibodies to smooth muscle and/or mitochondria, no evidence of HepB infection

Alternate Classification for Chronic Hepatitis

The traditional CPH, CLH, CAH terminology has several problems: subject to sampling error, little correlation with tendency for progression, misleading to clinicians

Increasing knowledge of the nature of hepatitis C infection has further damaged the utility of the traditional classification: with chronic hepatitis C infection, the histologic picture fluctuates between CPH and mild CAH, and can progress to cirrhosis, often suddenly, without "significant" piecemeal necrosis; hepatitis B may behave similarly

Proposed alternate classification scheme has three parts:

• Etiology: viral, autoimmune, drug induced, idiopathic
• Grade: mild, moderate, severe, based on portal and/or lobular activity
• Stage (degree of fibrosis): none, portal, bridging, cirrhosis

GRANULOMATOUS HEPATITIS

Often misused term because most cases show only granulomas but no hepatitis

Granulomas seen in 3–10% of all liver biopsies, usually portal

Most common causes: infection (viral, rickettsial, mycobacterial, fungal); lipogranulomas; sarcoidosis, intrinsic liver disease (primary biliary cirrhosis [PBC]), lupus, Crohn's

Drug-induced causes: phenylbutazone, sulfonamides

DRUG-INDUCED HEPATITIS

Response of liver to toxic injury is markedly variable—any pattern can be seen

Many responses are idiosyncratic (not related to dosage)

• Microvesicular fat: tetracycline (more marked in pregnancy)
• Cholestasis (no inflammation): contraceptives, anabolic steroids
• Cholestatic hepatitis: phenothiazines

• Chronic active hepatitis: oxyphenisatin, isoniazid, methyldopa
• Zonal hepatic necrosis: yellow phosphorus (zone 1), carbon tetrachloride (zone 3), acetaminophen (zone 3); zone 3 has highest concentration of P-450 oxidase
• Panlobular hepatitis: methyldopa, halothane, monoamine oxidase (MAO) inhibitors, anti-TB agents, mycotoxins of *Amanita phalloides*

ALCOHOLIC LIVER DISEASE

Most common cause of liver disease in the United States (by far)

Variety of changes seen—can never conclusively diagnose alcoholic etiology

Fatty change most common, usually macrovesicular; only finding in 40%; accumulates first in centrilobular area (zone 3); may involve entire lobules

Pericentral vein fibrosis initially involves just the wall, but then progresses to occlusion and insinuates into surrounding parenchyma in a *chicken-wire* pattern, encasing individual and groups of hepatocytes

Alcoholic hepatitis develops in 20–25% of heavy drinkers: includes inflammation and hepatocellular degeneration, predominantly in centrilobular area, with:

• Mallory bodies: refractile condensation of PAS+ material (keratin) in cells—not pathognomonic
• Neutrophilic infiltrate (attracted to Mallory bodies)
• Giant mitochondria: like Mallory bodies; PAS−

Most common cause of cirrhosis in U.S. (although only ~25% of heavy drinkers show progression to cirrhosis); initially large, fatty, micronodular, then progresses to shrunken, nonfatty, macronodular liver

NONALCOHOLIC STEATOHEPATITIS

Note: True microvesicular fat is too small to be seen on H&E (unlike mixed microvesicular and macrovesicular fat, which usually indicates waxing or waning macrovesicular fat deposits)

Nonalcoholic steatohepatitis can be indistinguishable from alcoholic, including the presence of hepatitis, Mallory bodies, neutrophils, central sclerosis, fibrosis, and cirrhosis, in addition to the steatosis

Obesity/rapid weight change, diabetes (often see glycogen nuclei), tuberculosis, ulcerative colitis, Reye's syndrome, anoxia

TOTAL PARENTERAL NUTRITION (TPN)-ASSOCIATED LIVER DISEASE

Seen in patients, esp. neonates, on prolonged TPN

Pathogenesis not understood: probably combination of toxic effects of amino acids, increased hepatic lipoprotein synthesis, and bowel rest with lack of luminal hormone secretion

Increased transaminases seen at 5 days

Steatosis and canalicular cholestasis begin within 2 wk

Moderate to severe portal fibrosis after 90 days

ACUTE FATTY LIVER OF PREGNANCY

Usually 30th–40th week, usually primigravidas

Grossly, pale-yellow small liver

Microvesicular steatosis involving zone 3, sometimes 2 and 3, sometimes panacinar or zonal

Marked ballooning of hepatocytes also seen

May see intrahepatic cholestasis, liver cell necrosis

Resolves following delivery

NONSPECIFIC REACTIVE HEPATITIS

Nonspecific reaction to variety of infections/toxins; frequently seen in AIDS patients

Mild intralobular ± portal inflammation, mild proliferation of bile ducts, rare necrotic hepatocytes

Usually spares some portal tracts

May be variant of chronic lobular hepatitis

LESIONS AFFECTING PRIMARILY BILE DUCTS

Note: Bile duct proliferation is also seen as a secondary process in a number of hepatic diseases

Bile plugs strongly suggest obstruction at some level

Bile plugs in regenerating ducts seen in sepsis, cholangitis, post-transplantation

Regenerating ducts (small, no lumen, peripherally located in triads) are chemotactic for neutrophils—not indicative of infection unless neutrophils are within the ducts

Copper accumulates in hepatocytes in all chronic cholestatic diseases (normally secreted in bile)

Cholestasis produces feathery degeneration of periportal hepatocytes (cholate injury)

INTRAHEPATIC BILIARY ATRESIA

(See earlier under Genetic/Childhood Disorders)

EXTRAHEPATIC BILIARY ATRESIA

(See later under Gallbladder; Congenital Abnormalities)

EXTRAHEPATIC BILIARY OBSTRUCTION

Acute cholestasis produces bile pigment accumulation initially in zone 3 (pericentral vein), which later extends toward the periportal canaliculi

Initially "bland" (i.e., no inflammation) centrilobular cholestasis (intrahepatocyte and canalicular)

Bile "infarct": not really an infarct; rupture of duct with local spillage of bile, resulting in hepatocellular ballooning degeneration *only* in areas of cholestasis; may form small bile lakes; pathognomonic for large duct obstruction

Acute "cholangitis" with periductal edema (predominantly large ducts), neutrophilic and mononuclear portal inflammation, ductular proliferation at periphery of triads (chemotactic for neutrophils; neutrophils should not be in the duct lumen unless associated with an ascending infection)

ACUTE CHOLANGITIS

Usually bacterial in nature (*E. coli, Klebsiella, Enterobacter*)

Almost never occurs without partial or complete biliary obstruction

Fever, chills, jaundice, sepsis, right upper quadrant pain

Distention of bile ducts with neutrophils in lumen of ducts; inflammation extends into periductal tissue

May progress to liver abscesses

PRIMARY BILIARY CIRRHOSIS

AKA: chronic nonsuppurative destructive cholangitis

Progressive, protracted destruction of small bile ducts

Middle age female (male : female = 1 : 9)

Elevated alkaline phosphatase with normal transaminases

Increasing incidence recently; normal life expectancy

Antimitochondrial antibodies found in 90–95% (also seen in 20% of patients with chronic active hepatitis); four types of antimitochondrial antibodies are seen, most commonly against pyruvate dehydrogenase subunit on inner membrane

Patients frequently have polyclonal IgM peak in serum

Associated with HLA-DR8

Four stages: Schuer (Ludwig)
I   Florid duct lesion (portal)
II Ductular proliferation (periportal)
III Scarring (bridging fibrosis)
IV Cirrhosis

Patchy distribution and asynchronous progression: may see areas of stage I–III in same biopsy

Florid duct stage: pathognomonic—lymphocytic and plasma-cell infiltrate centered on the bile ducts; degeneration of ductal epithelium, foamy macrophages, granulomas, minimal extension of inflammation into surrounding parenchyma with "cholate injury" (mildly pale swelling) to surrounding hepatocytes

Decrease in number of ducts, proliferation of ductules

Later, fibrosis, eventually cirrhosis

May be difficult to distinguish from chronic active hepatitis because may see piecemeal necrosis in PBC and bile duct injury in CAH

Copper accumulation suggests PBC (normally secreted in bile)

Granulomas, generally poorly formed, may indicate a favorable prognosis

Associated autoimmune disorders unfavorable

Treatment: liver transplantation

PRIMARY SCLEROSING CHOLANGITIS

Progressive inflammatory destruction of the extrahepatic and later intrahepatic biliary system, leading to biliary cirrhosis

Rare disorder; unknown etiology, most likely autoimmune

Male : female = 2 : 1, usually <45 yr

Involves intrahepatic and left, right, and common hepatic bile ducts (10% are intrahepatic only; none are extrahepatic only)

Patients present with progressive fatigue, pruritus, jaundice

Cholangiogram shows focal strictures, producing an apparent beading

Early lesion: pericholangitis

Later: uneven thickening of extrahepatic ducts by fibrosis and sparse mixed inflammatory infiltrate; spares epithelium

Late: fibrous obliteration of intrahepatic ducts with replacement of duct segments by solid cords of connective tissue, leading ultimately to biliary cirrhosis

Ulcerative colitis (UC) seen in 60–90% patients; UC usually develops first; PBC more common in P-ANCA positive UC

Association with UC suggests PBC may be caused by draining of bacterial or other products through the portal system

Also seen in association with Riedel's thyroiditis, retroperitoneal fibrosis, orbital pseudotumor

Associated with HLA-B8 and DR3

Increased risk of cholangiocarcinoma

Differential diagnosis: schistosomiasis (involves veins, not ducts); cholangiocarcinoma, CMV

PERICHOLANGITIS

May not be unique entity; may be early stage of pseudomembranous colitis (PSC)

Chronic inflammatory infiltrate of portal tracts surrounding bile ducts with duct damage

CIRRHOSIS

Scarring of the *entire* liver with diffuse fibrosis, loss of lobular architecture, and nodular regeneration

Final common pathway for many diseases—often, the specific etiology cannot be determined histologically

Vascular reorganization with formation of abnormal arteriovenous connections is common

Ductular proliferation is seen regardless of etiology; does not necessarily indicate PBC

It is important to evaluate the level of activity: look for ongoing necrosis at border between septa and parenchyma

MICRONODULAR CIRRHOSIS
Almost all parenchymal nodules ≤3 mm diameter
Fibrous septa are thin (2 mm) and uniform
Nodules lack portal tracts and hepatic veins
Regularity suggests a uniform pathogenesis
Used to be referred to as Laënnec's, portal, or nutritional cirrhosis; these terms are no longer used because their etiologic implications are not always accurate
Associated with alcoholism and chronic biliary obstruction

MACRONODULAR CIRRHOSIS
Many nodules >3 mm diameter; some up to 3 cm
Broad fibrous septa as well as some delicate septa
Nodules contain portal tracts and hepatic veins
Variability suggests irregular preceding insult
May evolve from micronodular cirrhosis
Greater association with hepatocellular carcinoma
Incomplete septal fibrosis: subtype with delicate septa forming portal–portal connections

MIXED CIRRHOSIS
Combination of micro- and macronodular cirrhosis
May represent livers in transition from micronodular to macronodular cirrhosis

LIVER DISEASE IN PREGNANCY
Portal hypertension, chronic active hepatitis, Dubin-Johnson syndrome are diseases exacerbated by pregnancy

ACUTE FATTY LIVER OF PREGNANCY (see earlier)
VIRAL HEPATITIS
Most common cause of jaundice in pregnancy (as well as in nonpregnant women of childbearing age)
Treatment of newborn with hyperimmune serum and HBV vaccine will decrease risk of acute infection, chronic carrier state, hepatocellular carcinoma

INTRAHEPATIC CHOLESTASIS OF PREGNANCY
Second most common cause of jaundice in pregnancy
May occur anytime during gestation—more common later
Pruritus and jaundice persist till delivery
Bland cholestasis, predominantly zone 3
Presumably related to pregnancy-associated steroids
Greater risk is to fetus: fetal distress, premature delivery, fetal death in utero

LIVER DISEASE IN TOXEMIA (PRE-ECLAMPSIA) OF PREGNANCY
Usually 3rd trimester, usually primigravida
May see diffuse or confluent hemorrhage, parenchymal or capsular
Areas of infarction common—may be massive
Hemorrhage, fibrin deposition, hepatocellular necrosis in periportal regions
May also see sinusoidal fibrosis, steatosis, portal lymphoplasmacytic infiltrate, bile inspissation in canaliculi

HELLP SYNDROME
Severe form of toxemia
Combination of Hemolysis, Elevated Liver tests, Low Platelets (HELLP)
May result in hepatic rupture

CYSTIC LIVER DISEASE
ADULT POLYCYSTIC LIVER DISEASE
Autosomal dominant
Multiple variable-sized cysts (mm's to >10 cm) usually (90%) lined by a cuboidal epithelium
Do *not* communicate with biliary tree
Frequently accompanied by medullary renal cysts
Usually asymptomatic

CAROLI'S DISEASE
AKA: communicating cavernous biliary ectasia
Autosomal recessive
Multiple, large, ectatic ducts communicating with biliary tree
Patients may have recurrent cholangitis
Often seen in conjunction with congenital hepatic fibrosis or choledochal cysts

SOLITARY NONPARASITIC CYST
Etiology unclear—probably retention cyst of bile ductule origin; flattened cuboidal epithelial lining

ECHINOCOCCUS CYST
AKA: hydatid cyst
Rare in U.S., frequent in Iceland, Australia, South America
Caused by larval or cystic stage of dog tapeworm, most commonly *Echinococcus granulosus*
Liver and lung most common sites for cysts
Eosinophilia present while parasite is alive
When parasite dies, wall of cyst collapses and calcifies
Rupture into peritoneum can cause death by anaphylaxis
Usually unilocular cyst, 1–7 cm diameter; 75% right lobe
Cyst filled with colorless fluid, daughter cysts
Wall has outer chitinous (fibrous) layer and inner germinal layer—inner layer calcifies

ABSCESS (AMEBIC/PYOGENIC)
Originally, used to be more common in young adults, caused by ameba or secondary to pylephlebitis
Now, more commonly seen in older patients, usually enteric bacteria
30–80% mortality
Amebic cysts: odorless "anchovy paste" composed of necrotic hepatic tissue
Pyogenic cysts: foul-smelling contents with necrosis and neutrophils
Predisposing factors: biliary tract obstruction/infection, bacteremia, direct extension, trauma, pylephlebitis
Multiple lesions seen in 50% pyogenic, 25% amebic

MESENCHYMAL HAMARTOMA
(See later under Neoplasia, Other)

LIVER TRANSPLANTATION
First one performed in 1963
Indications: idiopathic cirrhosis, primary biliary cirrhosis, sclerosing cholangitis, biliary atresia, alpha$_1$-antitrypsin deficiency
~75% recipients have one or more episodes of rejection
~15% require retransplantation because of graft failure
Graft rejection most common reason for failure; usually occurs 1–4 wk after transplant; earlier failure usually caused by technical problems; later more commonly infectious
Harvesting/reperfusion injury: microsteatosis, ballooning degeneration, central canalicular cholestasis; later: acidophil bodies, hemorrhage, increased numbers of Kupffer cells; finally: centrilobular necrosis
Hyperacute rejection (necrotizing arteritis) very unusual; immediate graft failure usually secondary to occlusive or nonocclusive ischemia or infection
Acute rejection: triad—mixed lymphocytic-neutrophilic portal infiltrate, bile duct injury, endotheliitis:
• Grade I: <50% bile ducts damaged, endotheliitis
• Grade II: >50% bile ducts damaged, ± endotheliitis
• Grade III: larger vessel arteritis
Treated rejection: mononuclear cell infiltrate disappears first, leaving acute inflammation
Chronic rejection: obliterative endarteritis, portal fibrosis with bridging, paucity of bile ducts, cirrhosis, foam cell accumulation within intima of large vessels

Acute vanishing bile duct syndrome: irreversible loss of bile ducts within 100 days following transplantation caused by a destructive cholangitis

Lymphoproliferative disorder: affects 3–4% of patients

HYPERPLASIA/NEOPLASIA

NODULAR REGENERATIVE HYPERPLASIA
AKA: nodular transformation

Formation of cirrhosis-like nodules but without intervening fibrosis; nodules separated by compressed atrophic "normal" liver

May represent compensatory hyperplasia following diffuse chronic injury, such as ischemia or chemical injury

Cell plates usually two cells thick, indicating regeneration

Generally involves the entire liver

PARTIAL NODULAR TRANSFORMATION
Variant in which changes are confined to the area of the porta hepatis

Probably an early stage of nodular transformation

FOCAL NODULAR HYPERPLASIA
Any age, usually 20–40s, but all ages; female : male = 4 : 1

Asymptomatic in 80%; multiple in 20%

Arteriographically: hypervascular with centrifugal filling and a dense capillary blush

Grossly: gray-white, unencapsulated, solid mass (usually <5 cm) beneath capsule, sometimes pedunculated; often central fibrosis with radiating, stellate bands of fibrosis

Histology: all components of the normal liver lobule present; may have eccentrically thickened vessels in septa secondary to fibromuscular hyperplasia; septa may divide lesion into lobules, simulating cirrhosis

Arteriolar occlusion in central scar often seen: presumably etiologic: small area infarcts and scars; surrounding areas undergo compensatory hyperplasia

LIVER CELL ADENOMA
Usually female (male : female = 1 : 9), 20–40s; definite relationship to oral contraceptives (80–90%), often regress when discontinued

Most are solitary, right lobe, usually >10 cm at presentation

More often symptomatic; hemorrhage common: 25% present with hemoperitoneum

Well-defined capsule, well-differentiated hepatocytes with abundant cytoplasm, two cell layers thick, but *no* portal triads, central veins, or fibrosis, and no bile ducts or connection with the biliary system

Largest vessels are at the periphery and show intimal thickening and smooth muscle proliferation

Absence of vascular invasion differentiates from carcinoma; also, hepatoma often shows "nodule within nodule," infiltrative growth pattern, thick cords to sheets of cells

MULTIPLE HEPATOCELLULAR ADENOMATOSIS
Male = female; no association with contraceptives, patients are older

Usually >10 nodules of varying size

May be a *very* well-differentiated hepatocellular carcinoma

MACROREGENERATIVE NODULE
AKA: adenomatous hyperplastic nodule

Small numbers of nodules, usually >1 cm, usually occurring in the setting of cirrhosis, with a thin fibrous rim

Two types:
• Nodules similar to surrounding smaller nodules
• "Dysplastic nodule" with small cell dysplasia, a basophilic cytoplasm, monomorphous histology; borderline lesion; nodule within nodule appearance suggests hepatoma

HEPATOCELLULAR DYSPLASIA
Controversial subject

Even when correctly diagnosed, no clear indications for therapy

LARGE CELL DYSPLASIA
Isolated large cells with enlarged nuclei but normal N : C ratio

Normal nuclear contours

Commonly seen in cirrhosis

No evidence for premalignant condition

SMALL CELL DYSPLASIA
Clusters of normal-sized cells with larger nuclei (increased N : C ratio) and irregular nuclear contours

Architecture reasonably normal

DNA ploidy shows an increased number of peaks, most centered around 2n and 4n

Proliferating cell nuclear antigen and Ki-67 are both increased, although not as much as in hepatocellular Ca

Premalignant

HEPATOCELLULAR CARCINOMA
AKA: hepatoma

Any age; male > female, esp. when associated with cirrhosis

Usually presents with abdominal pain, ascites, hepatomegaly

Alpha-fetoprotein (AFP) levels often elevated in serum

Predisposing factors: cirrhosis, hepatitis B and C, Thorotrast (thorium dioxide), anabolic or progestational steroids (may be adenomas), alcohol, radiation, alpha₁-antitrypsin deficiency, aflatoxins from fungus *Aspergillus flavus*, ataxia-telangiectasia syndrome, hemochromatosis

May be single large mass ("massive"), multiple discrete masses ("nodular"), or numerous small nodules scattered throughout the liver ("diffuse")

May be encapsulated, pedunculated, any size

Histologic patterns: trabecular (most common), solid, pseudoglandular (acinar), pelioid, giant cell, sarcomatoid, clear cell

Network of sinusoidal vessels surrounds tumor cells

Stroma usually scanty

Hepatocytes may be well differentiated to very bizarre

Vascular invasion common

Portal vein thrombosis found in a large percentage of cases

Intranuclear pseudoinclusions, Mallory's hyaline, bile pigment, even significant clear cell change can all be seen

AFP, AAT, transferrin, Cam 5.2 positive; CEA, AE1 negative

Prognosis poor: 10% survival at 5 yr

Good prognosis: low stage, encapsulation, single lesions, absence of cirrhosis, perhaps those associated with oral contraceptives

No effect on prognosis: tumor size, age, sex, presence of HBV

SCLEROSING HEPATIC CARCINOMA

3% of primary hepatic tumors; male = female; usually in 60s

Two thirds of patients have hypercalcemia and hypophosphatemia without bone metastases

Only 50% of cases associated with cirrhosis

Cords of tumor cells in a dense fibrotic stroma

Most show hepatocellular histology; one third show partial to complete cholangiocarcinoma histology

Aggressive: mean survival = 6 months

FIBROLAMELLAR VARIANT

AKA: polygonal cell type; oncocytic type

Predominantly young patients (~25 yr); male = female; two thirds in left lobe

1–2% of hepatomas, but ~40% of the under 40 yr population

No association with cirrhosis or hepatitis virus

Fibrosis arranged in a lamellar fashion around polygonal, deeply eosinophilic hepatocytes (packed with mitochondria), which form sheets and occasional trabeculae

Calcification may be seen on plain films

More amenable to resection (60%)

Cure rate of 50 much better than conventional hepatoma

Staging

Stage	Number of Tumor Masses	Size	Vascular Invasion
T1	1	<2 cm	−
T2	1	<2 cm	+
	Multiple in 1 lobe	<2 cm	−
	1	>2 cm	−
T3	1	>2 cm	+
	Multiple in 1 lobe	<2 cm	+
	Multiple in 1 lobe	>2 cm	+/−
T4	Multiple lesions of any size in multiple lobes or involving major vessels		
N1	Regional lymph nodes involved		
M1	Distant metastases		

Stage	T1	T2	T3	T4
N0	I	II		IVA
N1			III	
M1			IVB	

HEPATOBLASTOMA

Almost exclusively in children, usually in first 3 yr; may be congenital; may be familial

Single, usually encapsulated

Can be associated with Wilms' tumor, glycogen storage disease, hemihypertrophy, virilization (ectopic steroid production), Beckwith-Wiedemann syndrome, polyposis coli

Tumor cells reactive for EMA, keratin, vimentin, AFP, CEA

Immunohistochemistry suggests the small "anaplastic" cells mature first to embryonal cells, which may then undergo ductular differentiation or progress to fetal-type cells

Locally invasive; metastases to regional lymph nodes (LNs), lung, brain

40–70% are unresectable at diagnosis

Prognosis better than hepatocellular carcinoma (esp. for the fetal type) but is still <40% long term survival

PURE (EPITHELIAL) TYPE (75%)

Fetal: small monotonous hepatocytes arranged in irregular two-cell thick cords with sinusoids, recapitulating fetal liver; extramedullary hematopoiesis common

Embryonal: predominantly solid growth pattern with ribbons, rosettes, and papillary formations; cells smaller, immature, usually more mitoses, higher N : C ratio; may represent ductular differentiation

Macrotrabecular type: resembles hepatocellular carcinoma

MIXED TYPE (25%)

Epithelial cells plus primitive stromal component, which may be undifferentiated or develop into bone or cartilage

ANAPLASTIC TYPE (RARE)

AKA: undifferentiated, small cell

Sheets of loosely cohesive small blue cells

BENIGN BILE DUCT TUMORS

BILE DUCT HAMARTOMA

AKA: von Meyenburg complex, Moschowitz complex, ductal plate anomaly

Multiple small, white nodules scattered throughout the liver

Focal (usually periportal) disorderly collection of bile ducts and ductules, slightly dilated and containing bile, surrounded by abundant fibrous stroma

Some may be ischemic in origin

May be associated with adult polycystic hepatorenal disease

BILE DUCT ADENOMA

Firm, white, discrete subcapsular nodules, usually <1 cm

80% of true adenomas are single; almost never bile stained

Multiple small cuboidal epithelium-lined ducts with small lumens, without bile, in a scant to abundant connective tissue stroma

CEA, EMA, keratin positive

BILIARY CYSTADENOMA

Multilocular cysts with mucinous or clear fluid lined by a simple cuboidal to columnar epithelium

Usually right lobe; 25–30 cm in diameter; female >> male

Malignant transformation can occur: pleomorphism, anaplasia, stromal infiltration

BILIARY PAPILLOMATOSIS

Dilated intrahepatic or extrahepatic ducts with exophytic, papillary proliferations of duct lining cells on fibrovascular cores

Although cytologically benign, often recurrent, progressive, and ultimately fatal

CHOLANGIOCARCINOMA

5–30% of primary hepatic malignancies

Most seen >60 yr of age; male = female

Some arise within congenitally dilated intrahepatic bile ducts, after Thorotrast, anabolic steroids, intrahepatic lithiasis, primary sclerosing cholangitis

No relationship with cirrhosis

Marked heterogeneity of neoplastic cells within same gland

Tendency to spread between hepatocyte plates and along ducts and nerves, and to invade lymphatics

Usually marked desmoplastic response

Mucin stains usually positive; occasionally signet ring cells

Keratin (Cam 5.2 and AE1), EMA, CEA positive; AFP negative

Klatskin's tumor: cholangiocarcinoma arising at confluence of left and right hepatic ducts

Adenosquamous and mucoepidermoid variants have been described

Staging is same as for hepatocellular carcinoma

VASCULAR TUMORS

HEMANGIOMA

Most common benign tumor of liver; usually cavernous

Male : female = 1 : 5; may enlarge during pregnancy

INFANTILE HEMANGIOENDOTHELIOMA
Solitary or multiple
Two histologic types:
- Type I: small, well-formed vessels with plump endothelial lining cells; may progress to cavernous hemangioma
- Type II: marked nuclear pleomorphism, mitoses, papillary projections of endothelial cells into lumen of cystic spaces

High mortality, often due to hepatic failure or CHF

EPITHELIOID HEMANGIOENDOTHELIOMA
Mostly adult females, perhaps related to oral contraceptives
Tumors often multiple, involving entire liver
Dendritic and epithelioid tumor cells infiltrate sinusoids and veins
Abundant stroma, which is variably myxoid to sclerotic; dystrophic calcification can be seen
Better prognosis than angiosarcoma; 28% metastasize, but does not preclude long-term survival

ANGIOSARCOMA
AKA: malignant hemangioendothelioma
Freely anastomosing vascular channels; varying degrees of differentiation
Usually factor VIII immunoreactive
Increased risk factors: cirrhosis, vinyl chloride exposure, thorium dioxide exposure, arsenic exposure
Most patients die within 6 months of liver failure or abdominal hemorrhage

OTHER TUMORS

FOCAL FATTY CHANGE
Not a tumor
Steatosis confined to a discrete area of the liver from a few millimeters to 10 cm in diameter
No clinical significance, but often mistaken at ultrasound or computed tomography (CT) for something more ominous

MIXED/COMBINED HEPATOCELLULAR AND CHOLANGIOCARCINOMA
Both malignant hepatocytes and malignant bile duct cells
<5% of primary hepatic carcinomas
Presumably arise from common precursor cell (both the bile ducts and hepatocytes arise from same precursors)

MESENCHYMAL HAMARTOMA
Usually infants
Solitary, spherical, reddish nodule 5–20 cm in diameter; may be pedunculated; may show cystic accumulation of fluid in stroma
Well-vascularized, loose, mature connective tissue intermixed with irregular, elongated, branching bile ducts, vessels, occasional islands of hepatocytes or hematopoiesis
Looks like breast fibroadenoma at low power

MALIGNANT MESENCHYMOMA
AKA: undifferentiated sarcoma, embryonal sarcoma
Usually children 6–10 yr old; present with abdominal swelling
Highly atypical mesenchymal cells with entrapped hyperplastic and dilated bile ducts near periphery
Large, solitary, well-circumscribed, necrosis, hemorrhage
Very poor prognosis

ANGIOMYOLIPOMA
Generally solitary, 1–20 cm, tan to yellow, well demarcated
Hematopoietic islands seen in two thirds

CARCINOID TUMOR
TERATOMA

METASTATIC TUMORS
Most common malignant tumor in liver (>90%!; drops to <50% in cirrhotic livers)

Frequent primary sites include gallbladder, bile ducts, pancreas, stomach, large bowel, lung, breast, kidney
Leukemias and lymphomas often involve the liver
Sarcomas also frequently metastasize to liver

GALLBLADDER

NORMAL
In 60–70% of individuals, common bile duct joins the pancreatic duct and empties into duodenum at a single site
Gallbladder has no muscularis mucosa or submucosa; mucosal lining and lamina propria directly above muscularis
Some glands penetrate into wall
Bile is 97% water
Liver secretes 0.5–1.0 l bile/day; gallbladder can hold 50 ml—concentrates bile 5- to 10-fold
Bile acids (cholates, deoxycholates, chenodeoxycholates) make up 70% of solutes in bile, phospholipids 22%, cholesterol 4%, bilirubin 1%
Most bile salts excreted into duodenal lumen are reabsorbed in the small intestine and colon: enterohepatic circulation

CONGENITAL ABNORMALITIES

EXTRAHEPATIC BILIARY ATRESIA
Partial/total absence of permeable bile ducts between porta hepatis and duodenum; may have fibrous cords without patent lumen
1/20,000 live births; most common cause of persistent neonatal cholestasis
Etiology may be developmental (persistence of solid stage of duct development) or acquired (in utero destruction of duct system by viral/other injury)
Intrahepatic ducts initially proliferate (peaks at 205 days), fibrose, then regress (most rapid at ~400 days)
- Correctable (10%): patent proximal ducts; perform biliary enteric anastomosis
  Type I: involves only common bile duct
  Type II: common bile duct and hepatic duct absent
- Uncorrectable (type III) (90%): no patent portion of the extrahepatic system; two thirds will have no gallbladder, one third will have patent gallbladder and cystic duct, but no ducts between liver and cystic duct; performing Kasai procedure (hepatic porto-enterostomy) before 10 wk of age can restore bile flow, but large failure rate—presence of bile ducts larger than 200 μm in diameter in resected portion is a positive prognostic sign

CHOLEDOCHAL CYST
Most common cause of obstructive jaundice in children beyond infancy
Focal fusiform or diverticular dilatation of common bile duct
May secondarily obstruct extrahepatic biliary tree
Cyst wall fibrous, sometimes calcified, with 1–2 L of bile
Increased incidence of carcinoma

HETEROTOPIC TISSUE
Gastric mucosa, intestinal, pancreas, adrenal, thyroid
Most occur as well defined nodules in neck of cystic duct

CHOLELITHIASIS

Only 10% of gallstones are pure:
- Pure cholesterol stones: pale yellow, round/ovoid, granular surface, often single, crystalline core, radiolucent
- Pure calcium bilirubinate stones (pigment stones) are black oval, numerous; associated with cirrhosis and hemolytic disorders; when develop in setting of infection, brown rather than black and softer

80% of all gallstones are mixed with varying combinations of cholesterol, calcium bilirubinate, and calcium carbonate; usually multiple and laminated

Some designate any stone with >70% cholesterol as a cholesterol stone and any with <30% cholesterol as a pigment stone

Combined stones (10%) have either pure nucleus with a mixed shell or vice versa

~20% of stones have enough calcium to be radiopaque

Bile salts and, to a lesser extent, lecithin (phospholipid) increase solubility of cholesterol in bile

Lithogenesis promoted by excess of cholesterol relative to amount of bile salts, followed by nucleation precipitation and then growth of aggregates

Biliary sludge with mucus and small crystals usually precedes stone formation

Risk factors: female, age >40, obesity, multiple pregnancies; any drugs or hormones that increase cholesterol excretion or decrease bile salt levels promote stones

Inflammatory Disorders

ACUTE CHOLECYSTITIS

90% of cases caused by impaction of gallstone in neck of gallbladder or cystic duct ("calculous cholecystitis")

Often sudden onset; surgical emergency

E. coli or other gram-negative bacilli can be cultured from bile in 80% of cases; probably secondary event

Acalculous cholecystitis much less common; seen more frequently in men and in association with previous surgery, bacteremia, trauma, systemic arteritis, diabetes, prolonged labor, intravenous hyperalimentation

Grossly, gallbladder enlarged and tense; may be bright red

Serosa may be coated by fibrin

Contents may be turbid with fibrin or pus

Wall thickened and edematous, but in severe cases may be gangrenous—infiltrated by neutrophils

In rare cases, may heal by calcifying → porcelain gallbladder

CHRONIC CHOLECYSTITIS

Virtually always associated with cholelithiasis; female : male = 3 : 1

May result from repeated mild acute inflammatory events, but usually seen in absence of history of acute events

Wall often has some degree of chronic inflammation, but may be minimal; subserosal fibrosis, entrapped epithelial crypts (cholecystitis glandularis), dystrophic calcification

Acute and chronic features may be seen together

FOLLICULAR CHOLECYSTITIS

Lymphoid follicles present transmurally

EOSINOPHILIC CHOLECYSTITIS

Large number of mature eosinophils

XANTHOGRANULOMATOUS CHOLECYSTITIS

OTHER NON-NEOPLASTIC DISORDERS

CHOLESTEROLOSIS

No clinical significance

Yellow flecks studding mucosal surface

Mucosa usually congested ("strawberry gallbladder")

Focal accumulation of lipid-laden macrophages in the lamina propria at the tips of mucosal folds

ADENOMYOMA AND ADENOMYOMATOSIS

Proliferation of both glandular and smooth muscle elements with extension of the surface epithelium deep into the wall

INFLAMMATORY POLYPS

Fibrous stroma covered by a usually intact epithelium, creating a sessile mucosal projection; stroma infiltrated with chronic inflammatory cells

MUCOCELE (HYDROPS)

When outflow obstructed by a stone but acute inflammation does not develop

Gallbladder distended with clear, watery, mucinous secretion

Wall often becomes stretched and atrophic

Neoplasms

BENIGN LESIONS

PAPILLOMAS AND ADENOMAS

Rare

Localized benign overgrowths of lining epithelium

Papilloma usually has stalk-like connection; adenoma connected via broad base

PARAGANGLIOMA

GRANULAR CELL TUMOR

CARCINOMA OF GALLBLADDER

More frequent in females (3–4 : 1)

90% of patients >50 yr old

May be diffuse (70%) or polypoid (30%) mass

80–90% of cases also have gallstones

Diffuse form may be grossly indistinguishable from chronic cholecystitis

Most are adenocarcinomas; may be papillary, usually deeply invasive, poorly differentiated cytologically

Keratin and CEA positive

Focal intestinal metaplasia common

Squamous metaplasia can give rise to adenoacanthoma or adenosquamous carcinoma

Undifferentiated (anaplastic, pleomorphic, sarcomatoid) histology also exists

Most have invaded the liver by time of diagnosis (stage V); uniformly fatal

Staging

NEVIN SCHEME

Stage	Description	5 Yr Survival
I	Intramucosal	90%
II	Mucosa and muscularis	55%
III	Full thickness of wall	15%
IV	Cystic lymph node	15%
V	Liver or other organs	3%

AMERICAN JOINT COMMITTEE ON CANCER

T1a	Mucosal
T1b	Muscularis
T2	Perimuscular connective tissue

T3	Perforates serosa or extends into adjacent organ (if liver, <2 cm)	
T4	>2 cm into liver, or into two or more adjacent organs	
N1	Cystic duct, pericholedochal, or hilar LNs	
N2	Peripancreatic, periduodenal, periportal, celiac, or superior mesenteric LNs	

Stage	T1	T2	T3	T4
N0	I	II	III	IVA
N1	III	III	III	IVA
N2	IVB	IVB	IVB	IVB

CARCINOMA OF EXTRAHEPATIC BILE DUCTS
AKA: cholangiocarcinoma

Equal frequency in males and females; usually >60 yr

90% present with jaundice

In order of frequency, most common sites in biliary tree are gallbladder, papilla of Vater, common bile duct, left or right hepatic ducts, common hepatic duct

Can be polypoid or superficial, but most are nodular or sclerosing with deep penetration into wall

Heterogeneity of cells within the same gland, increased N:C ratio, nucleolar prominence, and stromal and perineural invasion

Choledochal cysts, cholangitis, and *Giardia* predispose

Overall survival rate <10%

EMBRYONAL RHABDOMYOSARCOMA
Usually in children <5 yr old

Arise in extrahepatic bile ducts (>75% in common bile duct); patients present with obstruction and jaundice

Botryoid morphology with cambium layer subjacent to the bile duct epithelium

15

PANCREAS

NORMAL ANATOMY

Averages 15 cm length, 60–140 g in adult

Close proximity to duodenum, ampulla of Vater, common bile duct, superior mesenteric artery, portal vein, spleen and its vessels, stomach, transverse colon, left lobe of liver

Large reserve of function, so damage detected only when advanced or when involves surrounding structures

At birth, the islets represent a greater fraction of the whole gland than in the adult, because with age the exocrine pancreas "overgrows" the endocrine pancreas

EXOCRINE

Acini separated by scant connective tissue stroma

Ductal system: centroacinar cells, then cuboidal, columnar

Duct cells are mucin secreting; intercalated ducts to intra-lobular to interlobular, etc.

Main ducts: Wirsung (main) and Santorini (accessory)

In 60% of adults, major pancreatic duct does not empty into the duodenum directly but rather into the common bile duct

Secretion occurs in response to secretin from duodenum

ENDOCRINE

Islets of Langerhans (10^6); more in tail; 1–1.5 g total

Cell types	Granules by Electron Microscopy
Alpha (20%; peripheral; glucagon)	Round with gray halo
Beta (70%; central; insulin)	Rectangular, halo, matrix
Delta (5–10%; somatostatin: suppresses insulin + glucagon)	Large, pale, no halo
PP cell (1–2%; pancreatic polypeptide; also in exocrine pancreas)	Small, dark
D1 cells (P cells); vasoactive inhibitor peptide	
EC cells (serotonin)	

Dorsal-derived islets have more alpha cells than PP cells; ventral-derived islets have abundant PP cells

EMBRYOLOGY

Both exocrine and endocrine pancreas form from endoder-mally derived tubules

Islets form from cells that separate from tubules (~9 wk)

Arises from two duodenal buds: dorsal and ventral pancreas

Ventral (uncinate process and inferior portion of head) arises near the entry of the common bile duct and grows more slowly, eventually swinging around posteriorly with the bile duct as the duodenal C-loop forms (5–6 wk) to fuse with the larger dorsal portion (body and tail)

Wirsung's duct formed from ventral duct and distal portion of the dorsal duct; the proximal portion of the dorsal duct, if it persists, becomes Santorini's (accessory) duct

In 10%, the ducts fail to fuse—double duct system persists

HETEROTOPIA

Approximately 2% incidence

Most common sites are duodenum, stomach, jejunum, Meckel's diverticulum, gallbladder, large bowel

Firm, yellow, lobulated; often central umbilication

Islet tissue found in only one third

May become inflamed or neoplastic

ANNULAR PANCREAS

Rare malformation; more prevalent in males

May result from growth of bifed ventral bud, both anterior and posterior to the duodenum, each fusing with dorsal bud

May cause duodenal obstruction shortly after birth

CONGENITAL ISLET HYPERPLASIA

Children of diabetic mothers

Islets infiltrated by eosinophils

Also see asymmetric septal hypertrophy and sacral agenesis

Nesidioblastosis: diffuse beta cell hyperplasia both within islets and throughout the pancreas

INFLAMMATORY/NON-NEOPLASTIC DISORDERS

ACUTE PANCREATITIS

Etiology controversial: most likely transient/partial obstruc-tion (calculus or sphincter spasm) resulting in bile reflux into pancreatic duct system with activation of pancreatic enzymes and subsequent tissue destruction

80% of cases are associated with either biliary tract disease (male : female = 1 : 3) or alcoholism (male : female = 6 : 1)

Postoperative pancreatitis, usually related to surgical trauma

10–20% of patients with parathyroid adenoma/carcinoma develop acute pancreatitis—hypercalcemia?

Other etiologies include idiopathic hypercalcemia, thia-zides, furosemide, and estrogen use

Acinar cell homogenization, ductal dilatation, diffuse edema, acute inflammation, fibrosis, fat necrosis, calcification

May result in large abscess formation

Severe form referred to as *acute hemorrhagic pancreatitis* or *acute pancreatic necrosis*

20% mortality (10–15% for swollen, edematous gland; 50% if hemorrhagic and necrotic gland)

CHRONIC PANCREATITIS
AKA: chronic relapsing pancreatitis
Usually not associated with acute pancreatitis
Duct and islets are spared initially

CHRONIC OBSTRUCTIVE PANCREATITIS
Narrowing or occlusion of the duct, usually from carcinoma or stone, most commonly cholelithiasis
Less severe changes than calcifying form, with relative sparing of the duct epithelium
With large duct obstruction, pancreatic damage is relatively uniform throughout the gland

CHRONIC CALCIFYING PANCREATITIS
Most commonly seen in alcoholics
Damage is irregular and patchy: dilatation of ducts with squamous metaplasia and intraluminal protein plugs (which often calcify), acinar dilatation and atrophy, interlobular fibrosis
Pseudocyst formation common
Calcifications range from microscopic to stones several centimeters in diameter

COMPLICATIONS
Widespread metastatic fat necrosis: presumably related to release of lipase—involves subcutaneous tissue, mediastinum, pleura, pericardium, liver, etc.
Erythema nodosum–like panniculitis
Initially a marked proliferation of islet cells, and then later a preferential loss of insulin-secreting cells
Avascular bone necrosis

CYSTIC LESIONS OF THE PANCREAS

CONGENITAL CYSTS
Anomalous development of pancreatic ducts
Related to similar diseases in liver and kidney
May be single or multiple, microscopic or large
Von Hippel-Lindau disease: pancreatic cysts associated with angiomas in the retina, cerebellum, brain stem

CYSTIC FIBROSIS
AKA: mucoviscidosis
Cysts form secondary to duct obstruction with thick, tenacious secretions
(See also Congenital Syndromes outline)

PSEUDOCYSTS
Account for >75% of all cystic lesions in the pancreas
Seen in pancreatitis, trauma, and occasionally neoplastic duct obstruction
Amylase-rich fluid in cysts
Can extend well beyond pancreas; multiple in 15%
Cysts characteristically have no epithelial lining or connection with the duct system
Complications include rupture, hemorrhage, erosion into surrounding structures (e.g., splenic artery)

DIABETES MELLITUS
Most common disease process affecting the pancreas
Islets may be normal but may see amyloid deposition (40%), fibrosis (25%), or vacuolation/destruction of beta cells
Other associated findings:
• Microangiopathy
• Retinopathy (nonproliferative [exudative] and proliferative types)
• Nephropathy (nodular Kimmelstiel–Wilson glomerulosclerosis, pyelonephritis, papillary necrosis)
• Neuropathy (usually symmetric polyneuropathy)

Primary
TYPE I
AKA: juvenile onset, insulin dependent; ketoacidosis prone

Genetic susceptibility (50% concordance among identical twins)
Autoimmune destruction of islets
Increased association with rubella and coxsackie viruses, and with cow-milk allergy

TYPE II
AKA: adult onset, non–insulin dependent
Obese and non-obese subtypes
90% concordance among identical twins
Decreased secretion of insulin without loss of islets

Secondary
Hemochromatosis, drugs, tumors, chronic pancreatitis

OTHER
HEMOCHROMATOSIS
Hemosiderin deposition in acinar and islet cells leads to brown discoloration ("bronze diabetes")
FATTY INFILTRATION (LIPOMATOSIS)
Nondestructive infiltration—no clinical significance

PANCREATIC ATROPHY
If ischemic, will affect both endocrine and exocrine
Obstruction of ducts (ligation) can cause complete destruction of exocrine pancreas with sparing of islets (allowed the initial isolation of insulin)

PANCREAS TRANSPLANT
Sparse inflammatory infiltrate (lymphocytes) always seen
For rejection, need to have patchy inflammation in acinar tissue and ducts, with cell dropout, interstitial fibrosis, cellular atypia, and a capillaritis
Chronic rejection shows endarteritis with foam cell accumulation

NEOPLASMS

Tumors of Exocrine Pancreas

Staging

T1	Limited to pancreas
Ia:	≤2 cm
Ib:	>2 cm
T2	Extension to duodenum, bile ducts, soft tissue
T3	Extension to stomach, spleen, colon, major vessels
N0	No regional nodes
N1	Positive regional nodes

	T1	T2	T3
N0	I	I	II
N1		III	
M1		IV	

INFANTILE PANCREATIC CARCINOMA
AKA: pancreatoblastoma
Common pancreatic tumor in children, but not only kind

Well-formed glands arranged around solid nests of cells, which may have squamoid features

Looks like islet cell tumor or carcinoid, but no granules by electron microscopy (EM)

Actually an acinar cell tumor

Relatively favorable prognosis but can be large, direct extension, metastases

PAPILLARY AND SOLID EPITHELIAL NEOPLASM

AKA: papillary-cystic carcinoma, cystic-solid papillary carcinoma (depending on proportion of components)

Probably begins as a solid tumor; degeneration of cells far from vessels with sparing of the perivascular cells leads to a pseudopapillary pattern and cystic spaces

Most cases in young women (20s)

Usually large and hemorrhagic/necrotic on cut section

Solid areas are very cellular, simulating islet cell tumor; cells have ovoid nuclei with folds, indistinct nucleoli, few mitoses; cytoplasmic PAS+ hyaline globules

Papillae: thick, edematous (sometimes mucinous with foamy cells), fibrovascular cores covered by a multilayered epithelium

Can see focal reactivity for a number of antigens, most commonly NSE; usually vimentin positive, keratin negative

Ultrastructure: features of acinar, ductal, and endocrine differentiation

Most likely tumor of primitive cells with the capacity for dual differentiation

Excellent prognosis

MICROCYSTIC CYSTADENOMA

AKA: glycogen-rich, serous cystadenoma

Patients usually elderly; usually head of pancreas

Associated with von Hippel-Lindau syndrome

Large; numerous small cysts (most <1 cm), lined by flat cuboidal cells with abundant glycogen, minimal mucin, microvilli; myoepithelial cells still present

Prominent vascularization, central scar (may be calcified); islet cells in trabeculae

Invariably benign

MUCINOUS CYSTIC TUMORS

AKA: mucinous cystadenocarcinoma

Younger age group (40s), female predominance

More commonly body or tail; may be confused with pseudocyst

Large, often encapsulated, with multilocular or unilocular cysts, tall mucin-producing cells; may have intermixed endocrine or Paneth cells

Cellular stroma (similar to ovary), often calcification in wall; hypovascular

Invasion of wall or frank anaplasia indicates malignancy, but *all mucinous tumors are potentially malignant*

Overall 5 yr survival 50%

DUCTAL ADENOCARCINOMA

85% of all pancreatic malignancies, even though duct cells account for only 4% of pancreatic mass

4th most common cancer killer in U.S.

Increased incidence in Peutz-Jeghers syndrome, exposure to beta-naphthylamine or benzidine, cigarette smoking (2×), diabetes, gastrectomy

Most patients are elderly, slight male predominance

Two thirds of cases in head of pancreas; one third in body or tail

Multiple tumors found in 20%

Poorly delineated, firm, white/yellow

Well to poorly differentiated; occasionally papillary

Well-differentiated tumors can be very difficult to diagnose; look for nuclear pleomorphism (size variation >4 : 1), loss of polarity, incomplete glandular structures, disorganized duct distribution, prominent nucleoli, mitoses

Diagnosis by cytology even more problematic: success rate varies with source: pancreatic secretions, 50–85%; duodenal secretions, 66%; percutaneous or intraoperative fine needle aspiration (FNA), 90%; transduodenal biopsy avoids the risk of fistula formation

Desmoplastic stromal reaction common

Immunoreactive for keratin, EMA, CEA, CA19-9, laminin

Carcinoma in situ present in 20–30%; often far from tumor mass—may be at surgical margin

Obstruction of the duct can lead to a background of chronic pancreatitis

Islet tissue preserved longest, but when destroyed creates diabetic picture clinically

Trousseau's syndrome: migratory peripheral thrombophlebitis seen in 10–25% of patients

MICROSCOPIC VARIANTS

Adenosquamous, oncocytic, clear cell, signet ring, mucinous (colloid) carcinoma

SPREAD

Perineural invasion in 90%; beware of benign epithelial inclusions

85% of cases are beyond pancreas at the time of diagnosis

88% to peripancreatic lymph nodes (LNs); 33% to more distant nodes

Liver, peritoneum, lung, adrenal, bone, skin, CNS

Liver metastases most common in tumors of body or tail

PROGNOSIS

10% 1 yr survival; 2% 5 yr survival

Even T1 lesions have only a 15% 5 yr survival

ACINAR CELL CARCINOMA

1–2% of all pancreatic cancers

May arise from acinar hyperplasia, benign form may exist

Generally solid mass obliterating architecture without duct dilatation; occasionally multicystic

Acinar cells with numerous zymogen granules, often prominent nucleoli, usually immunoreactive for trypsin

May be associated with widespread subcutaneous fat necrosis

Very poor prognosis

ANAPLASTIC CARCINOMA

7% of non-endocrine pancreatic malignancies

Most involve body or tail

Most patients >50 yr; male predominance

Extremely poor prognosis

Three subtypes:

• Pleomorphic: bizarre multinucleated giant tumor cells

• Sarcomatoid: spindle cells

• Undifferentiated: small cell

GIANT CELL TUMOR

Two cell types: uniform spindle cells with atypical features and multinucleated osteoclast-like giant cells (not atypical)

Prognosis more like ductal than anaplastic

Tumors of the Endocrine Pancreas

General
Much less common than tumors of the exocrine pancreas
Mostly adults, some in infants (even newborns)
Most commonly body or tail (more islets)
May arise from pleuripotential precursor (terminal ducts) rather than islets themselves
May be nonfunctioning or secrete one or several peptides: if multiple tumors, each may be same peptide, different peptide, or mixture
Gross: solid, pink, vascular, may show extensive fibrosis, calcification, bone; may be partially cystic
Generally, monotonous proliferation of small cells with central nuclei, occasional small nucleoli, and a finely granular cytoplasm; grows in one of four patterns:
• Solid (A, I): most common pattern; any cell type
• Gyriform (B, II): alpha or beta cells
• Glandular (C, III): G or VIP cells
• Nondescript (D, IV)
Amyloid may be seen in stroma of insulin-secreting tumors
Cells generally immunoreactive for NSE, chromogranin, synaptophysin, and neurofilament, plus specific peptides (may be focal), including insulin, glucagon, somatostatin, pancreatic polypeptide, serotonin, vasoactive intestinal peptide (VIP), adrenocorticotropic hormone (ACTH), antidiuretic hormone (ADH), melanocyte-stimulating hormone (MSH), calcitonin, parathormone, growth hormone (GH)

MALIGNANCY
Stromal invasion, vascular invasion, metastases best criteria
Nuclear pleomorphism and mitoses common in benign lesions
Malignant tumors are more likely to be functional—may also secrete chorionic gonadotropin
Beta cell tumors usually benign, all others usually malignant
Slow-growing tumors—resection of unresectable tumors or metastases (liver most common site) is warranted

BETA CELL TUMOR
AKA: insulinoma
Most common functioning islet cell tumor
Clinically, Whipple triad
• Mental confusion, weakness, fatigue, convulsions
• Fasting blood sugar <50 mg%
• Symptoms relieved by glucose
>90% are solitary; 0.3–1.5 cm in diameter
Use angiography to localize—70% successful
Microscopy: solid or gyriform; glands usually *not* seen
EM: dense-core granules ± crystalline material
Immunohistochemistry: insulin (less than normal islets); minimally reactive for chromogranin
In children: may see nesidioblastosis (direct transformation of ductal epithelium into neoplastic islet tissue)
Only 10% are malignant

ALPHA CELL TUMOR
AKA: glucagonoma
Glucagonoma syndrome
• Mainly adult females (perimenopausal)
• Abnormal glucose tolerance test
• Normocytic normochromic anemia
• Skin rash: necrolytic migratory erythema
• Weight loss, depression, deep vein thromboses (DVTs), frequent infections

ASSOCIATED WITH GLUCAGONOMA SYNDROME
Large, solitary
Nondescript microscopic pattern, atypical granules by EM
Focal reactivity for glucagon
Usually malignant

NOT ASSOCIATED WITH GLUCAGONOMA SYNDROME
Small, multiple
Gyriform growth pattern, typical granules by EM
Strongly reactive for glucagon
Nearly always benign

G-CELL TUMOR
AKA: gastrinoma
Zollinger-Ellison syndrome: gastric hyperacidity with gastric, duodenal, jejunal ulcers; diarrhea in one third of patients
Located in pancreas in 75%, duodenum in 23%, stomach rarely
Without other endocrine abnormalities, usually solitary and malignant; as component of multiple endocrine neoplasia (MEN) I (see Endocrine outline), often multiple, benign
Non-neoplastic pancreas usually shows islet cell hyperplasia
If localized tumor, remove; otherwise, remove stomach

OTHERS
DELTA CELL TUMOR
AKA: somatostatinoma
May present with diabetes, steatorrhea, hypochlorhydria (somatostatin is inhibitory of other islet cells)
Psammoma bodies common

VIP-PRODUCING TUMORS
AKA: vipoma
Watery diarrhea without gastric hypersecretion (hypokalemia, achlorhydria)
Indistinguishable histologically from G-cell tumor—use immunohistochemistry (may also be positive for PP, calcitonin, alpha human chorionic gonadotropin)

PP CELL TUMOR
Rare if count only those exclusive for PP
Pancreatic polypeptide common in other islet tumors

CARCINOID TUMOR
Similar to carcinoid tumors elsewhere
Probably arise from Kultschitsky cells in exocrine ducts

SMALL CELL CARCINOMA
Similar to counterpart in lung
May secrete ACTH or parathyroid hormone

16

KIDNEY

ANATOMY/PHYSIOLOGY

~150 g each in adult; left higher than right
Unit of function: nephron (1.3 million/kidney)
Receives 20–25% of the cardiac output (1700 l/day)
Arteries: renal, interlobar, arcuate, interlobular, afferent, glomerular capillaries, efferent, etc.
Renal lobules demarcated by interlobular arteries, contain medullary ray (collecting ducts)
Renal columns of Bertin between renal pyramids
Lobe: pyramid plus overlying cortex (6–18 lobes/kidney)
10–25 papillary ducts (of Bellini) per papilla

JUXTAGLOMERULAR APPARATUS

- JG cells (modified smooth muscle cells within afferent arterioles)
- Macula densa (specialized region of distal convoluted tubule where it adjoins its parent glomerulus)
- Lacis (nongranular) cells (mesangial-like cells situated between afferent arteriole, macula densa, and glomerulus

Ultrafiltration

Glomerular capillaries composed of fenestrated endothelium
Filtration barrier: glomerular basement membrane (~3.5 nm, negatively charged matrix: polyanions and acidic glycoproteins)
180 L filtrate/day; ~1 L final excretion/day

Reabsorption

FIRST THIRD (PROXIMAL CONVOLUTED TUBULES)

65% reabsorbed—output isotonic
All glucose + amino acids via Na symport
Secretion of acids; bicarbonate reabsorption

MIDDLE THIRD (LOOP OF HENLE)

15% reabsorbed—output hypotonic
Descending: low salt permeability, high water
Ascending: high salt permeability, low water
Thick ascending: active NaCl transport establishes countercurrent multiplier

DISTAL THIRD (DISTAL CONVOLUTED, COLLECTING TUBULES)

Output variable
NaCl transport controlled by aldosterone
Water permeability controlled by antidiuretic hormone (ADH)

Hormones

ALDOSTERONE

Increases NaCl transport
98% resorbed routinely—modulates remaining 2%
Can vary urine secretion by up to 3 l/day

ANTIDIURETIC HORMONE (VASOPRESSIN)

Increases water permeability of distal one third
Diabetes insipidus: no ADH—lose 10 l/day

Syndrome of inappropriate secretion of ADH (SIADH): high ADH—oliguric

RENIN

Secreted by juxtaglomerular apparatus (JGA) in response to hypotension; macula densa cells may provide JGA with information about the content of fluid in the distal tubule
Converts hepatic angiotensinogen to angiotensin I
Angiotensin converting enzyme (ACE) in lung converts angiotensin I to angiotensin II
Angiotensin II increases aldosterone production and causes vasoconstriction

NATRIURETIC HORMONE

Uncharacterized agent to explain how nephrons increase glomerular filtration rate (GFR) to compensate for nephron destruction

ERYTHROPOIETIN

Source not precisely known
Secreted in response to low oxygen tension, either as a result of low flow or low oxygen concentration

CLINICAL TERMINOLOGY

Clearance: amount of plasma cleared of a substance per minute to account for appearance in urine; $C = $ (mg/ml in urine $\times$ ml/min urine)/mg/ml in plasma
Azotemia: increased blood urea nitrogen (BUN)/creatinine (Cr); may be prerenal, renal, postrenal
Uremia: azotemia + clinical signs/symptoms; Sine qua non of chronic renal failure
Selective proteinuria: low molecular weight proteins
Acute renal failure: abrupt oliguria/anuria with rapidly progressive azotemia (increase in blood urea/ammonia)
Nephrotic syndrome: massive proteinuria (>3.5 g/day), hypoalbuminemia, severe edema (anasarca), lipiduria, hyperlipidemia
Nephritic syndrome (i.e., acute glomerulonephritis): acute hematuria, RBC casts, mild proteinuria, hypertension, edema, oliguria
Rapidly progressive glomerulonephritis: acute hematuria, profound oliguria, renal failure in weeks

EMBRYOLOGY

PRONEPHROS (FOREKIDNEY)

Wolffian duct based
Nonfunctional kidneys, but most of the ducts are retained to form collecting system

MESONEPHROS (MIDKIDNEYS)

Analogous to kidneys of fish and amphibians
Appear in 4th wk
Function for a while in rabbit, cat, pig, . . . human?
Form complete nephron-like tubules, but degenerate

METANEPHROS (HINDKIDNEYS)

Begin to form in 5th wk, function by 11–13 wk

Metanephric diverticulum (ureteric bud) forms ureter, pelvis, calyces, and collecting tubules, penetrating into the metanephric mesoderm, which forms the metanephric vesicles, then tubules (S-shaped)—proximal ends invaginated by glomeruli to form nephron

CONGENITAL ANOMALIES
RENAL AGENESIS
Bilateral: rare; severe oligohydramnios, early death
Unilateral: 1/1000; other kidney hypertrophies
HYPOPLASIA
Usually unilateral
Term collectively refers to true insufficient development (minority of cases) and to small kidneys secondary to vascular/infectious insult
True hypoplasia will show decreased number of lobules (<5 vs. >10)
ECTOPIC KIDNEYS
Usually pelvic, malrotated, smaller
HORSESHOE KIDNEY
1/600 persons
Fusion of upper (10%) or lower (90%) poles, anterior to the great vessels
MISCELLANEOUS
Malrotation; multiple renal vessels; duplications of the upper urinary tract

CYSTIC "DISEASES"

CYSTIC RENAL DYSPLASIA
"Multicystic kidney"; Potter's types 2 and 4
Sporadic (nonhereditary)
Developmentally abnormal kidney, with persistence within the kidney of undifferentiated mesenchyme, immature and cystically dilated collecting ductules, and, most diagnostically, cartilage (20%; pathognomonic)
Can be unilateral (60–70%) or bilateral (30–40%)
Enlarged, usually cystic organ, often irregular contour, with disorganized parenchyma; can't distinguish cortex from medulla grossly or histologically
90% of cases are associated with (may be caused by) outflow obstruction from ureteral atresia or urethral valves

AUTOSOMAL RECESSIVE POLYCYSTIC DISEASE
"Infantile"; Potter's type 1, perinatal, juvenile
Cysts usually begin to develop at 19–20 wk gestation
Most present in utero or neonatally; some in childhood
When severe, may result in pulmonary hypoplasia secondary to compression during development
Bilateral
Multiple small cysts derived from saccular or cylindrical dilatation of the *collecting ducts,* which completely replace the medulla and cortex
Associated with some form of hepatic cysts, bile duct proliferation (actually collapsed but interconnected sacs) and "congenital hepatic fibrosis"

AUTOSOMAL DOMINANT POLYCYSTIC DISEASE
"Adult"; Potter's type 3

Relatively common (1/500)
Always bilateral eventually (may be unilateral or focal early)
Symptoms (flank pain, hematuria, renal failure) usually appear in 30s–40s, although may range from early childhood to 70s or 80s
Urine concentrating defect is an early marker
Huge kidneys, almost entirely replaced by cysts, although some functioning nephrons may remain
Cysts have a variable lining (arise from *all parts of nephron*)
Two types:
• Type I (90%): linked to mutation in gene on chromosome 16p13.3(PKD1); 100% penetrance
• Type II (10%): no linkage to 16p; linked to gene on chromosome 4q(PKD2); milder form; later onset
Accounts for 5–8% of renal transplants
50–60% will have asymptomatic hepatic cysts; cysts may also occur in pancreas, spleen, lungs, ovary
Floppy mitral valve commonly seen
One sixth will have berry aneurysms
One third die from renal failure, one third from hypertension

MEDULLARY SPONGE KIDNEY
Multiple cystic dilatations restricted to collecting ducts
Usually asymptomatic, but increased risk of infection, calcifications, calculi
Cysts lined by cuboidal or transitional epithelium

UREMIC MEDULLARY CYSTIC DISEASE
AKA: familial juvenile nephronophthisis, hereditary tubulointerstitial nephritis
Often hereditary (65%: juvenile onset, autosomal recessive; 15%: adult onset, autosomal dominant)
Onset in childhood—progressive (5–10 yr to renal failure)
Renal insufficiency results from tubulointerstitial damage
Contracted, granular; medullary cysts, most prominent at cortical-medullary junction; tubular atrophy, thickening of basement membranes, interstitial fibrosis

SIMPLE CYSTS
Very common
Probably result from isolated dilatation of a single nephron
May be hemorrhagic, but always avascular

ACQUIRED POLYCYSTIC DISEASE
Seen in chronic dialysis patients (3–4 yr)
In most florid extent, may resemble adult polycystic kidney disease
Flattened epithelium with foci of papillary hyperplasia

HYDRONEPHROSIS
Obstruction of urinary outflow leading to cystic dilatation of the ureter, pelvis, and calyces
When occurs early in gestation, invariably produces some degree of cystic renal dysplasia
In adults, get progressive atrophy of renal cortex until only a thin rim remains

GLOMERULAR DISEASES

Glomerulonephritis: renal disease in which the major pathologic changes are confined to the glomeruli

Diffuse: involves all glomeruli (vs. focal)

Global: involves entire glomerulus (vs. segmental)

Major pathogenic mechanisms:

- Deposition of preformed immune complexes in glomeruli
- Formation of immune complexes by interaction of circulating antibodies with antigens deposited in the glomeruli
- Direct interaction of circulating antibodies with glomerular components

Focal involvement suggests secondary renal involvement in a systemic disease

Glomerular hypercellularity more common in nephritic patients (post-streptococcal, membranoproliferative, crescentic) than in nephrotic patients (minimal change disease, diffuse mesangial proliferative, focal and segmental, membranous)

"Primary" Glomerular Diseases

Note: minimal change disease, diffuse mesangial proliferative, and focal and segmental glomerulosclerosis may be all part of a spectrum of the same disease process (significant clinical and pathologic overlap)

MINIMAL CHANGE DISEASE

AKA: lipoid nephrosis, nil disease, foot process disease, primary nephrotic syndrome

10–15× more common in children than adults (>80% children with nephrosis vs. 20% adults)

Incidence increased in Hodgkin's disease

Selective proteinuria (nephrotic syndrome) usually without hematuria, hypertension, or loss of renal function

Generally responsive to glucocorticoid therapy

Some require immunosuppression (e.g., cyclosporin)

Relapsing or polycyclic course; 70–80% will completely remit, 1–2% will die

Light microscopic (LM) appearance: essentially normal; tubules may show hyaline droplets

Immunofluorescence (IF) localization of immune complexes: usually negative (occasionally, complement and fibrinogen in peripheral capillary walls)

Electron microscopy (EM): foot process "fusion" (actually represents loss of foot processes with swelling of those remaining); microvillus transformation of epithelial cells

DIFFUSE MESANGIAL PROLIFERATIVE

IDIOPATHIC FORM (IgM NEPHROPATHY)

Probably variant of minimal change (similar clinical course) but may be seen in lupus or Henoch-Schönlein purpura

Clinical presentation varies with etiology

LM: mild mesangial hypercellularity and sclerosis

IF: occasional IgM and C3 in small mesangial deposits; IgG seen in postinfectious or latent form

EM: mesangial sclerosis; occasional small mesangial deposits; foot process fusion

BERGER'S DISEASE (IgA NEPHROPATHY)

Different clinical entity: recurrent hematuria, mild proteinuria, elevated IgA; chronic and persistent course

LM and EM: as in idiopathic form

IF: IgA and C3 in mesangial distribution

FOCAL AND SEGMENTAL GLOMERULOSCLEROSIS

10% of childhood and 15% of adult nephrotic syndrome

80% have nephrotic syndrome, although proteinuria usually nonselective

Etiology: reflux?, obstruction, hypertension, radiation, aging; also associated with heroin use

Not a specific disease entity but rather a pattern of response

When present early in clinical course, bad prognosis

When present late in clinical course, not always bad

Usually steroid resistant, hematuria, hypertension

50% will die within 10 yr of diagnosis

Often recurs in patients receiving allografts

LM: Segmental sclerosis of focal glomeruli, more common in juxtamedullary glomeruli; focal tubular atrophy with interstitial fibrosis

IF: IgM and C3 in sclerotic segments (nonspecific; only occasionally seen)

EM: Foot process fusion; mesangial sclerosis with increased matrix; collapsed glomerular capillary loops

SPECIAL FORM SEEN IN AIDS

Seen more commonly in black intravenous drug abusers (IVDAs)

Rapid progression to renal failure

LM: large hyalin casts in tubules; active interstitial nephritis; marked hyperplasia of glomerular epithelial cells

EM: tubuloreticular structures in endothelial cells

MEMBRANOUS GLOMERULONEPHROPATHY

25–40% of adults with nephrotic syndrome

<5% of nephrotic syndrome in children

Idiopathic, but almost certainly an immune complex glomerulonephritis (GN)

Associated with malignancies, viral hepatitis, malaria, parasites, penicillamine, nonsteroidals, heavy metals (gold, mercury), autoimmune diseases (rheumatoid arthritis, Hashimoto's thyroiditis, myasthenia gravis, lupus)

Can lead to persistent proteinuria; 50% will progress to renal failure over many years; corticosteroid therapy may help

Some will transform to anti-GBM–type picture: rapid progression to renal failure

LM: uniform diffuse capillary wall thickening (loops appear stiff); spike-and-dome silver stain pattern; varying degree of interstitial scarring

IF: granular peripheral capillary deposits: IgG > IgM > IgA; ±C3

EM: four stages:

- Stage I: scattered subepithelial deposits
- Stage II: more deposits with basement membrane material deposited in between (*spike and dome*)
- Stage III: intramembranous deposits
- Stage IV: dissolution of deposits, rarefaction, irregular thickening of glomerular basement membrane (GBM)

POSTINFECTIOUS GLOMERULONEPHRITIS

AKA: acute diffuse intracapillary proliferative GN

Most associated with certain strains of group A hemolytic *Streptococcus,* less commonly with protozoa (malaria, toxoplasmosis), viruses (hepatitis B, Epstein-Barr virus [EBV]), spirochetes, other bacteria (*Salmonella, Enterococcus, Staphylococcus*)

Immune complex mediated

Onset of renal symptoms 1–4 wk after "illness"; classically present with nephritic syndrome

Darkening of urine, malaise, oliguria, edema, proteinuria, occasionally nephrotic syndrome

Marked decrease in GFR with salt and water retention

Pale cortex with petechial hemorrhages

95% of children recover spontaneously (histology usually returns to normal in 6 months to 3 yr)

~60% of adults recover; some develop rapidly progressive GN

LM: diffuse global glomerular hypercellularity; partial capillary obliteration by endocapillary proliferation; mesangial and epithelial proliferation, with or without crescents

IF: granular ("lumpy-bumpy") deposition of IgG, C3 in peripheral loops; fibrinogen in a mesangial pattern

EM: *Subepithelial* "humps" (deposits); may have small subendothelial deposits early; foot process effacement over deposits

DIFFUSE CRESCENTIC GLOMERULONEPHRITIS

AKA: rapidly progressive, extracapillary proliferative GN

Oliguria, azotemia, proteinuria, hematuria, hypertension, unresponsive nephrotic syndrome; eventually, anuria, end-stage failure (a few stabilize)

Rapid, generally irreversible course

Steroids, cyclophosphamide, plasmapheresis do not help

Three Subtypes (same LM appearance)

Glomerular crescents (proliferation of parietal epithelium and infiltration of monocytes; later fibrin deposition, collagen); segmental necrosis, glomerular capillary collapse, atrophic tubules, interstitial inflammatory infiltrate

Crescents may be associated with focal disruption of the GBM and/or of Bowman's capsule

POSTINFECTIOUS (SEVERE)

Slightly better prognosis than other two variants

IF: granular IgG and C3

EM: subepithelial "humps," mesangial deposits, fibrin deposition associated with breaks in GBM

ANTI–GLOMERULAR BASEMENT MEMBRANE ANTIBODIES

With lung involvement = Goodpasture's syndrome

IF: diffuse linear staining of GBM with IgG > IgM > IgA, granular staining for C3; fibrinogen focally within glomerular capillary loops; linear staining of tubular basement membranes for immunoglobulins (Igs) may be seen

EM: fibrin associated with breaks in GBM; no deposits

IDIOPATHIC

AKA: pauci-immune crescentic GN

Occasionally associated with a vasculitis; many patients are anti-neutrophil cytoplasmic antibody positive (see later)

IF: no Ig staining; complement and fibrinogen may be present, associated with crescents

EM: as for anti-GBM

MEMBRANOPROLIFERATIVE GLOMERULONEPHRITIS

AKA: hypocomplementic (C3), lobular

Variable presentation, but typically acute nephritis, nephrotic syndrome, hypertension

Primarily affects children and young adults

Course generally progressive, with intermittent remissions and gradual loss of renal function

High recurrence in transplants (especially type II), but usually does not compromise graft function for a while

Three Subtypes (same LM appearance)

Glomerular enlargement with lobular accentuation; increase in mesangial cell number and matrix

Irregular thickening of capillary wall by interposition of mesangial cells between the endothelium and the basement membrane: "tram track" or "reduplication of the GBM"

Crescents seen in ~20%

TYPE I—"CLASSICAL," "MESANGIOCAPILLARY"

Two thirds of cases

IF: IgG, IgM, C3, ± IgA deposition—lumpy bumpy; granular fibrin deposition

EM: *subendothelial* and mesangial deposits; occasional subepithelial deposits; increased mesangial matrix; *mesangialization* of the capillary loops; foot process fusion

TYPE II—"DENSE DEPOSIT"

One third of cases

Familial, associated with partial lipodystrophy

Abnormal activation of alternate complement pathway

C3 Nef (C3 nephritic factor—antibody) in serum

Poorer prognosis than type I

IF: extensive C3 in mesangium and peripheral capillary loops; Igs usually absent; fibrin occasionally seen

EM: very dense deposits in *lamina densa* of GBM, forming a long ribbon of hazy material, which may be discontinuous

TYPE III—"MIXED"

Rare; probably an advanced form of type I (classical)

Both subendothelial and subepithelial deposits by EM

"Secondary" Glomerular Diseases

LUPUS NEPHRITIS

Renal involvement in 50–80%

Prognosis correlates with extent of renal disease

Subendothelial deposits correlate with renal failure

Tubulointerstitial infiltrate common: lymphocytes, plasma cells, eosinophils

Pathogenesis: deposition of DNA–anti-DNA complexes

World Health Organization (WHO) Classification

WHO CLASS I

No lesions, no symptoms

WHO CLASS II (MESANGIAL)

Mild to moderate proteinuria, good prognosis

LM: IIA, no significant changes; IIB, mild mesangial hypercellularity centered away from vascular pole

IF: mesangial IgG, C3; occasionally other Igs

EM: mesangial deposits

WHO CLASS III (FOCAL SEGMENTAL)

Proteinuria, sometimes aggressive course

LM: focal and segmental necrosis/proliferation (<50% involvement of <50% glomeruli); mild diffuse mesangial prominence; segmental capillary proliferation with obliteration of lumen; hyaline wire loops; focal crescents

IF: more diffuse involvement with granular capillary Ig and C3

EM: subendothelial deposits and mesangial deposits; occasionally subepithelial deposits

WHO CLASS IV (DIFFUSE PROLIFERATIVE)

Most common type

Most to all of glomeruli are involved

Worst prognosis, progressing to renal failure (unless treated)

LM: mesangial proliferation; membranoproliferative and/or crescents; condensed nuclear debris ("hematoxyphil body"); thickened wire capillary loops; 25% show lobular accentuation

IF: Ig, coarsely granular pattern in mesangium and capillary loops; "full house pattern": multiple Igs: IgG + IgM > IgA > IgE (presence of IgE associated with poorer prognosis)

EM: large subendothelial deposits—"fingerprint"; mesangial, subepithelial, and intramembranous deposits common; tubuloreticular structures seen in endothelial cells

WHO CLASS V (MEMBRANOUS)
Identical to lesions of idiopathic membranous
Indolent progression

WHO CLASS VI (SCLEROSING)
LM: global glomerulosclerosis, usually fibrous crescents, interstitial fibrosis, nephron loss with tubular atrophy
EM: irregular thickening of capillary basement membrane with intramembranous deposits

DIABETIC NEPHROPATHY
More common in early onset or poorly controlled diabetes
Recurrent proteinuria, often nephrotic, with slow progression to chronic renal failure
Papillary necrosis seen
Diffuse and nodular types
LM: diffuse thickening of capillary wall, nodular (Kimmelstiel-Wilson) sclerosis, arteriolar nephrosclerosis, "insudative" glomerular lesions (fibrin cap, capsular drop)
Global sclerosis (related to duration, not severity)
IF: diffuse thin linear staining for IgG, C3, and albumin
EM: diffuse even thickening of GBM (up to 5–10× normal!); increased mesangial matrix; ± subendothelial granular deposits

AMYLOIDOSIS
(See also Inflammation and Immunology outline, under Autoimmune Diseases)
Deposits of amyloid protein A (stains with Congo red)
Massive proteinuria (12–20 g/24 hr!)
Glucocorticoid therapy unsuccessful, outlook poor
LM: homogeneous deposits in glomeruli, tubular basement membranes, and vessel walls
IF: Ig may be present in nonspecific pattern
EM: amyloid fibrils (β-pleated sheet, 7–12 nm) widely present in mesangium and peripheral capillary basement membrane

LIGHT CHAIN DISEASE
7–10% of patients with multiple myeloma
LM: capillary wall thickening, nodular sclerosis; "amyloid" deposits of AL type
IF: monoclonal κ or λ light chain—linear deposition
EM: granular deposits in glomerular and tubular basement membrane

CRYOGLOBULINEMIA
Renal lesions seen in 50% of patients; can be seen in lymphoma
Anatomically, same as type I membranoproliferative (mesangiocapillary) GN
LM: diffuse proliferation/lobular accentuation/neutrophils; intraluminal eosinophilic occlusive thrombi; ± crescents
IF: large peripheral capillary deposits with IgG and IgM; granular staining for C3, C1, C4
EM: subendothelial and mesangial deposits, with parallel arrays of fibrils or tubules

HENOCH-SCHÖNLEIN PURPURA
Purpuric skin lesions (leukocytoclastic vasculitis), characteristically involving the extensor surfaces of the arms, legs, buttocks; also joint pain, melena, abdominal pain; episodic
Most common in children 3–8 yr old, but renal disease is more severe when occurs in adults
Renal involvement in 25%: nephritis to asymptomatic hematuria/proteinuria
Usually self-limited; morbidity/mortality caused by renal disease
Wide range of histopathology, most similar to IgA nephropathy, but often crescentic GN when severe
Healed lesions may be present (episodic nature)

Hereditary/Familial Nephropathies

ALPORT'S SYNDROME
Type I: dominant, associated with deafness, males sterile
Others: X-linked dominant, autosomal recessive, ± deafness
Appears to be some defect in GBM
May or may not progress to renal failure
Glomerulosclerosis, tubular atrophy, interstitial foam cells
IF: no specific staining; does *not* stain with anti-GBM
EM: thinning, thickening, and splitting of GBM in an irregular pattern

NAIL-PATELLA SYNDROME
Similar to Alport's syndrome
EM: thickening of GBM with fibrillar collagen

CONGENITAL NEPHROTIC SYNDROME
Autosomal recessive
Occur before 1 yr of age; often fatal
FINNISH TYPE
Premature, low birth weight infants
Enlarged placenta (one third of body weight)
Immature glomeruli with sclerosis
Tubular cyst formation = "microcystic disease"
Arteriolar medial hypertrophy
EM: obliteration of foot processes
FRENCH TYPE
Usually develops between 3 months and 1 yr
Renal insufficiency within 1–3 yr
Glomeruli show mesangial, then global, sclerosis
Tubular atrophy with interstitial fibrosis
Increased mesangial matrix

THIN GLOMERULAR BASEMENT MEMBRANE DISEASE
AKA: benign familial hematuria
Autosomal dominant; onset in childhood
Similar to Alport's syndrome clinically; usually no uremia or renal insufficiency; microscopic hematuria (persistent or intermittent); proteinuria is unusual
More common in women (thinner basement membrane to begin with)
LM: normal, except for hematuria
IF: small amounts of Ig and C3 deposited along basement membrane
EM: thin GBM (~200 nm vs. 300 nm in normal adults); focal capillary wall collapse with thickening; ± mesangial deposits

TUBULOINTERSTITIAL DISEASES

ACUTE INTERSTITIAL NEPHRITIS
Interstitial inflammation almost always involves the tubules to some extent, caused by the intimate interrelationship between the tubules and the interstitium

ACUTE PYELONEPHRITIS
Flank pain, fever, malaise, dysuria, pyuria
Gram negative bacilli of GI tract account for >85% of cases (*E. coli, Proteus, Klebsiella, Enterobacter*)
Most common in pregnant women and men with obstructive prostatic hypertrophy
Mechanism of infection:
- Hematogenous spread: predominantly corticomedullary junction; kidney usually resistant unless damaged
- Ascending infection: male : female = 1 : 8 in non-instrumented patients
- Vesicoureteral reflux (during micturition)
Patchy, often wedge-shaped suppurative inflammation, usually predominantly cortical, with *edema, neutrophils* in interstitium and tubular lumina, and areas of necrosis/abscess formation in cortex
Inflammation rapidly spreads throughout tubules; glomeruli, arterioles, and arteries are spared

PYONEPHROSIS
Caused by near-complete obstruction
Pus, unable to drain, fills kidney

ACUTE HYPERSENSITIVITY NEPHRITIS
AKA: drug-induced nephritis
Seen with beta-lactam antibiotics, nonsteroidal anti-inflammatory drugs (NSAIDs), diuretics, dilantin, rifampin, amphotericin, gentamicin
Non–drug-related causes include viral (hantavirus, EBV, herpes simplex virus [HSV], cytomegalovirus [CMV], adenovirus, HIV) and autoimmune disease (systemic lupus erythematosus [SLE], Sjögren's, rheumatoid arthritis)
Predominantly interstitial inflammation with edema, lymphocytes (mostly helper T cells), macrophages, *eosinophils*, plasma cells; may have granulomas
Tubular epithelial damage with regeneration, tubulitis; glomeruli and vessels usually normal
With NSAIDs, also get glomerular foot process fusion

RENAL PAPILLARY NECROSIS
Most common in obstructed patients with diabetes (synchronized lesions), alcoholism, sickle cell disease, analgesic abusers (usually affects papilla of upper and lower pole; lesions at various stages; seen with acetaminophen, phenacetin, aspirin, codeine)
Three stages of progression:
- I: Papillae firm with gray streaks, interstitial homogenization, thickening of basement membranes, focal cell necrosis, fine calcification; cortex normal
- II: Papillae shrunken, brown; confluent necrosis, focal tubular atrophy in overlying cortex
- III: Kidneys decrease in weight, total papillary necrosis, extensive calcification (may have metaplastic bone), overlying tubular atrophy and interstitial fibrosis (cortical changes more marked if papillae fail to slough)

CHRONIC INTERSTITIAL NEPHRITIS
Hallmark of chronic injury is interstitial fibrosis

Often the etiology cannot be unequivocally determined once fibrosis is extensive; most common causes are obstruction, vesicoureteral reflux, and idiopathic (nonobstructive)
Irregular, asymmetrical scarring involving the calyces and pelvis as well as the cortex
Get predominantly tubulointerstitial damage with "normal" glomeruli; *tubular atrophy* or dilatation, thyroidization; *fibrosis,* periglomerular fibrosis; predominantly lymphocytes in interstitium

DRUG INDUCED
Interstitial fibrosis and tubular atrophy
Seen with lithium (nephrogenic diabetes insipidus), cyclosporin (see later under Renal Transplantation), and analgesics

XANTHOGRANULOMATOUS PYELONEPHRITIS
Large yellow-orange nodules replace normal renal parenchyma; can mimic renal cell carcinoma
Infiltrate of foamy macrophages and giant cells, plus granulomas, lymphocytes, plasma cells
Associated with *E. coli, Proteus, Staphylococcus aureus* (urea-splitting organisms)

MALAKOPLAKIA
AKA: megalocytic interstitial nephritis
Confluent yellow-tan nodules replacing renal parenchyma
Few lymphocytes, many histiocytes
Michaelis-Gutmann bodies (partially digested bacteria, calcified) in stroma and in cells

TUBERCULOSIS
Frequently unilateral
May be miliary (numerous small tubercles scattered throughout the cortex) or isolated to urinary tract, with progressive destruction of the renal parenchyma

PELVIC LIPOMATOSIS
Replacement of pelvis by adipose tissue following atrophy

ASK-UPMARK KIDNEY
Extensive scarring of a kidney lobule, resulting in apparent focal hypoplasia

ACUTE TUBULAR NECROSIS (ATN)
Major cause of acute renal failure (<400 ml urine/24 hr)
Complete anuria rare
Acute renal failure probably due to tubular obstruction by debris
Four clinical phases:
- Onset (36 hr)
- Oliguric (days–weeks): fluid overload, uremia, hyperkalemia
- Early diuretic: steady increase in urine volume, hypokalemia, electrolyte imbalance, increased vulnerability to infection
- Late diuretic: recovery of function
Gross: swollen and pale kidneys

ISCHEMIC
AKA: tubulorrhectic, shock kidney, hemoglobinuric nephrosis
Proximal tubules and thick portion of the ascending limb are most vulnerable to ischemic injury (greatest ATPase activity)
Usually following hypotension secondary to bacteremia, burns, etc.; unusual following hemorrhage alone
Focal tubular necrosis at multiple points along the nephron with skip lesions
Basement membrane rupture (tubulorrhexis)
Casts in distal tubules (eosinophilic and granular; contain Tamm-Horsfall protein)

Interstitial edema, leukocytes in dilated vasa recta

Later, epithelial regeneration with flattening of tubule cells

Can also be seen following massive hemolysis or massive rhabdomyolysis: "pigment associated ATN"

NEPHROTOXIC

Usually involves proximal convoluted tubules, sparing distal

No basement membrane destruction

Seen with heavy metals, organic solvents, sulfonamides, neomycin, methicillin, anesthetics

Can have non-oliguric ATN

Ethylene glycol not truly nephrotoxic; large accumulation of calcium oxalate crystals in tubules

CHRONIC RENAL FAILURE

Volume regulation: dehydration early, then systemic edema (anasarca): lose concentrating ability, then filtration rate

Acid/base: metabolic acidosis, Kussmaul breathing

GI: nausea/vomiting, bleeding?

Cardiovascular: congestive heart failure (CHF), hypertension (increased volume, renin, or both)

Hematopoietic: anemia (decreased erythropoietin + bleeds)

Bone metabolism: decreased Ca, increased PO_4, elevated parathyroid hormone (PTH) → renal osteodystrophy

NEPHROLITHIASIS

1% of all U.S. population will develop a kidney stone

"Primary" = occurs without renal abnormality or infection

Four kinds of stones, all with an organic matrix of mucopolysaccharides comprising <5% of stone weight

65–75% are calcium oxalate and Ca phosphate (sarcoidosis, hyperparathyroidism, excess Vitamin D, multiple myeloma)

5–20% are uric acid, xanthine (gout, Lesch-Nyhan, glycogen storage disease, excess dietary protein)

15% are magnesium ammonium phosphate ("triple stones" or "struvite stones")

1–2% are cysteine

May form at area of ulceration on surface of papillae

MISCELLANEOUS

OSMOTIC NEPHROSIS

Foamy clearing of cytoplasm of the proximal tubular epithelium secondary to sucrose or mannitol injection

No clinical significance

HYALINE CHANGE

Proximal tubular epithelium contains cytoplasmic eosinophilic PAS+ droplets

Seen in patients with marked proteinuria; represents reabsorption of filtered proteins

HYPOKALEMIC (VACUOLAR) NEPHROPATHY

Secondary to chronic protein depletion (e.g., GI disease)

Coarse "vacuolization" of tubule cells, mainly proximal, caused by dilatation of intercellular spaces

URATE NEPHROPATHY

Precipitation of uric acid crystals in renal tubules, principally collecting ducts

Common in leukemia/lymphoma patients on chemotherapy

MYELOMA KIDNEY

Insidious and progressive renal failure, or acute renal failure caused by precipitation of Bence Jones protein in tubules with obstruction

Normal to shrunken and pale kidneys, with pink to blue amorphous casts, giant cells, tubular necrosis, interstitial inflammation ± granulomas

NEPHROCALCINOSIS

Calcification in renal parenchyma, typically on tubular basement membranes and in interstitium, associated with hypercalcemia and hypercalciuria

Tubular atrophy, interstitial fibrosis, periglomerular fibrosis

VASCULAR LESIONS

BENIGN NEPHROSCLEROSIS

Always associated with hyaline arteriolosclerosis

Fine, even granularity to cortical surface

Cortical narrowing with mildly decreased renal mass

Focal tubular atrophy, interstitial fibrosis

Fibroelastic hyperplasia: reduplication of elastic lamina of interlobular and arcuate arteries, with fibrosis of media

MALIGNANT NEPHROSCLEROSIS

Associated with malignant hypertension (rapidly rising blood pressure, with diastolic pressure >130 mmHg, developing over 3 months to 2 yr, usually ending in death)

Fibrinoid necrosis of arterioles, often with inflammatory infiltrates in vessel wall (necrotizing arteriolitis)

Hyperplastic arteriolitis: intimal thickening by proliferation of concentric smooth muscle cells ("onion skinning")

RENAL ARTERY STENOSIS

70% caused by atheromatous plaque at origin; male > female

Fibromuscular dysplasia of renal artery accounts for many of the remaining cases, especially those occurring in younger patients (see Vessels outline); female > male

Diffuse ischemic atrophy of ipsilateral kidney with minimal arteriolosclerosis

Enlargement of contralateral kidney, often with marked arteriolosclerosis

INFARCTS

Usually embolic in origin (look for cholesterol crystals)

Wedge shaped, with base at capsule

Typically pale-white with hyperemic rim

With time, replaced by fibrous tissue—forms contracted scar

VASCULITIS

Hypersensitivity response to antigens (drugs) and various clinical syndromes (e.g., Wegener's granulomatosis, polyarteritis nodosa)

Distinction based on other organ involvement

LM: focal and segmental necrotizing to diffuse crescentic GN; can see granulomas in Wegener's, extending through Bowman's capsule into the interstitium

Tubulointerstitial infiltrate with eosinophils

IF: mesangial and subendothelial fibrin, ± IgG, IgM, C3

EM: mesangial deposits, fibrin in capillaries, capillary rupture

ANTINEUTROPHIL CYTOPLASMIC ANTIBODIES
Cytoplasmic (C-ANCA) pattern seen in Wegener's
Perinuclear (P-ANCA) pattern seen in small vessel vasculitides, polyarteritis nodosa, rheumatoid disorders

HEMOLYTIC UREMIC SYNDROME
Microangiopathic hemolytic anemia, thrombocytopenia, and acute renal failure
More common in children
75% of patients infected with verocytotoxin producing *E. coli*
Adults: postpartum women, oral contraceptive users
Prognosis better in children
LM: thrombi in glomeruli; focal necrosis without leukocyte infiltration; bloodless glomeruli; fragmented RBCs; thickening of capillary walls (tram tracks); myointimal proliferation in small arterioles
IF: fibrin, occasional Igs
EM: separation of endothelium from BM with light granular material in the new subendothelial space

THROMBOTIC THROMBOCYTOPENIC PURPURA
Identical to hemolytic-uremic syndrome (HUS), with perhaps more prominent platelets

RENAL TRANSPLANTATION

PRESERVATION INJURY
Swelling of tubular epithelial cells with occlusion of the lumen by cytoplasmic "blebs"; necrosis
EM: mitochondrial and lysosomal swelling

HYPERACUTE REJECTION
Minutes to hours after transplant; rarely may take 1 wk
Mediated by preformed antibodies vs. donor endothelium
Fibrin thrombi in glomeruli and other vessels, infarction, tubular necrosis, widened/congested interstitial capillaries, interstitial hemorrhage

ACUTE IMMINENT REJECTION
Occurs in 1st month; usually due to preservation injury
≥3 neutrophils in glomerular capillaries; dilated intertubular capillaries (with mononuclear cells)
Edematous interstitium, swollen tubular epithelium and vascular endothelium
Suggests graft will likely be rejected within 3 months

ACUTE REJECTION
May occur at any time after ~7 days (including years)
INTERSTITIAL (CELLULAR)
Interstitial edema and chronic inflammatory cell infiltrate, initially at the corticomedullary junction with immunoblasts, lymphocytes, plasma cells, and scattered neutrophils and eosinophils; lymphocytes often migrate into the tubular epithelium
Predominantly T cells, both CD4+ and CD8+ cells
Reversible with immunosuppression; in particular, OKT-3, a monoclonal antibody to T cells, is quite effective at reversing cellular rejection
VASCULAR (HORMONAL)
Endothelial cell swelling, subendothelial inflammatory cells (predominantly chronic), interstitial hemorrhage, infarcts

Severe cases: necrotizing arteritis, fibrinoid necrosis
Less easily reversible

CHRONIC REJECTION
Several months to years after transplantation
Clinically, slow gradual decrease in renal function
Glomeruli, vessels, interstitium, and the tubules are all involved
VASCULOPATHY
Myointimal proliferation of vessels
Interstitial scarring
Tubular atrophy or loss
Mononuclear cell infiltration
GLOMERULOPATHY
Glomerular hypercellularity, sclerosis, irregular basement membrane thickening, ischemic glomerular capillary collapse

CYCLOSPORIN TOXICITY
ACUTE
Related to high levels
May have no lesions or mild tubular and vascular changes (tubular degeneration with vacuolization and eosinophilic inclusions, peritubular capillary congestion)
Vacuolization of endothelial and smooth muscle cells
CHRONIC
Stripes of interstitial fibrosis, atrophic tubules in cortex, tubular dedifferentiation, glomerulosclerosis

RECURRENCE OF GLOMERULONEPHRITIS
Occurs in 10–20%; accounts for 2% of graft failures
Most commonly seen in patients with focal and segmental GN, but greatest frequency of recurrence is with membranoproliferative glomerulonephritis

KIDNEY TUMORS

Pediatric Cortex/Medulla

NEPHROGENIC RESTS
Predominantly to exclusively epithelial cells forming disorganized structures
Considered abnormal development rather than a neoplasm
Presumably, all Wilms' tumors arise from nephrogenic rests
• Perilobar rests:
  At periphery of renal lobe
  Found in 30–40% of kidneys with Wilms' tumors
  Type seen in Beckwith–Wiedemann syndrome
  Associated with *synchronous* bilateral Wilms' tumors
• Intralobar rests:
  Inner portions of cortex or medulla
  Seen with Wilms' tumors presenting at younger age
  Associated with *metachronous* bilateral Wilms' tumors

Both types of rests may be further subclassified:
- Dormant: no change for many years; older patients
- Regressing/sclerosing: maturing; most common subtype for perilobar rests
- Obsolescent: primarily hyalinized stroma
- Hyperplastic: macroscopic; may progress; if Wilms' tumor arises within one, causes a spherical expansion

NEPHROBLASTOMATOSIS
Multiple nodules or diffusely distributed nephrogenic rests

Single/multifocal, unilateral/bilateral, usually subcapsular; may be limited to a small region

Perilobar, intralobar, combined, and panlobar types

Found in 1% of neonatal kidneys

Similar to Wilms' histologically

WILMS' TUMOR (NEPHROBLASTOMA)
50% occur <3 yr of age, 90% <10 yr

Only rarely congenital, but 15–30% are associated with genitourinary malformations and genetic syndromes (e.g., deletion of 11p13 [WT-1]: Wilms' with aniridia; deletion of 11p15 [WT-2]: Beckwith-Wiedemann syndrome)

5–10% bilateral; can also occur outside the kidney

Presentation: abdominal mass (rarely as hematuria, hypertension, proteinuria)

Large, white, well-circumscribed, solid, hemorrhage, necrosis

Three components histologically; can have one, two, or all:
- Epithelial tissue: embryonic tubular structures (with or without glomeruli) to small, round cell rosettes
- Undifferentiated blastema: cellular, small round-oval primitive cells, scanty cytoplasm
- Mesenchymal tissue: spindle cell (fibroblast-like); may differentiate toward smooth or skeletal muscle (if large amount of skeletal muscle, always young children, 50% bilateral)

"Teratoid Wilms' tumor": differentiation to ganglion cells, adipose tissue, bone, etc.

Grade histology as "favorable" or "unfavorable"; unfavorable histology requires (must have all three): anaplasia (nuclei 3× size of neighbors); hyperchromasia; abnormal mitoses

Spread: local to perirenal soft tissue, adrenal, bowel, liver; renal pelvis or ureter invasion rare

Metastases: regional lymph node (LN) in 15%; distant: lungs, liver, peritoneum

Therapy depends on stage: chemotherapy ± radiation; therapy induces massive necrosis of the immature component but spares the mature portions

Prognosis: overall cure for unilateral: ~90%; survivors have increased risk for second neoplasm; unfavorable histology (seen in ~5%) increases mortality from 5% to 50%

Good prognostic signs: age <2; low stage, no anaplastic regions, tubular differentiation

Pure blastemal tumor may have worse prognosis

Pure rhabdomyomatous tumors do very well

CLINICAL STAGING
T1	Unilateral, intact, ≤80 cm², including kidney
T2	Unilateral, intact, >80 cm², including kidney
T3	Unilateral, ruptured
T4	Bilateral
N1	Regional LNs
M1	Metastases

Clinical

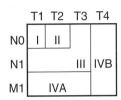

PATHOLOGIC STAGING
T1	Confined to kidney, capsule intact
T2	Beyond kidney, but completely excised
T3a	Microscopic residual tumor
T3b	Macroscopic residual tumor or ruptured
T3c	Not resected
T4	Bilateral
N1a	Regional LNs, resected
N1b	Regional LNs, incompletely resected
M1	Metastases

Pathologic

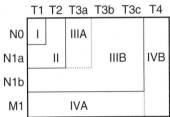

MULTICYSTIC NEPHROMA
AKA: multilocular cystic nephroma

Early infancy; nearly always unilateral

Presents as abdominal mass, ureteral obstruction

Sharply demarcated, 5–15 cm, coarsely nodular, white, serous cysts

Tubular epithelium lining cysts; hobnail cells; spindle cell stroma between cysts

Some refer to this entity as *multilocular cysts*—require the presence of blastemal cells in wall to diagnose multicystic nephroma

Probably just a well-differentiated variant of nephroblastoma

Curable by simple excision

MESOBLASTIC NEPHROMA
AKA: fetal, mesenchymal, or leiomyomatous hamartoma

<5% of pediatric renal tumors, but most common tumor before 1 yr (congenital: usually discovered before 6 months)

Solid, yellow-gray to tan, whirled configuration, usually infiltrative growth pattern (occasionally well circumscribed); no hemorrhage or necrosis

Spindled cells that look like smooth muscle cells; infiltrate and entrap tubules; no capsule

Usually benign, but will recur if not completely excised

Atypical variant: many mitoses, infiltrates pelvis or perirenal tissue, metastasizes

INTRARENAL NEUROBLASTOMA
Invades from adrenal or arises as primary

Can be confused with Wilms' tumor

(See Endocrine outline, Adrenal Medulla)

CLEAR CELL SARCOMA

AKA: bone-metastasizing renal tumor

4% of childhood renal tumors; peaks at 2–3 yr

Well demarcated, homogeneous tan, cystic; always unilateral

Small cells, round nuclei, clear cytoplasm in only 20%, prominent fibrovascular stroma

Growth patterns: epithelioid, spindled, sclerosing, myxoid, palisading, cystic, pericytoma-like, and pleomorphic

Very malignant

RHABDOID TUMOR

Young infants (median age 18 months)

Soft, solid, infiltrative margins

Monomorphic proliferation of medium-sized round/oval cells (can be spindled); large cytoplasmic eosinophilic globule displacing nucleus laterally; involves medulla and cortex

Looks like rhabdomyosarcoma (negative for muscle markers)

Should *not* find well-differentiated skeletal muscle; if do, probably a Wilms' tumor

EM: whirled array of intermediate filaments in the cytoplasm

Strong association with medulloblastoma of brain

Very malignant: mortality >75%

Adult Cortex/Medulla

ADENOMA

Found in 20% of adult kidneys, generally <6 mm

May be tubular or papillary

Probably nodular hyperplasia vs. neoplasm

Some pathologists consider all proliferations of renal tubule cells in the kidney to be renal cell carcinomas, because lesions as small as 1 cm have metastasized; others prefer to use the "3 cm rule," calling lesions with low-grade histology that are <3 cm adenomas

RENAL CELL CARCINOMA (RCC)

AKA: renal adenocarcinoma, hypernephroma

Median age 55–60 yr; male : female = 2–3 : 1; bilateral 1%

Account for 85–90% of all renal malignancies; 2% of all cancers in adults

RCC may develop in setting of von Hippel-Lindau (multiple and cystic tumors), acquired cystic disease (secondary to long-term dialysis), adult polycystic disease (or multicystic nephroma)

Patients present with a triad of hematuria (59%), flank pain (41%), abdominal mass (45%); also weight loss (28%), anemia (21%), fever (7%)

Often produce hormones resulting in polycythemia, hypercalcemia, hypertension, feminization, Cushing's syndrome

Well demarcated, centered in cortex, often extending outside kidney but extending to pelvis only late in course; golden-yellow; fibrous capsule; hemorrhage, necrosis, calcification, cystic change; multiple nodules in 5%

Cystic changes can be extensive; any multicystic lesion with hemorrhage needs to be thoroughly sampled

Large, optically clear ("clear cell") or granular ("granular cell") cytoplasm; may have hyaline droplets, central nuclei

Clear cells contain fat, glycogen, few organelles

Tubular, papillary, solid, alveolar, or trabecular pattern

Believed to be a tumor of the renal tubular epithelial cell

Immunohistochemistry: reactive for keratin, vimentin, EMA (adrenal cortical tumors are EMA negative), ± CEA

Often see deletion/rearrangement of chromosome 3p (except in papillary renal cell carcinoma—see later)

Occasionally regresses without treatment

Most common recipient of metastasis into a tumor (most common donor is lung)

SPREAD/METASTASES

One third have invaded perinephric fat or regional LNs

Renal vein and inferior vena cava invasion common

One third have distant metastases: lung, bones (pelvis, femur), adrenal gland, liver

Frequently solitary metastases

Metastases may develop years after primary removed

Rare in tumors <3 cm in diameter

GRADING

1   Small, round, uniform nuclei

2   Larger nuclei, small nucleoli

3   Even larger nuclei, prominent nucleoli

4   Pleomorphic/multilobated nuclei, cells may be spindled

STAGING

T1   Confined to kidney, ≤2.5 cm

T2   Confined to kidney, >2.5 cm

T3a Extends to adrenal or soft tissue

T3b Extends into renal vein or lower inferior vena cava

T3c Extends into inferior vena cava above diaphragm

T4   Beyond Gerota's fascia

N1   Single LN, ≤2 cm

N2   Single LN, 2–5 cm or multiple LNs, all <5 cm

N3   Any LN >5 cm

M1   Metastases

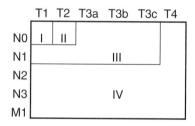

PROGNOSIS

5 yr: I, 60–80%; II, 40–70%; III, 10–40%; IV, 5%

Metastases most important bad sign

Tumor size (<3 cm best, prognosis decreases with size up to 10 cm, then plateaus)

Clear cell less aggressive than granular cell

Special Histologic Types of Renal Cell Carcinoma

TUBULOPAPILLARY RENAL CELL CARCINOMA (5–15%)

Predominantly papillary (>75%); hypovascular on arteriography; necrosis, inflammation, cyst formation

Cores of papillae often have foamy macrophages

Papillary adenomas may also be present

Does not show changes in chromosome 3p; instead, see gains of chromosome 7 or 17 and, in men, loss of Y chromosome

If pure, usually localized to kidney: better overall prognosis

CHROMOPHOBE RENAL CELL CARCINOMA (<5%)

Sharply defined cell borders, lightly staining cytoplasm but not completely clear

Low nuclear grade, well-defined nuclei
Will stain with colloidal iron, alcian blue
Vimentin negative; keratin and EMA positive
EM: peculiar vesicles
Better overall prognosis

ONCOCYTIC RENAL CELL CARCINOMA
Similar to oncocytoma but higher nuclear grade or mixed with other histologic patterns

COLLECTING DUCT CARCINOMA (1–2%)
Differentiates toward collecting (Bellini's) ducts
Centered in medulla, tubulopapillary, desmoplastic reaction

SARCOMATOID CARCINOMA (1%)
AKA: spindle cell, anaplastic, carcinosarcoma
Spindle and/or pleomorphic giant cells; simulate sarcoma
Cytology: grade 4 (by definition)

ONCOCYTOMA
Mahogany-brown, solid, central stellate scar; may be large (>10 cm)
Solid sheets or nests of regular cells with abundant acidophilic granular cytoplasm (mitochondria—often swollen); small, round, regular nuclei
Must be grade 1–2 with no other histologic patterns and no necrosis; otherwise, diagnose as RCC with oncocytic change
Some multicentric, few bilateral
May be a tumor of the collecting duct cells
Most are negative for vimentin
Lack the cytogenetic abnormalities of RCC
Invasion of capsule or renal vein possible, although most behave in a benign fashion, regardless of size
Some pathologists do not make the diagnosis of oncocytoma, preferring instead to call all of these lesions "renal cell carcinoma, oncocytic variant"

JUXTAGLOMERULAR CELL TUMOR
Presents with hypertension, secondary to renin production
Looks like hemangiopericytoma with oval to spindle cell background, small vessels, ± tubules
EM shows characteristic large rhomboid crystals in membrane-bound granules
Usually benign

ANGIOMYOLIPOMA
Rare; may be hamartomas rather than neoplasms
<1–20 cm in size; well circumscribed, yellow to gray-tan; frequently multifocal, 15% bilateral; may be confused grossly with RCC
Mixture of fat, thick-walled tortuous blood vessels without elastic lamina, and smooth muscle; marked variability in appearance, based on relative proportions of each component; spectrum includes capsular leiomyoma
Cells are HMB-45 positive with a granular staining pattern
PAS+ crystalloid structures in some cells
20–50% of cases are associated with tuberous sclerosis; also with lymphangiomyomatosis (often multiple)
Capsular invasion in one quarter; local recurrences
Does not metastasize (LN involvement = multifocality)
Sometimes fatal hemorrhage
Can coexist with RCC

MEDULLARY FIBROMA
AKA: renal medullary interstitial cell tumor

Probably hamartomatous rather than neoplastic
Usually <1 cm; gray-white; composed of fibroblast-like cells and collagenous tissue; cells are derived from medullary interstitial cells
May "trap" small cords of tubular cells
Benign

OTHER TUMORS
Benign: hematoma, teratoma, lipoma, leiomyoma, hemangioma
Malignant: carcinoid, sarcomas (various types), lymphoma, plasmacytoma
Metastatic tumors usually bilateral

Tumors of the Pelvis and Ureter

TRANSITIONAL CELL CARCINOMA
Mostly in adults
One quarter of cases have history of analgesic abuse and/or renal papillary necrosis
Associated with Thorotrast, cyclophosphamide
Presentation: hematuria
Soft, white to grayish red masses with glistening surfaces
Histology can show glandular or squamous metaplasia (see later), or can acquire sarcomatoid appearance
May have small pools of mucin
May diffusely involve entire pelvis; can involve parenchyma
Frequently multicentric; 40% have tumors elsewhere in urinary tract

EPIDERMOID CARCINOMA (5–10%)
Associated with squamous metaplasia (leukoplakia)

ADENOCARCINOMA (<1%)
Reserve for rare tumors with mucin and well-formed glands
Related to glandular metaplasia of transitional epithelium secondary to longstanding chronic inflammation

URETER

NORMAL
Approximately 30 cm in length, 5 mm in diameter
Three points of narrowing:
• Ureteropelvic junction
• Where cross anterior to the iliac vessels
• Entry into the bladder

CONGENITAL ANOMALIES
2–3% of all autopsies

DOUBLE (BIFED) URETERS
Usually accompanied by partial or complete duplication of the renal pelvis

URETEROPELVIC JUNCTION OBSTRUCTION
Usually males, more commonly on left

Abnormal organization of and/or excess stromal deposition of collagen between smooth muscle bundles
Results in hydronephrosis
DIVERTICULA

INFLAMMATION
Changes arise only in longstanding ureteritis
URETERITIS FOLLICULARIS
Accumulation of subepithelial lymphoid aggregates, imparting a fine granularity to the mucosa

URETERITIS CYSTICA
1–5 mm fine cysts protruding from luminal mucosa
Dilated Brunn's nests with clear contents

TUMORS
Very rare; most tumors are metastases
Primary tumors are of same type as seen for the renal pelvis and urinary bladder

17

BLADDER

NORMAL

Epithelium derived from endoderm of urogenital sinus; epithelium of renal pelvis and ureter are mesodermally derived

Only the most superior/anterior aspect is covered by peritoneum

Urothelium is a transitional epithelium, usually 5–8 cells thick, divided into three layers:
- Superficial zone: single layer of large, flattened cells that cover relatively large areas—"umbrella cells"
- Intermediate zone: 4–5 layers when maximally stretched, 6–8 layers when fully contracted
- Basal zone: single layer of small cells, cylindrical to flattened

Lamina propria is juxtaposed to the muscularis propria; there is no submucosa

Electron microscopy (EM) shows scalloped concave rigid membrane plaques (asymmetric unit membrane plaque); cytoplasmic "fusiform vesicles" contain similar plaques—this allows increase in surface area of membrane

CONGENITAL AND ACQUIRED MALFORMATIONS

EXSTROPHY

Developmental defect of closure of the anterior wall of the abdomen and the bladder so that the bladder communicates with the exterior of the body through a large defect or as an open sac

Often associated with other abnormalities of genitourinary (GU) tract

Increased incidence of malignancy (adenocarcinoma)

URACHUS

5–6 cm vestigial structure located between the apex of the bladder and the umbilicus

In the embryo, this connected the bladder to the allantois

Tubular urachal remnants are found in 32% of individuals; lining may be transitional or columnar

CYSTOCELE

Protrusion of the bladder into the vagina, creating a pouch

Caused by relaxation of the pelvic support in females, leading to uterine prolapse; this pulls the bladder floor downward

DIVERTICULA

Pouchlike evaginations of the bladder wall

Congenital: caused by focal muscular defect; some muscle is retained within the wall

Acquired: more common; arise following persistent urethral obstruction; only mucosa and lamina propria in the pouch (no muscle); more commonly multiple; posterior wall above trigone most common location

Diverticula represent sites of urinary stasis, with potential for infection

CYSTITIS

General Acute and Chronic Cystitis

Frequently precedes pyelonephritis

Most common organisms: *E. coli,* then *Proteus, Klebsiella, Enterobacter;* also tuberculosis, *Candida albicans, Cryptococcus,* schistosomiasis, adenovirus, *Chlamydia, Mycoplasma*

Also seen following cytotoxic antitumor drugs, radiation, or trauma

Present clinically with frequency, lower abdominal pain, dysuria (pain or burning on urination)

HEMORRHAGIC CYSTITIS

Often following radiation or chemotherapy; also adenovirus

Marked epithelial atypia (more bizarre than carcinoma)

SUPPURATIVE CYSTITIS

Accumulation of large amounts of pus in lumen

GRANULOMATOUS CYSTITIS

Frequently seen following bacillus Calmette-Guérin (BCG) therapy for papillary transitional cell carcinoma (TCC)

Also seen with TB

CHRONIC CYSTITIS

More extreme heaping of mucosa

Red, friable, granular, sometimes ulcerated surface

Lymphoplasmacytic infiltrate

Fibrous thickening of the muscularis

CYSTITIS FOLLICULARIS

Variant of chronic cystitis with aggregation of lymphocytes into follicles

Special Forms of Cystitis

INTERSTITIAL (HUNNER'S) CYSTITIS

Persistent, chronic cystitis, most frequent in middle-aged women (male : female = 1 : 10), very painful hematuria, urgency; unresponsive to medical (antibiotic) therapy

Clinical-pathologic correlation required; histology may be normal

Inflammation and fibrosis of all layers of the wall

Localized ulcer is often present

Lamina propria shows edema, hemorrhage, granulation tissue, mononuclear inflammation, often perineural

Often, numerous mast cells are present beneath the ulcer, *within the detrusor muscle,* and between the epithelial cells in the mucosa

EOSINOPHILIC CYSTITIS

Two clinical settings:
- Women and children, associated with allergic disorders and eosinophilia
- Older men after bladder injury

Dramatic, recurrent episodes of frequency, dysuria, and hematuria

Grossly: broad-based polypoid growths

Chronic cystitis with dense inflammation, abundant eosinophils in lamina propria (numbers decrease with increasing fibrosis), fibrosis, muscle necrosis, occasionally giant cells; overlying epithelium often metaplastic or proliferative

POLYPOID CYSTITIS
Benign, inflammatory process that simulates neoplasm
Usually dome or posterior wall, secondary to catheter trauma
Stromal edema, congestion, chronic inflammation, normal epithelium without atypia

EMPHYSEMATOUS CYSTITIS
Occurs most frequently in diabetics (50% of cases)
Gas bubbles in the submucosal connective tissue, presumably caused by gas-forming bacteria
Giant cells surround gas bubbles

TUBERCULOSIS
Most frequent cause of granulomatous cystitis
Usually secondary infection from kidney; initially involves the area around the ureteral orifices

MALAKOPLAKIA
Soft yellow 3–4 cm mucosal plaques composed of closely packed, large, foamy macrophages with occasional giant cells and interspersed lymphocytes
Macrophages contain basophilic PAS+ granules filled with bacterial debris
Michaelis-Gutmann bodies: laminated mineralized concretions within and between macrophages
Most likely represents a defective host response to bacterial infection, usually from gram-negative bacilli
Probably same as xanthogranulomatous cystitis

MISCELLANEOUS
OBSTRUCTION
Usually due to prostatic hypertrophy in males, cystocele in females
Other causes: congenital urethral narrowing, inflammatory strictures, mechanical obstructions, neurogenic paralysis
Thickening of wall caused by hypertrophy of smooth muscle, resulting in marked trabeculations of the wall
With time, crypts between muscle bundles may form diverticula (see above)

LITHIASIS
Bladder calculi much more common in men than women
Most are solitary and composed of phosphate salts

AMYLOIDOSIS
May be part of a systemic process or nodular and localized to the bladder (amyloid tumor)
Deposits in interstitium of lamina propria, often penetrating into the muscularis
Minimal inflammation unless ulcerated
Can also be seen in the ureter, renal pelvis, or urethra
Most are AL type (light chain) amyloid protein

ENDOMETRIOSIS

PROLIFERATIVE/METAPLASTIC LESIONS
Occur in setting of longstanding chronic inflammation
BRUNN'S NESTS, CYSTITIS CYSTICA, AND CYSTITIS GLANDULARIS
Invagination of transitional epithelium into the underlying lamina propria (Brunn's nests)
May lose connection with the surface and become cystic with a flattened transitional to cuboidal lining (cystitis cystica)
Cyst lining may undergo metaplasia to columnar, mucus-secreting cells (cystitis glandularis)
Probably not premalignant

SQUAMOUS METAPLASIA
Nonkeratinizing: most commonly seen in trigone of women; responsive to estrogen
Keratinizing: seen secondary to trauma, diverticula, bladder stones, or schistosomiasis

BLADDER TUMORS

TUMOR-LIKE LESIONS
AMYLOID TUMOR
(See earlier discussion)
INFLAMMATORY PSEUDOTUMOR
AKA: plasma cell granuloma
Well-defined mass; may be encapsulated
Lymphocytes, histiocytes, plasma cells
SPINDLE CELL (PSEUDOSARCOMATOUS) NODULE
Occurs following instrumentation (transurethral resection [TUR])
Small, sessile, friable nodule; ulceration of overlying epithelium, hemorrhage
Simulates sarcoma (usually leiomyosarcoma) with high cellularity, high mitotic activity; may "invade" and destroy muscle
No pleomorphism, ulcerated surface, RBC extravasation, and history distinguish from true sarcoma

Benign Tumors

CONDYLOMA ACUMINATUM
HPV-induced papillomas, almost always associated with lesions of the perineum

INVERTED PAPILLOMA
AKA: Brunnian adenoma
Most commonly adults, males, located in trigone, neck, or prostatic urethra; usually solitary
May be a reactive lesion
Presents with hematuria and/or obstruction
Often a polypoid, usually sessile mass, showing invagination of the epithelium without atypia, without papillae, few mitoses, normal maturation
Must distinguish from TCC involving Brunn's nests

NEPHROGENIC ADENOMA
AKA: adenomatoid tumor, mesonephric adenoma
May be localized or diffuse metaplasia rather than neoplasm
Occurs in response to chronic infection, calculi, prolonged catheterization; 20% multiple
Papillary, polypoid, or sessile; generally small
Small tubules (microcysts) lined by cuboidal and hobnail cells, often with a prominent basement membrane

No atypia, not premalignant
Differential diagnosis: mesonephroid (clear cell) adenocarcinoma

OTHER BENIGN TUMORS
PARAGANGLIOMA (EXTRA-ADRENAL PHEOCHROMOCYTOMA)
Can occur as a primary bladder lesion, localized within wall
Patients present with fainting during micturition
Not all are necessarily benign
LEIOMYOMA
HEMANGIOMA
GRANULAR CELL TUMOR
NEUROFIBROMA

Malignant Tumors

TRANSITIONAL CELL CARCINOMA
90% of all primary tumors of the bladder; 3% of cancer deaths
Most patients >50 yr old; male:female = 3:1; present with hematuria
Risk factors: exposure to aniline dyes (esp. benzidine), *smoking* (4× relative risk), cyclophosphamide ingestion, phenacetin, schistosomiasis
75% arise from trigone region; partial or complete ureteral obstruction common
Papillary and nonpapillary (in situ or "flat") forms; >70% of patients have multiple recurrences of papillary TCC before progression to a more invasive lesion; some patients present with high-grade lesion from the start
Foci of glandular or squamous metaplasia common
Immunoreactive for keratins, CEA (esp. high grade), Leu-M1
Tumors can be graded on scale of I–IV or 0–III, where lowest grade is essentially equivalent to benign papilloma
Many of these tumors, esp. higher grade, are multifocal; most common in presence of dysplasia

GRADING

Grade I	Papillary structures, uniform cells, >7 layers
Grade II	Pedunculated or sessile; more crowding/layering of cells; enlargement of nuclei, more than occasional mitosis
Grade III	Sessile or cauliflower-like, often with necrosis and ulceration, smaller masses of cells, many mitoses
Grade IV	Most sessile with necrosis; marked atypia and pleomorphism, frequent mitoses, often atypical

STAGE

AJCC		Alternate Staging
Ta	Noninvasive, papillary (stage 0a)	
Tis	Noninvasive, flat (stage 0is)	
T1	Subepithelial connective tissue	A
T2	Superficial muscle (<50%)	B1
T3a	Deep muscle (>50%)	B2
T3b	Perivesicle fat	C
T4a	Prostate, uterus, vagina	D1
T4b	Pelvic wall, abdominal wall	D2
N1	Single LN, <2 cm	
N2	Single LN 2–5 cm or multiple LNs <5 cm	
N3	Any LN > 5 cm	

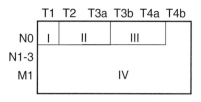

	T1	T2	T3a	T3b	T4a	T4b
N0	I	II		III		
N1-3	IV					
M1						

LN metastases in 25%; distant sites: lung, liver, bone

TREATMENT
Carcinoma in situ: total cystectomy—usually multifocal
Grade I–II: transurethral resection
Grade III–IV or any grade with stage >A: radical cystectomy
Radiation works well for papillary component but has little effect on invasive component
BCG therapy has been effective at decreasing recurrence rates

PROGNOSIS
Poor: high stage (muscle invasion), LN involvement, grade, dome or anterior wall, dysplasia elsewhere in bladder, vascular invasion
Good: young patient, inflammatory response

SQUAMOUS CELL CARCINOMA
~5% of primary bladder tumors
Association with schistosomiasis, chronic irritation (e.g., calculi)
male:female = 3:2
More commonly fungating and invasive
Somewhat worse prognosis than TCC, but probably caused by higher stage at presentation

ADENOCARCINOMA
Rare (~2% of primary bladder tumors)
Develop in setting of cystitis glandularis, exstrophy, or in urachal remnant
Unlike TCC, most are solitary lesions
Generally deeply invasive
Restrict term to pure adenocarcinomas; focal glandular changes or mucin production by a TCC is still a TCC
Poor prognosis

Variants
CLEAR CELL (MESONEPHRIC, MESONEPHROID) TYPE
Usually papillary
Mixture of glands, ducts, papillae, cysts, solid areas
Cells have abundant cytoplasmic glycogen and a hobnail morphology
Marked pleomorphism, infiltration, and mitoses distinguish from adenomatoid tumor
SIGNET RING CELL CARCINOMA
Diffuse infiltration of wall (linitis plastica pattern)

SMALL CELL CARCINOMA
As with its pulmonary counterpart, frequently shows some neuroendocrine features
May be pure or combined with invasive TCC
Extremely aggressive

SARCOMATOID CARCINOMA
AKA: carcinosarcoma
High-grade tumor: epithelial component (transitional, glandular, squamous, or undifferentiated) and sarcomatous

component (spindle cell to specific types of differentiation)
Generally, even sarcomatoid regions are keratin positive

RHABDOMYOSARCOMA
ADULT FORM
Usually >40 yr old
Similar to rhabdomyosarcoma of skeletal muscle

SARCOMA BOTRYOIDES
Generally infants and children
Embryonal rhabdomyosarcoma
Grows as large grapelike polypoid projections into lumen

LEIOMYOSARCOMA
More common in adults
Usually well circumscribed, may protrude into lumen, may ulcerate

18

TESTIS, PROSTATE, AND PENIS

TESTIS

NORMAL

Adult: 12–18 g; 5 × 3 × 3 cm
Capsule composed of three layers:
• Tunica vaginalis (outer serosa)
• Tunica albuginea (fibrous capsule)
• Tunica vasculosa
250 lobules, each with up to four seminiferous tubules (each ~200 μm long)
Germ cell : Sertoli cell ratio usually 13 : 1
Sertoli cells form the blood–testis barrier; basal spermatogonia are on the blood side of the barrier
Spermatogenesis: spermatogonia (two types: pale, dark), primary spermatocytes, secondary spermatocytes, spermatids, spermatozoa
Approx. half of germ cells should be in late spermatid stage
Spermatogenesis stimulated by follicle stimulating hormone (FSH); Leydig cells produce testosterone in response to luteinizing hormone (LH)
Leydig cells contain Reinke's crystalloid (hexagonal prisms by electron microscopy (EM), tapered ends, moderately electron dense)

DEVELOPMENT

Three phases of development:
• Static (birth to age 4—seminiferous tubules compactly filled with small undifferentiated cells; Leydig cells present in newborn, but then disappear)
• Growth (4–10 yr: minimal growth, lumen forms, increased tortuosity of tubules)
• Development and maturation (age 10 to puberty: gonadotropin-driven growth; mitoses, Leydig cells reappear; primary and secondary spermatocytes appear at age 8–11, spermatids by age 12)

FAILURE OF PUBERTAL MATURATION

Hypogonadotropic eunuchoidism (60%): low LH + FSH levels, small tubules, few Leydig cells
Klinefelter's syndrome (30%): XXY, fibrosis of tubules, prominent basement membrane thickening, Leydig cell hyperplasia, increased incidence of breast carcinoma
Testicular aplasia (10%): absent testicular tissue; elevation of urinary LH and FSH

CONGENITAL/ACQUIRED MALFORMATIONS

CRYPTORCHIDISM

In 10% of males at birth: 80% inguinal, 20% abdominal
90% descend in 1st yr, leaving <1% cryptorchidism
Should be corrected by age 2–3 yr (earlier if bilateral)
Unilateral: 100% fertile if corrected before age 10
Bilateral: 50% fertile if corrected before age 5

If uncorrected by puberty:
Small, brown testis with atrophic tubules, thickened basement membrane, foci of Sertoli cell hyperplasia, prominent interstitial cells
10–50× more likely to develop malignancy (usually seminoma) unless corrected by age 6; some increased risk persists even after correction
Increased incidence of malignancy in contralateral testis of patient with unilateral cryptorchidism

ECTOPIC SPLEEN

Splenogonadal fusion syndrome: congenital malformation occurring when two organs are in close proximity
Always left sided
Continuous variant: cord of fibrous or splenic tissue
Discontinuous variant: no connection

POLYORCHISM

ADRENAL CORTICAL RESTS

EPIDERMOID CYSTS

Intraparenchymal keratin-filled cysts with squamous lining
Squamous metaplasia or monodermal teratoma—unknown
Sample thoroughly for adnexal structures (rule out teratoma)

HYDROCELE

Accumulation of fluid in tunica vaginalis
May occur following trauma or epididymitis

SPERMATOCELE

Cystic dilatation of efferent ducts, lined by tall ciliated cells

VARICOCELE

Abnormal dilatation of veins in the spermatic cord
90% occur on left
Often results in decreased fertility

TORSION

SPERMATIC CORD

Peak incidence in 1st yr, 2nd peak near puberty
Enlarged, painful
Intense congestion to hemorrhagic infarction (veins occlude first; arteries may or may not occlude)
Usually minimal inflammation (impaired blood flow)
If reduce within 6 hr, usually no infarction; if >24 hr, almost always infarcted

APPENDIX TESTIS OR EPIDIDYMIS

Pain well out of proportion to size of structure
• Testis: paramesonephric duct remnant (92%)
• Epididymis: mesonephric duct remnant (8%)

CAUSES OF INFERTILITY

AZOOSPERMIA

• Germ cell aplasia (Sertoli cell only syndrome) (29%): thickening of basement membrane (BM) with fibrosis
• Spermatocytic arrest (26%): usually at primary spermatocyte; Leydig cells normal

167

- Generalized fibrosis (18%)
- Normal spermatogenesis (27%): total bilateral obstruction causing secondary spermatocytic arrest with sloughing of immature spermatocytes into the lumen

OLIGOSPERMIA
- Incomplete arrest
- Spermatogenic hypoplasia (no specific arrest, just decreased production)
- Regional (incomplete) fibrosis
- Tubular hyalinization (e.g., Klinefelter's syndrome)
- Normal spermatogenesis: partial obstruction

TESTICULAR ATROPHY
(Note: if elastic fibers present, puberty was reached before disease developed)
- Atherosclerosis
- Hypopituitarism
- Irradiation
- Chemotherapy (esp. cyclophosphamide)
- End-stage inflammatory orchitis (e.g., postpubertal mumps)
- Exogenous estrogen or gonadotropin-releasing hormone (GnRH) for prostatic carcinoma
- Exhaustion atrophy following persistent elevated FSH
- Hepatic cirrhosis (increased endogenous estrogens, not metabolized by liver)
- Uncorrected cryptorchidism
- Semen outflow obstruction
- Generalized malnutrition

INFLAMMATORY ORCHITIS
MUMPS
Orchitis occurs in 20% of postpubertal patients
Edema of tunica albuginea and the interstitium, with vascular congestion, necrosis of spermatocytic cells (largely sparing the Sertoli cells), interstitial lymphocytic aggregates, neutrophils
10% of postpubertal patients with orchitis become infertile

PYOGENIC EPIDIDYMO-ORCHITIS
Congestion, edema, neutrophils (interstitium, then tubules)
May lead to venous thrombosis, septic infarction
E. coli most commonly (for children and men >35 yr); when sexually active: *Neisseria gonorrhoeae, Chlamydia*
Other infections agents: *Toxoplasma,* fungi, parasites, syphilis, TB (hematogenous or via prostate; former usually spares tail of epididymis), atypical mycobacteria
Most infectious agents (especially TB) infect epididymis first, then spread to testis; however, syphilis usually begins in testis

NONSPECIFIC GRANULOMATOUS ORCHITIS
Solid, nodular enlargement of testis
History of trauma usually present
Granulomatous inflammation surrounding the seminiferous tubules; probably secondary to acid-fast products of disintegrating sperm
Can be secondary to sarcoid or infectious
Noninfectious autoimmune form also exists

MALAKOPLAKIA
Abscess formation, tubular atrophy
Michaelis-Gutmann bodies (intracellular and extracellular round bodies that stain for iron and calcium)
Bacterial in origin, usually *E. coli*

OTHER NON-NEOPLASTIC LESIONS
Juvenile xanthogranuloma
Sinus histiocytosis with massive lymphadenopathy

TESTICULAR TUMORS

Germ Cell Tumors

Account for 90–95% of all testicular tumors
Arise from germinal epithelium; 60% are mixed tumors
Most common malignancy in males 25–29 yr
Increased risk in patients with cryptorchidism, a positive family history, previous germ cell tumor, intersex syndrome, or oligospermic infertility
Presents usually with painless unilateral enlargement
1–3% bilateral (15% if both undescended); usually metachronous
Many germ cell tumors (80%), regardless of type, show isochromosome 12p
Histologic types: originally it was thought that these tumors followed either a seminomatous or a nonseminomatous pathway; it is now known that the sequence appears to be intratubular germ cell neoplasm, then seminoma, then others, usually via embryonal; however, can progress to others without an embryonal or even a seminoma stage, and most of the subtypes appear to be able to interconvert

SPREAD
Lymphatic: first, periaortic and iliac nodes (80% ipsilateral, 20% bilateral), then mediastinal, left supraclavicular nodes; inguinal nodes involved only if skin or scrotum invaded
Blood: lungs, liver, brain (esp. choriocarcinoma), bone (esp. seminoma)
Histology of metastases may be completely different from that of the primary tumor

STAGING
Tis   Intratubular tumor
T1   Limited to testis
T2   Beyond tunica albuginea or into epididymis
T3   Spermatic cord involvement
T4   Scrotal involvement
N1   Single lymph node (LN) <2 cm
N2   Single LN 2–5 cm or multiple LNs all <5 cm
N3   Any LN >5 cm

	Any T
N0	I
N1–3	II
M1	III

THERAPY AND PROGNOSIS
Initially, inguinal orchiectomy; get histology, then:
- Seminoma: radiation of retroperitoneum (very sensitive)
- Nonseminomatous germ cell tumor (NSGCT): lymphadenectomy if vascular invasion identified; chemotherapy if metastases present
Prognosis: cure rate is >95% without LN involvement; 40–90% with positive LNs (except choriocarcinoma, which is almost always fatal)
If alive at 2 yr, 90% chance of cure; at 6 yr, ~100%
Bad prognostic signs: extension into spermatic cord, Leydig cell hyperplasia in residual testis, vascular invasion
Follow serum: human chorionic gonadotropin (HCG) elevated in 72% (may present as gynecomastia), alpha-fetoprotein (AFP) elevated in 75%

INTRATUBULAR GERM CELL NEOPLASIA (IGCN)

Seen in 80% of testes with invasive malignancy
Can be seen in contralateral testis
Histology is usually independent of the histology of the invasive component

IGCN, UNCLASSIFIED

Atypical germ cells at base of otherwise normal seminiferous tubules, with clear cytoplasm (glycogen), placental alkaline phosphatase (PLAP)+
Thickened lamina propria with hyalinization

IGCN WITH EXTRATUBULAR EXTENSION ("MICROINVASIVE")

Atypical germ cells in interstitium
Invasion? vs. ectopic germ cell elements

INTRATUBULAR SEMINOMA

INTRATUBULAR EMBRYONAL CARCINOMA

IGCN, OTHER FORMS

SEMINOMA

30–40% of all testicular tumors
Most common type in men >60 yr
Rare in prepubertal male
Tend to remain localized a long time before metastasizing

Classic Seminoma (95%)

Mean age 42 yr
Solid, homogeneous, light yellow; often replaces entire testis; may show some necrosis; cystic changes or hemorrhage suggest nonseminomatous component
Clear cells (abundant glycogen) with sharp borders, central hyperchromatic nuclei with one or two prominent nucleoli; cells arranged in sheets, nests, trabeculae, or dispersed throughout the interstitium; nests are surrounded by fibrous bands infiltrated by inflammatory cells (lymphocytes, plasma cells, granulomas)
20% show no inflammatory response (may have worse prognosis)
Serum shows elevated PLAP in 40–50%
May occur in extratesticular sites (pineal, anterior mediastinum, retroperitoneum); worse prognosis
Immunoreactive for PLAP, vimentin; generally *negative for keratin*

SEMINOMA WITH TROPHOBLASTIC GIANT CELLS

10–20% of classic seminomas contain isolated or syncytial masses of large cells, often perivascular, with associated hemorrhage
Cells contain chorionic gonadotropin, ± elevation in serum
May be more aggressive
If serum HCG does not fall after orchiectomy, suggests there are metastases with the same histology or that the patient has choriocarcinoma

ANAPLASTIC SEMINOMA

Initially defined as >3 mitoses/high power field (HPF); need other pleomorphism
Poorly defined; unclear significance

SPERMATOCYTIC SEMINOMA (5%)

Mean age 65 yr (older age group)
Never occurs in combination with teratoma; never occurs outside of testis; no association with cryptorchidism or IGCN
Soft, pale gray, homogeneous; ~10% are bilateral
Three cell types (small, medium, and large), all with perfectly round nuclei (medium-sized cells predominate)
Cells have dense cytoplasm, numerous mitoses
Prominent intratubular growth pattern at periphery
Few lymphocytes

Excellent prognosis unless sarcomatous transformation

NONSEMINOMATOUS GERM CELL TUMORS

Mean age 30 yr; rare beyond 60 yr of age

Embryonal Carcinoma

Metastasize early: poor prognosis
Heterogeneous solid gray mass with foci of hemorrhage and necrosis
Sheets, glands, tubules, papillae, or alveolar nests of undifferentiated cells with vesicular nuclei, prominent nucleoli, numerous mitoses, pleomorphism
Immunoreactive for keratin, although may be only focal
When pure, AFP negative
Most occur mixed with other histologic types, only 3–7% pure

Teratoma (Mature, Immature)

5–10% of all testicular tumors
Heterogeneous tumor: multiloculated cysts, cartilage
Most common tissues: nerve, cartilage, epithelium
Immature components of unclear significance
In children, never metastasize
In adults, may have metastases, even if all mature

TERATOCARCINOMA

Teratoma plus embryonal carcinoma
Appearance depends on relative amounts of each
Can get sarcomatous elements

TERATOMA WITH MALIGNANT TRANSFORMATION

Malignancy (e.g., adenocarcinoma) arising in a mature component

PRIMITIVE NEUROECTODERMAL TUMOR

All immature neural tissue

Choriocarcinoma

5% of all testicular tumors
Usually very small, hemorrhagic, partially necrotic
Giant syncytial trophoblasts with large atypical nuclei intermixed with cytotrophoblasts (must have both) in a biphasic, plexiform pattern; no intermediate trophoblasts
Syncytial component positive for chorionic gonadotropin
Almost always disseminated at presentation, thus fatal
Primary may regress leaving only hemosiderin-laden scar

Yolk Sac Tumor

AKA: endodermal sinus tumor, juvenile embryonal carcinoma, embryonal adenocarcinoma, orchidoblastoma
Monomorphic teratoma mimicking embryonal yolk sac
Homogeneous, soft, microcystic, yellow-white, mucinous
Organoid intermingling epithelial and mesenchymal elements (microcystic, glandular, alveolar, papillary); hyaline intracytoplasmic inclusions, PAS+, diastase resistant
Perivascular Schiller-Duval bodies (endodermal sinuses: mesodermal core, central capillary, visceral and parietal layers; resembles primitive glomerulus)
Immunoreactive for keratin and AFP

PURE FORM

Infants and children (<2 yr old); excellent prognosis

MIXED FORM

Adults; worse prognosis

POLYEMBRYOMA

Multiple embryoid bodies (amnion-like cavity with embryo-like cellular invagination overlying a yolk sac–like structure)
Considered a mixed tumor with yolk sac, embryonal

DIFFUSE EMBRYOMA
Embryonal, yolk sac, and trophoblastic elements in orderly arrangement

Sex Cord–Stromal Tumors

~4% of all testicular tumors

LEYDIG (INTERSTITIAL) CELLS
Testosterone-producing cells
NODULAR LEYDIG CELL HYPERPLASIA
Usually multiple nodules, almost always <0.5 cm
Seen in cryptorchid testes
LEYDIG CELL TUMOR
3% bilateral
Presentation: mass or gynecomastia
Small (average 3 cm), sharply demarcated, dark brown
Well-defined cell borders, acidophilic to clear cytoplasm, round to oval nucleus, nuclear pleomorphism; solid growth, occasionally trabecular
EM: smooth endoplasmic reticulum (ER), Reinke's crystalloids (elongated, often tapered crystals; moderately electron dense)
10% metastasize (larger [7.5 cm], other malignant features)

SERTOLI CELLS
SERTOLI CELL HYPERPLASIA
AKA: hypoplastic tubules, tubular adenomas
Seen in half of the cryptorchid testes and in 20% of patients with testicular tumors
Frequency decreases with age
SERTOLI CELL ADENOMA
Not uncommon in testicular feminization syndrome
Elongated tubules lined by Sertoli-like cells
SEX CORD TUMOR WITH ANNULAR TUBULES
Closely related to Sertoli cell adenomas
Seen in patients with Peutz-Jeghers syndrome
SERTOLI CELL TUMORS
AKA: androblastoma
One third associated with gynecomastia
Well circumscribed, white or yellow, firm, focally cystic
Sertoli cells form tubules or solid sheets
10% behave malignantly—metastasize
SCLEROSING SERTOLI CELL TUMOR
Mean age 35
Well circumscribed, firm, white
Solid and hollow tubules in a hypocellular fibrous stroma
Generally well behaved
LARGE CELL CALCIFYING SERTOLI CELL TUMOR
Usually <20 yr old; frequently bilateral or multifocal
Associated with Leydig cell tumors, pituitary tumors, adrenal cortical hyperplasia, cardiac myxomas, Peutz-Jeghers
Sheets to cords of tumor cells with abundant cytoplasm separated by abundant fibrous tissue with calcifications

OTHER SEX CORD–STROMAL TUMORS
Granulosa cell tumor (juvenile form in infants <6 months; abnormal chromosomes and ambiguous genitalia)
Counterparts of ovarian surface epithelial tumors (serous, mucinous, endometrioid, clear cell, Brenner tumor)

Other Testicular Tumors

GONADOBLASTOMA
Mixed germ cell–sex cord–stromal tumor

Arises in individuals with underlying gonadal disorder, usually chromosomal abnormality, with occasional exceptions
Calcifications; hyaline bodies surrounded by malignant cells

LYMPHOMA
5% of all testicular malignancies; 50% of the bilateral tumors
Most common testicular tumor in elderly
Large cell type most common (noncleaved, immunoblastic)
If primary, good prognosis; if not, bad prognosis
Involvement interstitial with relative sparing of the seminiferous tubules, especially at periphery

LEUKEMIA
Usually acute lymphoblastic leukemia (ALL); similar pattern to lymphoma
Clinically evident in 8% children with ALL, microscopically evident in 20%—often first sign of relapse

OTHERS
CARCINOID TUMOR
Well-circumscribed, firm yellow masses
Orchiectomy usually curative
SPINDLE CELL TUMOR
May have islands of squamous metaplasia
PARATESTICULAR RHABDOMYOSARCOMA
Most common nongerminal tumor of scrotal contents in children and adolescents
Nearly always of embryonal type
Metastases to retroperitoneal nodes in 40%
METASTATIC TUMORS
Most common primaries: lung or prostate

Epididymal Tumors

ADENOMATOID TUMOR
Most common type; 20–30 yr peak incidence
Presents as mass with or without pain
Small (~2 cm), solid, firm white, occasional small cysts
Unencapsulated, cords of flattened to cuboidal epithelium, often with vacuolated cytoplasm, with dilated channels and prominent stroma with smooth muscle and elastic fibers
Hyaluronidase-sensitive mucin staining
Immunoreactive for keratin and EMA; negative for CEA, factor VIII
Histogenesis unclear—may be special form of mesothelioma
Invariably benign

MESOTHELIOMA
Usually fibrous type
Arises from tunica vaginalis testis
Differential includes adenocarcinoma of rete testis

PAPILLARY CYSTADENOMA
Unilateral or bilateral
Familial incidence: part of von Hippel-Lindau syndrome
1–5 cm, well circumscribed, cystic or solid

Papillary infoldings with clear cytoplasm
Malignant counterpart, rare

PROSTATE

Normal
Approximately 20 g in normal adult
Retroperitoneal; encircles neck of bladder
No distinct capsule
Classically, five lobes: posterior, middle, anterior, two lateral
Urethra enters from bladder on superior surface of gland and exits anteriorly
Glands lined by two cell layers: low cuboidal basal layer and cuboidal to columnar secretory layer
Epithelial cells immunoreactive for prostate-specific antigen (PSA), prostate-specific acid phosphatase (PAP), keratin, Leu7, EMA (80%), CEA (25%)
Basal cell layer immunoreactive for keratin 903 (difficult stain to do correctly)

PROSTATITIS
ACUTE BACTERIAL PROSTATITIS
Usually a localized process involving small number of ducts or acini
Formerly, gonorrhea most common cause
Now, *E. coli* infection associated with some degree of urinary obstruction and urinary retention is most common
Abscess formation can be seen
Usually not biopsied
CHRONIC PROSTATITIS
Can be bacterial or nonbacterial
Lymphocytes, plasma cells, macrophages
Can result in mild elevations of PSA
TUBERCULOSIS
Prostate involved in ~10% of patients with systemic infection
Usually lateral lobes, usually bilateral
Confluent foci of caseous necrosis common
Some cases occur following treatment with bacillus Calmette-Guérin (BCG) therapy for transitional cell carcinoma (TCC); these cases tend to remain localized
NONSPECIFIC GRANULOMATOUS PROSTATITIS
Firm prostate with dense fibrosis and granulomas
No necrosis
Unknown etiology; probably duct rupture and leakage of contents
EOSINOPHILIC PROSTATITIS
MALAKOPLAKIA
Usually associated with similar disease in bladder

NODULAR HYPERPLASIA
AKA: benign prostatic hypertrophy
Often results in some degree of urinary obstruction
Occurs in 50% of men by 40s, 75% by 70s; ~4% of men over 70 have prostates larger than 100 g
Intact testes required, because hormonal stimulation necessary
Average size is 100 g; up to 800 g has been reported
Begins on inner portion of gland (periurethral)
Both glandular and stromal (fibrous and smooth muscle) hyperplasia
Inspissated secretions, calcifications, calculi (7%), corpora amylacea, infarction (20–25%)
BASAL CELL HYPERPLASIA
Small, generally solid nests of benign-appearing epithelial cells with a somewhat clear cytoplasm
Can mimic prostatic intraepithelial neoplasia (PIN), but generally is *not* papillary
Always an accompanying usual hyperplasia
Keratin 903 positive
May be ischemic in origin

TUMOR-LIKE CONDITIONS
SARCOMA-LIKE NODULES
Usually few weeks to months following transurethral resection (TUR) procedure
Exuberant stromal reaction
May have high mitotic activity, extreme cellularity
MELANOSIS
Can occur in epithelium or in stroma (blue nevus)
URETHRAL POLYPS
Tall columnar cells—cause hematuria in young
AMYLOID NODULE
SCLEROSING ADENOSIS
AKA: fibroglandular nodule
Relatively well-circumscribed aggregate of smaller glands in the middle and larger glands to the periphery
Nucleoli generally present but small
S-100 stains myoepithelial cells in this lesion, but not elsewhere (i.e., not in normal prostate)
ATROPHY
Small basophilic glands with open lumina, often lined by a single cell layer, but cells are flattened (atrophic)
Sclerotic stroma
May be confused with adenocarcinoma

PROSTATIC INTRAEPITHELIAL NEOPLASIA
Identifiable on low power: glands with normal architecture but with papillary projections into the lumen and darker staining caused by hyperchromasia and enlargement of the nuclei with overlapping and stratification; cells may contain pigment
Almost exclusively confined to peripheral zones
Four histologic patterns: micropapillary, tufted, cribriform, flat
Graded as PIN I, II, or III; some use low (I) and high (II or III)
Prominent nucleoli make PIN II (at least)
PIN I or II can be found in 70% of "normal" patients
Keratin 903 staining may be scanty
PIN III indicates up to a 70% chance of a coexisting adenocarcinoma elsewhere in the gland

ADENOCARCINOMA
Second most common malignancy in men in U.S.
Responsible for 10% of cancer deaths
Black : white = 2 : 1; hormonally related
Unlike benign prostatic hypertrophy (BPH), most carcinomas arise peripherally
75–85% are multifocal
Most arise from peripheral ducts and acini; a few arise in the larger primary ducts
Gray or yellowish grossly
Variable growth patterns: cribriform, diffuse, glandular, papillary, etc.

Morphologic variants include small cell, mucinous (more aggressive; less responsive to hormonal therapy), squamous, adenoid, cystic, and large duct adenocarcinoma (papillary or cribriform; prostatic, endometrioid, transitional cell, mixed)

10–25% show protein crystals in glandular lumina; strong indicator of malignancy; crystals are deeply eosinophilic, often rhomboid, and are immunoreactive for Ig light chain (κ or λ)

Other indicators of probable malignancy: necrosis in secretions, deeply eosinophilic secretions, basophilic mucinous secretions

When nucleoli exceed 3 μm, always malignant; 1–3 μm is suggestive of carcinoma

Can use keratin 903 to look for presence of basal cell layer; because of the variability in staining, absence does not necessarily mean carcinoma

SPREAD
Marked propensity for perineural invasion
"Capsular" invasion very common
Seminal vesicles involved in 30%
Metastases most commonly to bone and lymph nodes (LNs)
Bone lesions usually multiple, osteoblastic, or osteoclastic
LN involvement is first pelvic, then retroperitoneal

CLINICAL STAGING
A: No palpable lesion	A1: <5%
	A2: >5% or high grade
B: Confined to prostate	B1: One lobe
	B2: Both lobes
C: Periprostatic	C1: <70 g
	C2: >70 g tumor or seminal vesicle
D: Metastatic	D1: Pelvic LNs
	D2: Distant

35% of males >50 and 60% >80 have stage A1 disease
<10% of individuals with stage A1 disease progress
30–50% stage A2 lesions progress within 5 yr, 20% fatal
75% patients are stage C or D when present clinically

PATHOLOGIC STAGING
T1a	Not palpable; ≤5% of resected tissue
T1b	Not palpable; >5% of resected tissue
T1c	Not palpable; positive needle biopsy
T2a	Confined to prostate; ≤1/2 lobe
T2b	Confined to prostate; 1/2–1 lobe
T2c	Confined to prostate; both lobes
T3a	Unilateral extracapsular extension
T3b	Bilateral extracapsular extension
T3c	Involves seminal vesicle
T4a	Bladder neck, external sphincter, rectum
T4b	Levator muscles, pelvic wall
N1	Single LN, <2 cm
N2	Single LN, 2–5 cm; or multiple LNs, all <5 cm
N3	Any LN >5 cm

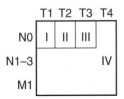

Note: T1a, grade 1 lesions are considered stage 0

GRADING (GLEASON)
Score two most predominant patterns
1: Single, separate, uniform glands, closely packed, round, well delimited
2: Single, separate, less uniform glands, loosely packed, less well delimited
3a: Single, separate, variable glands, irregularly separated, poorly delimited
3b: Like 3a, but very small glands or tiny cell clusters
3c: Cribriform tumor, well circumscribed
4a: Raggedly outlined, infiltrating, fused glands
4b: Large pale cells (hypernephroid)
5a: Comedocarcinoma pattern
5b: Anaplastic cell masses or single cells

THERAPY AND PROGNOSIS
Stage A1 lesions are treated conservatively (followed)
Radiotherapy or radical prostatectomy for A2
Radical prostatectomy for B
Stage C and D are treated with radiation and anti-androgen therapy
Stage and grade most important prognostic indicators
Age is *not* a factor in prognosis
Weak reactivity for PSA and PAP may indicate a more aggressive tumor

FLUTAMIDE THERAPY
Flutamide is an antiandrogen that blocks peripheral conversion of estrogens to androgens (primary stimulation for prostate growth is androgens from the adrenal gland)
(Note: patients treated with flutamide are often given Lupron (leuprolide acetate), a LHRH agonist, to maintain testicular function)
Flutamide induces atrophy of both the normal and malignant prostatic glands
Prominent basal cell layer, immature squamous metaplasia, shrinking of secretory layer with vacuolization of cells, which may become difficult to find; pigment may be present
May need keratin stain to find residual tumor
Don't give a Gleason grade to treated tumor—inaccurate
Same histologic changes are seen in LN metastases

ENDOMETRIOID CARCINOMA OF THE PROSTATE
Arises from utricle
Usually papillary
Generally does not metastasize to bone; normal serum acid phosphatase level
May have relatively good prognosis

PENIS

Normal
Erectile tissue: two corpora cavernosa, one corpus spongiosum containing the urethra and extending into the glans
Urethral meatus normally at the central ventral glans
Covered by a squamous epithelium, nonkeratinized on the glans

CONGENITAL AND ACQUIRED MALFORMATIONS

ABNORMALITIES OF SIZE
Almost always associated with other abnormalities of the genitourinary tract
Aphalalia: penile agenesis (very rare)
Hypoplasia
Hyperplasia
Diphalalia: duplication of penis

ABNORMALITIES OF URETHRAL MEATUS
Epispadias: opens on dorsum of glans
Hypospadias: opens on ventral surface of penis
Accessory urethral canals

PHIMOSIS
Orifice of prepuce too small to allow normal retraction
May be caused by congenital anomaly or chronic infection
Paraphimosis: prepuce retracted but too tight to be re-extended
Treated with circumcision

INFECTIONS
(See also Infectious Agents outline)

BALANOPOSTHITIS
Infection of glans and prepuce
Most commonly seen in uncircumcised newborns
Streptococcus, Staphylococcus, Neisseria gonorrhoeae, Gardnerella vaginalis, Trichomonas
Inflammation is nonspecific

SYPHILIS
Usually on glans
Initially firm, erythematous papule that ulcerates (hard chancre)
Plasma cells and lymphocytes underlying ulcer, with endothelial cell proliferation and capillaritis
Secondary syphilis: condyloma lata (flat maculopapule)
Tertiary syphilis: gummas (granulomas)

LYMPHOGRANULOMA VENEREUM
Chlamydia trachomatis
Short-lived painless papule or ulcer, followed by suppurative inflammation of the inguinal lymph nodes

OTHERS
Granuloma inguinale, herpes, molluscum contagiosum

MISCELLANEOUS INFLAMMATORY LESIONS

BALANITIS XEROTICA OBLITERANS
Equivalent to lichen sclerosus et atrophicus of the vulva
Gray-white geographic areas of atrophy, which histologically show loss of lamina proprial structures, thinning of the epidermis, and diffuse fibrosis
Predominantly lymphocytic infiltrate deep

BALANITIS CIRCUMSCRIPTA PLASMACELLULARIS
AKA: Zoon's balanitis
Unknown etiology; usually uncircumcised men
Epidermal atrophy; plasma cell–rich inflammation, histiocytes with hemosiderin pigment

PEYRONIE'S DISEASE
Fibrous thickening of the tissue between the corpora cavernosa and tunica albuginea, limiting the movement of these structures past each other during an erection (curvature toward side of lesion)
Histology is that of fibromatosis
May be inflammatory in etiology
May lead to ossification

NONINVASIVE SQUAMOUS LESIONS

CONDYLOMA ACUMINATUM
Sexually transmitted disease caused by human papilloma virus, most commonly types 6 and 11
Accounts for approx. one third of all polypoid lesions of the male urethra
Most commonly urethral meatus or fossa navicularis
Exophytic, fungating wartlike lesion
Hyperkeratosis, hypergranulosis, acanthosis, koilocytosis

BOWENOID PAPULOSIS
Occur in patients <35 yr, usually skin of the shaft or glans
Multiple, small, rapidly developing shiny erythematous lesions, which histologically are very similar to squamous cell carcinoma in situ but with slightly more orderly background, and some maturation toward the surface
80% of cases have been shown to have HPV-16
Often spontaneously disappear without treatment

BOWEN'S DISEASE
AKA: squamous cell carcinoma in situ
Usually shaft or scrotum of patient >35 yr
Slowly enlarging, sharply demarcated, single lesion, scaly
Full-thickness dysplasia with hyperchromasia, mitoses
5–15% will progress to invasive squamous cell carcinoma
Nearly one third of patients will have some "unrelated" visceral malignancy (lung, GI tract, or urinary tract)

ERYTHROPLASIA OF QUEYRAT
AKA: squamous cell carcinoma in situ of the glans
Asymptomatic, well-defined shiny-red lesions of the glans and foreskin of uncircumcised men
Histology same as Bowen's disease
No association with visceral malignancy

SQUAMOUS CELL CARCINOMA
1% of male cancers in U.S.; much higher elsewhere; appears to be significantly decreased incidence among circumcised population
Patients usually 40–70 yr old; usually arises on glans
May be some association with HPV 16 and 18
Predominantly two growth patterns: exophytic papillary and ulcerating flat
Slow growing
~15% have metastasized at diagnosis
If limited to the glans, >95% survival; with involvement of shaft and regional LNs, survival at 3 yr <50%

STAGING
Tis   Carcinoma in situ
Ta   Noninvasive verrucous carcinoma
T1   Subepithelial connective tissue
T2   Corpus spongiosum or cavernosum
T3   Urethra or prostate
T4   Adjacent structures
N1   Single superficial inguinal LN
N2   Multiple or bilateral superficial inguinal LNs
N3   Deep inguinal or pelvic LNs

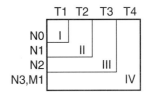

Histological Types

~50% of squamous cell carcinomas of the penis fall into the not otherwise specified (NOS) category

VERRUCOUS CARCINOMA

5% of penile cancers

Large, warty, exophytic growth

Extremely well-differentiated histology throughout, with pushing borders

Does not metastasize

Very good prognosis

SUPERFICIALLY SPREADING

VERTICAL GROWTH

MULTICENTRIC

BASALOID

INFLAMMATORY

SPINDLE CELL

19

OVARY AND FALLOPIAN TUBES

Normal Ovary

Follicles: primordial, primary, secondary, tertiary, graafian, atretic; also corpora lutea and corpora albicantia

Hilus cells (counterpart of Leydig cells) are intimately associated with nerves; more prominent in older women

Walthard's cell nests may be cystic or solid

Germ cells develop from endoderm; rest of ovary is mesodermal in origin

CONGENITAL MALFORMATIONS
MESONEPHRIC (WOLFFIAN DUCT) REMNANTS

Small ductlike structures at ovarian hilus

May become cystically dilated

Mesonephric ducts have cuboidal epithelium, predominantly nonciliated, on a well-developed basement membrane

(In contrast, paramesonephric [Müllerian] ducts are taller, contain a mixture of ciliated and nonciliated cells, and have an inconspicuous basement membrane)

GONADAL DYSGENESIS

May be "pure" or associated with Turner's syndrome

Ovaries represented by a streak of fibrous tissue

MIXED GONADAL DYSGENESIS

One streak ovary and the other with testicular tissue

Particularly prone to develop gonadoblastoma

INFLAMMATORY LESIONS
NONSPECIFIC INFLAMMATION

Usually ascending, practically always associated with salpingitis, resulting in a tubo-ovarian abscess (see later)

Heals with fibrous scarring and by conversion to a tubo-ovarian cyst

GRANULOMATOUS INFLAMMATION

TB, actinomycosis, schistosomiasis, *Enterobius vermicularis*

Sarcoidosis, Crohn's disease

TORSION

Usually secondary to inflammation or tumor of tube or ovary, but both are normal in 20% of cases

Hemorrhagic infarction

If reduce quickly enough, may be able to recover

Nonoperated cases may calcify

NON-NEOPLASTIC CYSTIC LESIONS
GERMINAL INCLUSION CYSTS

Small, multiple; probably invaginations of surface epithelium

Flattened epithelium, tubal metaplasia, psammoma bodies

FOLLICULAR CYSTS

Distention of developing follicles; may occur at any age

Generally called *follicular cyst* only if >2 cm; if smaller, simply a *cystic follicle*

Lined by theca layer, frequently luteinized, ± granulosa layer

CORPUS LUTEUM CYST

Reproductive age patients

Bright yellow convoluted thick rimmed hemorrhagic cyst

Lined by luteinized granulosa cells surrounded by theca lutein cells

May rupture into peritoneum

POLYCYSTIC OVARIES

3–5% of all women

Multiple subcapsular follicular cysts (usually <1 cm) covered by a dense fibrous capsule

Stein-Leventhal syndrome: polycystic ovaries, amenorrhea, and sterility

Follicular cysts produce androgens, which are converted to estrogens, which leads to endometrial hyperplasia and anovulation (by suppression of follicle stimulating hormone [FSH])

EPIDERMOID CYSTS

NON-NEOPLASTIC PROLIFERATIONS
ENDOMETRIOSIS

"Ectopic" proliferation of endometrial glands and stroma with hemosiderin

Ovary is most common site; associated with infertility

May be small focal lesions or convert entire ovary into a "chocolate cyst" from repeated hemorrhages

ENDOSALPINGIOSIS

Proliferation of tubal epithelium without stroma

Usually one cell layer, obvious lumen; cells may be ciliated

Increased frequency in presence of serous ovarian tumors

STROMAL HYPERPLASIA

Bilateral diffuse (single cells or clusters) or nodular proliferation within the cortex and medulla of plump ovarian stromal cells, often with patchy or extensive luteinization (hyperthecosis, diffuse thecomatosis)

True thecomas may develop in this background

HILUS CELL HYPERPLASIA

Multiple nodules, usually <2 mm each

ECTOPIC DECIDUAL REACTION
MASSIVE EDEMA OF THE OVARY

Patients present with pain and an abdominal mass

Usually unilateral, massively enlarged, soft, boggy ovary; may be in excess of 2 kg!

In addition to diffuse edema, cystic follicles usually present

Partial torsion may have an etiologic role

Differential diagnosis: ovarian fibroma

FIBROMATOSIS

Usually younger age group (13–40 yr) than fibroma

Firm, white cut surface with residual follicles

175

OVARIAN NEOPLASMS

General

5th leading cancer killer in women; most common cause of death from gynecologic malignancies

Predominantly disease of older white women

Pregnancy and oral contraceptives *decrease* risk

~10% of tumors in women <45 yr are malignant; ~50% in women >45 yr

Most common sites of spread: contralateral ovary, peritoneal cavity, pelvic lymph nodes (LNs), para-aortic LNs

Overall survival: 35% at 5 yr, 28% at 10 yr, 15% at 25 yr

Prognosis for borderline tumors generally good, even with involvement of the peritoneal cavity

FIGO STAGING

(Note: TNM staging same: T2c = FIGO IIc)

I: Limited to the ovaries
  Ia: One ovary, no ascites
    Ia1: Intact capsule, no tumor on surface
    Ia2: Tumor on external surface or ruptured capsule
  Ib: Both ovaries, no ascites
    Ib1: Intact capsule, no tumor on surface
    Ib2: Tumor on external surface or ruptured capsule
  Ic: Ascites or malignant washings
II: Pelvic extension
  IIa: Uterus or tubes
  IIb: Other pelvic tissues
  IIc: IIa or b with ascites or positive washings
III: Intraperitoneal metastases outside pelvis, retroperitoneal nodes, or small bowel or omentum
  IIIa: Microscopic peritoneal seeding
  IIIb: Implants larger, but <2 cm
  IIIc: >2 cm implants or positive lymph nodes
IV: Distant metastases or liver metastases

STAGE AND PROGNOSIS

Stage	Frequency	5 Yr Survival
I	26%	61%
II	21%	40%
III	37%	5%
IV	16%	3%

Surface Epithelial Tumors

Two thirds of ovarian tumors; ~90% of all malignant ovarian tumors

Believed to arise from the epithelium lining the outer surface of the ovary, variably termed *surface, coelomic* or *germinal* epithelium—continuous with the mesothelium

Actually, tumors probably arise from an invaginated portion of this epithelium

Not infrequently tumors can be mixture of multiple types

All of these tumors are divided into benign, borderline, and malignant categories

Borderline tumors also go by the terms *low malignant potential* or *indeterminate malignant potential*

Both borderline and malignant tumors are treated with total abdominal hysterectomy with bilateral salpingo-oophorectomy (TAH-BSO) and surgical staging; if preservation of fertility is desired and tumor is stage I and borderline, can limit surgery to unilateral salpingo-oophorectomy

In general, one tissue block per 1–2 cm of maximum tumor dimension is recommended

SEROUS TUMORS

Comprise 25–30% of all ovarian tumors, most in adults; 30–50% are bilateral

Usually cystic spaces with papillary formations protruding into the cavities, which are filled with a clear (sometimes viscous) fluid

Cuboidal to columnar cells line cyst wall and papillae

Psammoma bodies seen in 30%

Immunoreactive for keratin, EMA, sometimes vimentin

Negative for CEA (unlike mucinous tumors)

SEROUS CYSTADENOMA/CYSTADENOCARCINOMA

- Benign (~70%): single layer of cells, no atypia, no invasion
- Borderline (10–15%): stratification and glandular complexity, often with cytologic atypia and mitotic figures but *no* definite destructive stromal invasion (i.e., no associated stromal edema and reactive fibroblastic response)
- Malignant (15–20%): high mitotic rate, atypical cells, stratification, glandular complexity, branching papillary fronds, *destructive stromal invasion*

Bilateral in 10% of benign, 25% borderline, 70% malignant

Borderline lesions tend to occur in a slightly younger age group than carcinoma, and tend to be lower stage at presentation

CYSTADENOFIBROMA

Prominent fibrous stromal component surrounding benign glands

Solid, white lesion grossly

Malignant counterpart (cystadenofibrocarcinoma) is rare

SEROUS SURFACE PAPILLARY CARCINOMA

Grows exophytically on surface of ovary with little involvement of underlying ovary

Most are bilateral; rapidly spread throughout abdomen

MUCINOUS TUMORS

15–25% of ovarian tumors

Bilateral in 10–20% (most commonly when malignant)

Most common surface epithelial tumor in children, perhaps because of its unclear recurrent relationship with teratoma

Tend to grow larger than serous type

Usually at least partially cystic, most commonly multiloculated; cysts contain mucinous material

Papillae, solid areas, necrosis, hemorrhage more common in malignant form

Tall, columnar, nonciliated cells with intracellular mucin overlying basal nuclei

Tumors can be endocervical type or intestinal type (latter with goblet cells, Paneth cells, etc.)

Stroma often cellular, may be luteinized; stromal invasion is often difficult to assess because of gland complexity

Types:
- Benign: most common (80%)
- Borderline (15%): increased layering, but ≤4 cells
- Malignant (5%): cell atypia, increased layering of cells (>4 cells thick), complex glands, stromal invasion

Tendency to implant on peritoneal structures; if extensive, *pseudomyxoma peritonei;* may be impossible to distinguish from appendiceal primary when both involved

CEA positivity seen in 15% of benign, 80% of borderline, and 100% of malignant mucinous tumors

Not uncommonly seen concurrently with Brenner tumor or with teratoma

ENDOMETRIOID TUMORS
5–10% of ovarian tumors
10–20% have coexistent endometriosis
Generally large cystic mass with solid areas, often hemorrhagic, usually *without* papillary structures
Resemble endometrial adenocarcinomas
Areas of squamous metaplasia are common
Borderline variant exists, but it is very rare
Prognosis generally twice as good as serous or mucinous carcinoma, but because most are stage I and well differentiated

CLEAR CELL (MESONEPHROID) CARCINOMA
Usually 40s–50s
Spongy, often cystic appearance
Tubular-cystic, papillary, and solid growth patterns
Cores of papillae often hyalinized
Large tumor cells with clear cytoplasm and hobnail appearance; cytoplasm may be oncocytic
Probably a variant of endometrioid carcinoma
5 yr survival 40–50%

BRENNER TUMOR
1–2% of all ovarian tumors
Average age at presentation is 50 yr; three quarters over 40 yr
Usually unilateral, firm, white, solid
Solid and cystic nests of cells resembling transitional epithelium with distinct cell borders, oval nuclei with small but distinct nucleolus and longitudinal grooves
Stroma is dense and fibroblastic
Not infrequently seen with mucinous cystadenoma
METAPLASTIC BRENNER TUMOR
Prominent cystic formations with mucinous changes
PROLIFERATING BRENNER TUMOR
Presence of papillary fronds and nuclear atypia
Resembles papillary low-grade transitional cell carcinoma (TCC)
MALIGNANT BRENNER TUMOR
Stromal invasion, cytologically malignant (resembles high-grade TCC)

MIXED MESODERMAL TUMOR
BENIGN
Papillary adenofibroma
MALIGNANT
Same as counterpart in uterus
Carcinomatous component may be serous, endometrioid, squamous, or clear cell
Extremely poor prognosis, esp. heterologous type
Most common heterologous element is chondrosarcoma

Germ Cell Tumors

20–30% of all ovarian tumors
Most are seen in children or young adults; the younger the patient, the more likely tumor will be malignant
95% are benign cystic teratomas
~10% of germ cell tumors are of mixed type (most common is dysgerminoma and yolk sac tumor)

DYSGERMINOMA
<1% of all ovarian tumors; 5% of malignant ovarian tumors
80% of patients are under 30 yr old, 40% under 20 yr
Bilateral in 15%; when unilateral, more common on right
Female counterpart of classical seminoma
Large, encapsulated, smooth, often convoluted surface
Gray solid cut surface; foci of hemorrhage and necrosis may be seen, but not as commonly as in other ovarian tumors
Well-defined nests of tumor cells separated by fibrous stroma infiltrated by lymphocytes
Tumor cells have clear cytoplasm, oval uniform large nuclei, one or more prominent nucleoli
10% will have other germ-cell components—worse prognosis
Metastases most commonly to other ovary, retroperitoneal nodes, peritoneal cavity
When encapsulated, 95% 5 yr survival; 33% with metastases
DYSGERMINOMA WITH MULTINUCLEATED GIANT CELLS (3%)
Scattered human chorionic gonadotropin (HCG) positive syncytiotrophoblast-like cells
No change in prognosis
ANAPLASTIC DYSGERMINOMA
Marked mitotic activity (often >30 per high power field [HPF]!)

YOLK SAC TUMOR
AKA: endodermal sinus tumor
Tumor of children and young adults (mean age 19)
Serum alpha-fetoprotein (AFP) invariably elevated; HCG levels normal
Smooth, glistening surface
Reticular and microcystic growth patterns are most common; may also see papillary and solid
Schiller-Duval bodies: glomeruloid structures with bulbous pseudopapillary processes containing central vessels
Intracytoplasmic PAS+ hyaline droplets
Subclinical metastases common
3 yr survival was only 13%; multidrug chemotherapy has markedly improved this
POLYVESICULAR VITELLINE PATTERN
Small cystic structures with eccentric constrictions separated by a dense spindle cell stroma
When pure, good prognosis
HEPATOID PATTERN
Resembles hepatocellular carcinoma (large, polygonal cells in cords or sheets)
GLANDULAR PATTERN
May resemble endometrioid carcinoma

EMBRYONAL CARCINOMA
Rare in the ovary; median age 15 yr
Serum HCG levels always high; AFP levels often elevated
Solid sheets and nests of large primitive cells, often with abortive glandular formations, frequently admixed with syncytiotrophoblast-like giant cells
Necrosis, hemorrhage common
Poor prognosis

POLYEMBRYOMA
Very rare
Preponderance of embryoid bodies in various stages of development

CHORIOCARCINOMA

Most are metastases from uterine tumors

When primary to ovary, usually part of mixed germ cell tumor

Biphasic cell population with cytotrophoblasts and syncytio-trophoblasts

When pure, usually lethal

IMMATURE (MALIGNANT) TERATOMA

Mixture of embryonal and adult tissues from all three germ layers; main component usually neural

- Grade I: mostly mature tissues (immature neural tissue comprises <1 HPF), loose mesenchymal stroma, immature cartilage, occasional mitoses
- Grade II: fewer mature tissues, foci of neuroepithelium not exceeding 3 low power fields (LPF) on any one slide
- Grade III: little to no mature tissue; numerous neuroepithelial elements occupying 4+ LPF

When yolk sac pattern also present, worse prognosis

MALIGNANT NEUROECTODERMAL TUMOR

Nearly exclusively composed of neuroectodermal elements

EPENDYMOMA

MATURE CYSTIC TERATOMA

20% of all ovarian tumors; bilateral in 12%

Most occur in women <30 yr old

>98% are benign (unlike counterpart in testis)

Usually multiloculated with large cysts containing sebum, hair, keratin, teeth

Microscopic foci of immature tissue are allowed

Rokitansky's protuberance: central area containing bone and well-formed teeth

MATURE SOLID TERATOMA

Rare; young women

Predominantly solid mass grossly (may have small cystic areas microscopically)

Some prefer to refer to this as Grade 0 immature teratoma

Entirely adult tissue; excellent prognosis

EPIDERMOID CYST

Absence of other elements

Probably arises from epithelial cell nest

STRUMA OVARII

Dominant growth of thyroid component of teratoma

Can be seen in combination with mucinous cystadenoma, Brenner tumor, or carcinoid tumor

CARCINOID TUMOR

May be component of teratoma, primary tumor without other teratomatous components (good prognosis), or metastasis from some other primary (bad prognosis)

Most primary carcinoids are unilateral, often symptomatic

STRUMAL CARCINOID

Combination of carcinoid and thyroid elements

MUCINOUS CARCINOID

Analogous to the appendiceal tumor with goblet cell–like cells growing in nests or glands

Differential diagnosis: Krukenberg tumor

MALIGNANT TRANSFORMATION

Usually to squamous cell carcinoma, then carcinoid, then adenocarcinoma

Sex Cord–Stromal Tumors

5% of all ovarian tumors

GRANULOSA CELL TUMOR

5% before puberty, 40% postmenopausal

<5% are bilateral

Three quarters produce estrogen in excessive amounts; one quarter are associated with endometrial hyperplasia

Usually encapsulated, solid, lobulated, gray

May contain cysts with straw-colored fluid

Variable microscopic appearance: microfollicular, macrofollicular, trabecular, insular, solid

Call-Exner bodies: small gland-like "follicles" filled with acidophilic material; not always present

May have a thecal cell component; may luteinize, but less commonly than juvenile variant

Reticulin fibers surround groups of cells

Coffee-bean nuclei with folds or grooves

Can have bizarre multinucleated cells; probably degenerative rather than sign of malignancy

Immunoreactive for vimentin; usually keratin negative

Most are low stage (FIGO I) at presentation

Prognosis related to tumor size and stage; most deaths occur after 5 yr, so 5 yr survival rates are not meaningful

JUVENILE GRANULOSA CELL TUMOR

Nearly 80% of patients are <20 yr old; most present with isosexual precocity

Larger tumor cells, extensive luteinization, paucity of nuclear grooves, nuclear atypia, often high mitotic rate; Call-Exner bodies are rare

Cysts are usually larger than in conventional variety

Better prognosis than typical granulosa cell tumor

THECOMA/FIBROMA

Most patients are >40 yr old

Usually unilateral, well-defined, firm, solid

Thecoma is yellowish, fibroma white

Both have spindle cells with central nuclei and a moderate amount of cytoplasm

Oil red O staining of fresh (frozen) tissue can show intracytoplasmic fat in thecomas

Reticulin fibers surround individual cells

Differential diagnosis: massive edema, fibromatosis

CELLULAR FIBROMAS

High cellularity, ≤3 mitoses/10 HPF (if more, fibrosarcoma)

May recur

SCLEROSING STROMAL TUMOR

Younger age group (15–30 yr)

Gray-white to yellow variegated cut surface

Multiple pseudolobules of cellular stroma with prominent ectatic vessels separated by anastomosing hypocellular regions, which vary from fibrous to edematous

Dual cell population: collagen-producing spindle cells, round or oval cells with clear cytoplasm (lipid)

SERTOLI-LEYDIG CELL TUMOR

AKA: arrhenoblastoma; androblastoma

Uncommon; <0.2% of ovarian neoplasms

Young patients (average age 25 yr)

Despite name, electron microscopy (EM) shows that the Sertoli-like cells are actually more granulosa cell–like

Testosterone and estradiol are found in both cell types

Relatively good prognosis

WELL DIFFERENTIATED (MEYER TYPE I) (11%)
Tubules lined by Sertoli-like cells separated by fibrous stroma with variable numbers of Leydig-like cells
100% survival

INTERMEDIATE (MEYER TYPE II) (54%)
Cords, sheets, or other aggregates of Sertoli-like cells growing in lobules separated by spindled stromal cells and intermixed Leydig-like cells
~90% survival

POORLY DIFFERENTIATED (MEYER TYPE III) (13%)
Masses of spindled cells arranged in a sarcomatoid pattern
~40% survival

WITH HETEROLOGOUS ELEMENTS (22%)
Mucinous epithelium, liver, skeletal muscle, cartilage

RETIFORM (15%)
Occurs in children (10–25 yr)
May have papillary appearance grossly
Sertoli-Leydig elements mixed with irregular cleftlike spaces lined by low cuboidal cells, occasionally with blunted papillae (looks like rete testis)
20% die of disease

PURE SERTOLI CELL TUMOR
Rare; almost always at least some Leydig cell component
Solid and hollow tubules lined by Sertoli-like cells, which usually lack atypia
Abundant lipid may be present in the cytoplasm

GYNANDROBLASTOMA
Sex cord–stromal tumor with a mixture of similar amounts of granulosa-thecal elements and Sertoli-Leydig elements

LIPID CELL TUMORS
Include: Leydig (hilus) cell tumor, luteoma, etc.
Usually unilateral, yellow or yellow-brown nodules separated by fibrous trabeculae
Aggregates of large rounded or polyhedral cells with features of steroid hormone–secreting cells
~40% of these tumors are negative for intracellular fat
Most patients have a virilizing syndrome
When Reinke's crystals are visualized, subclassify as Leydig cell; if located at the hilus of the ovary (most common location), designate as hilus cell tumor
Almost all behave in benign fashion, esp. when less than 8 cm in diameter

SEX CORD TUMOR WITH ANNULAR TUBULES
One third of cases associated with Peutz-Jeghers syndrome
Growth pattern of Sertoli cells but cells appear more like granulosa cells—may be a variant of either
Simple and complex annular tubules containing eosinophilic, often calcified, hyaline bodies

Other Tumors

GONADOBLASTOMA
AKA: dysgenetic gonadoma
Combination of germ cell elements and sex cord–stromal elements
Usually nests containing multiple, small, round, glandlike spaces filled with hyaline material; nests surrounded by fibrous bands
Occurs almost exclusively in sexually abnormal individuals, most commonly XY gonadal dysgenesis and XO-XY mosaicism
Never seen in normal ovaries
36% are bilateral
Hyalinization and marked calcification common

GERM CELL–SEX CORD–STROMAL TUMORS, UNCLASSIFIED
Wastebasket diagnosis for mixed tumors that don't neatly fit into any of the well-characterized types

ENDOMETRIOID STROMAL SARCOMA
Proliferation of malignant stromal cells
Resembles endometrial stroma
Most cases represent spread from the uterus

SMALL CELL CARCINOMA
May be confused with granulosa cell tumor
Large, solid tumor with areas of necrosis and hemorrhage
Diffuse proliferation of small cells with small nuclei and minimal cytoplasm; clusters of larger, more pleomorphic cells may be present; follicle-like structures may be seen
Immunohistochemistry is variable: sometimes keratin, vimentin, laminin, all, none
Unknown histogenesis

HYPERCALCEMIC TYPE
Usually unilateral
Generally young women (mean age 22)
Patient has hypercalcemia, which resolves after resection of the tumor

PULMONARY TYPE
~50% are bilateral
Generally older women (mean age 59)

HEPATOID ADENOCARCINOMA
Hepatoid histology may occur in the absence of yolk-sac differentiation (similar tumor also seen in the stomach)
Most patients are older
Usually at least focally positive for AFP
Very aggressive

KRUKENBERG TUMOR
Metastatic adenocarcinoma, nearly always bilateral
Diffusely infiltrating signet ring cells with marked stromal proliferation
Primary sites include stomach, and also breast and large bowel

FALLOPIAN TUBES

Normal
Three distinct cell types: secretory, ciliated, intercalated (peg) Immunohistochemical stains for amylase are positive

Lymphatic drainage joins that of ovary and uterus; ampulla also drains via broad ligament to superior gluteal nodes

INFLAMMATION
ACUTE SUPPURATIVE SALPINGITIS (PELVIC INFLAMMATORY DISEASE [PID])
Common, usually ascending
Neisseria gonorrhoeae (~45%), *Chlamydia* (~20%)
May result in fusion of tubal plicae, obliteration of ostium, and subsequent infertility
Pyosalpinx: lumen filled with acute inflammation
Tubo-ovarian abscess: inflammation involves both fallopian tube and ovary; more commonly polymicrobial (enteric)
GRANULOMATOUS SALPINGITIS
Tuberculosis: hematogenous, therefore usually bilateral
Actinomycosis, schistosomiasis, fungal
Foreign bodies, e.g., lubricant or other therapeutic agents

OTHER NON-NEOPLASTIC ABNORMALITIES
TUBAL PREGNANCY
Incidence increased markedly following PID
Trophoblastic invasion of wall of tube occurs—vessels usually rupture, causing hematosalpinx
Significant hemorrhage if tube ruptures into peritoneum
WALTHARD CELL NESTS
Small collections of flat to cuboidal cells on the tubal serosa
Probably focal mesothelial hyperplasia
PARATUBAL CYSTS
AKA: hydatids of Morgagni, paraovarian cysts
Small, round, attached by pedicle, thin wall, serous contents
ENDOMETRIOSIS
Focal replacement of tubal epithelium by uterine mucosa
ENDOSALPINGIOSIS
Presence of tubal epithelium outside of fallopian tube
Most common site is ovary, close to fimbria of tube
SALPINGITIS ISTHMICA NODOSA
Usually young women (~25 yr), usually bilateral
Well-delimited nodular enlargement of isthmic portion
Cystically dilated glandlike formations surrounded by hypertrophied muscle and occasionally endometrial-like stroma; glands do connect to tube lumen

May be inflammatory or related to adenomyosis
Approximately 50% of patients are infertile

Tumors

ADENOMATOID TUMOR
Usually small, solid, firm, white, unencapsulated
Dilated channels lined by a flattened to cuboidal epithelium, often with vacuolated cytoplasm, and separated by a stroma rich in smooth muscle and elastic fibers
Immunoreactive for keratin and EMA; negative for CEA, factor VIII
Alcian blue positive, hyaluronidase sensitive mucin
Benign
Probably represents a special form of mesothelioma

CARCINOMA
Rare, <1% of gynecologic tract malignancies
One tenth as common as extension from endometrial primary
By convention, extensive involvement of uterus and tube is a uterine primary; ovary and tube is an ovarian primary
Most patients are postmenopausal
Usually invasive papillary adenocarcinoma, often solid areas
Any of the endometrial variants may also be seen
Prognosis determined more by stage than by grade
5 yr survival: stage I, 77%; II, 40%; III, 20%
FIGO STAGING
I: Confined to one or both tubes
  Ia: One tube, no ascites
  Ib: Both tubes, no ascites
  Ic: Ascites with malignant cells
II: Pelvic extension
  IIa: Involves uterus or ovary
  IIb: Involves other pelvic structures
III: Widespread intraperitoneal metastases
IV: Extraperitoneal extension

OTHERS
PAPILLARY CYSTADENOMA
TERATOMA
LEIOMYOMA
MALIGNANT MIXED MÜLLERIAN TUMOR
CHORIOCARCINOMA

20

UTERUS AND VULVA

UTERINE CORPUS

General
Uterus weighs 50 g, 8 cm long during reproductive life
Postmenopausally, atrophies to 5–6 cm
Zona basalis (deepest layer) is unresponsive to hormones
Zona functionalis (responsive layer) is subdivided into the superficial zona compacta and the deeper zona spongiosis

Embryology
During 6th wk, an invagination of the coelomic lining epithelium forms the paramesonephric (müllerian) ducts
Müllerian ducts form high on dorsal wall (8th–9th wk) and grow caudally, fusing caudally and extending to the urogenital sinus
Unfused portions form the fallopian tubes, fused portion forms the uterus and upper one third of vagina

ENDOMETRIAL DATING
Generally give a 2 day range
In normal cycle, the secretory phase is always 14 days
The proliferative phase is usually ~14 days, but may vary from individual to individual and from cycle to cycle (up to 2 days); therefore, secretory endometrium dated either based on a 14 day proliferative phase, or simply as *postovulatory day* (POD; e.g., POD 1 = day 15; POD 14 = day 28)

PROLIFERATIVE PHASE
Columnar cells, pseudostratified, with cigar-shaped nuclei with coarse (clumpy) chromatin, mitoses
Increasing tortuosity of glands as progress
- Early (4–7): short, narrow, straight glands, compact stroma
- Mid (8–10): peak stromal edema, numerous mitoses, curving, coiled glands
- Late (11–14): Tortuous glands with pseudostratification, moderately dense stroma

INTERVAL (DAY 15)
Subnuclear secretory vacuoles present, but in <50% of cells

SECRETORY ENDOMETRIUM
Single layer of cuboidal cells with round nuclei and fine chromatin; tortuous glands, secretions in glands
Day 16: Subnuclear vacuoles, pseudostratification
Day 17: Orderly row of nuclei, subnuclear vacuoles
Day 18: Vacuoles above and below nuclei, smaller
Day 19: Decreased number of vacuoles, orderly nuclei
Day 20: Peak secretion; ragged luminal border
Day 21: Early stromal edema; still significant secretion
Day 22: Peak stromal edema; "naked" stromal nuclei

Day 23: Spiral arterioles become prominent
Day 24: Periarteriolar cuffing of predecidua
Day 25: Predecidua beneath surface, inspissated secretions
Day 26: Coalescence of decidual islands, few neutrophils
Day 27: Many neutrophils, focal necrosis and hemorrhage
Day 28: Prominent necrosis and hemorrhage
Menstrual: stromal clumping, glandular breakup

OTHER ENDOMETRIAL PATTERNS
Arias-Stella reaction: hypersecretory glands with marked enlargement of nuclei with hyperchromasia; changes usually focal; cytoplasm cleared or eosinophilic
Estrogen therapy: proliferative endometrium, often to point of endometrial hyperplasia if unaccompanied by progestin
Progestational agents: decidualized stroma; initially glands are secretory, then with time become weakly proliferative

ABNORMAL BLEEDING
DEFINITIONS
Dysfunctional (anovulatory) uterine bleeding: excessive bleeding without demonstrable cause (e.g., estrogen breakthrough bleeding, estrogen withdrawal bleeding)
Menorrhagia: prolonged (>7 days) or excessive (>80 ml) bleeding at normal time in cycle
Metrorrhagia: bleeding at irregular intervals
Menometrorrhagia: prolonged or excessive bleeding outside of normal cycle
Luteal phase defect: histologic date >2 days behind clinical date
Dys-synchrony: >4 day variation between glands and stroma

CAUSES
Anovulation
Endometritis
Intrauterine device (IUD)
Leiomyoma
Carcinoma
Pregnancy related
Endometrial polyp or hyperplasia
Exogenous hormones
Thyroid dysfunction

ENDOMETRITIS
ACUTE ENDOMETRITIS
Usually seen following abortion, delivery, or instrumentation
Neutrophils predominate

CHRONIC ENDOMETRITIS
Lymphocytes and plasma cells (only need one plasma cell) in a stroma, which tends to be spindled and edematous
Usually vaginal bleeding and pelvic pain
May be accompanied by mucopurulent cervicitis or pelvic inflammatory disease

Do not attempt to date endometrium in endometritis (usually can't, which is a clue to the diagnosis)

IUD: induces chronic endometritis, sometimes with necrosis and squamous metaplasia; actinomycosis, *Entamoeba histolytica* infections common

ENDOMETRIAL METAPLASIA
SQUAMOUS METAPLASIA
- Adenoacanthosis: diffuse metaplasia
- Morules: berry-like aggregates of squamous cells without keratinization
- Ichthyosis uteri: rare; keratinization

Seen most commonly in women on exogenous estrogens

Often continuous with surface glands

CILIATED CELL (TUBAL) METAPLASIA
Scattered ciliated cells normally present in endometrium

When increased in number, resembles fallopian tubes (may have peg cells)

SYNCYTIAL PAPILLARY METAPLASIA
Papillary growth of an eosinophilic syncytium replacing the surface epithelium, associated with prolonged estrogen stimulation; nuclei are pyknotic; neutrophils common

MUCINOUS METAPLASIA
May be endocervical or intestinal type

EOSINOPHILIC (OXYPHILIC) METAPLASIA
HOBNAIL AND CLEAR CELL (MESONEPHROID) METAPLASIA
Common in gestational endometrium or in repair

STROMAL METAPLASIA
Rare; metaplasia is in the stroma rather than the epithelium

Islands of foam cells, smooth muscle, cartilage, bone

ADENOMYOSIS AND ENDOMETRIOSIS
Presence of islands of endometrial glands and stroma within the myometrium (adenomyosis) or outside of the uterus (endometriosis—can occur essentially anywhere)

Can both be present or occur independently

To make diagnosis, need two of glands, stroma, hemosiderin

Adenomyosis generally produces myometrial hypertrophy

When adenomyosis involves a leiomyoma, frequently referred to as an *adenomyoma*

Adenomyosis is generally nonfunctional basal type endometrium, whereas endometriosis is frequently functional and cycles similar to orthotopic endometrium

Pathogenesis still unknown; proposals include regurgitation, metaplasia, and lymphatic dissemination

ABNORMAL ENDOMETRIUM
ATROPHIC
Nonstratified, flattened to cuboidal cells, aligned pyknotic nuclei

Glands often cystically dilated

Stroma spindled

WEAKLY PROLIFERATIVE
Nonstratified to mildly pseudostratified columnar, thin, and elongate nuclei with coarse to dense chromatin

Low gland to stroma ratio

DISORDERED PROLIFERATIVE
Relatively common in perimenopausal women

Normal proliferative endometrium lining glands, which are cystically dilated or budding or show irregular branching

Endometrium may be stratified, but there should be no atypia

Gland to stromal ratio is normal (1 : 1) but there is nonuniformity from field to field

Stromal cells spindled with plump nuclei

ENDOMETRIAL HYPERPLASIA
Absolute increase in endometrial volume for the patient's age

Background endometrium is *proliferative*

Classified as simple (cystic) or complex (adenomatous) and with or without atypia

Adenomatous indicates branching or budding glands or tightly packed glands with loss of intervening stroma; occurs at older age than simple

Cytologic atypia: nuclear clearing (prominent euchromatin), irregular nuclear size and shape, prominent nucleoli, atypical mitoses

Architectural atypia: increased epithelial thickness, loss of radial orientation, glandular bridging

Risk of progression to carcinoma higher for complex and higher when cytologic atypia present:

Simple without atypia	5%
Complex without atypia	25%
Atypical	>50%

ENDOMETRIAL POLYPS
HYPERPLASTIC POLYP
Localized irregular hyperplasia of endometrium

Endometrium and stroma unresponsive to progesterone

Stroma composed of spindle, fibroblast-like cells with abundant extracellular connective tissue

Large blood vessels with thick walls

ATROPHIC POLYP
Involuted hyperplastic polyp; cystically dilated glands

SECRETORY (FUNCTIONAL) POLYP
Cycles with the surrounding endometrium

ADENOMYOMATOUS POLYP
Hyperplastic polyp with smooth muscle fibers separating the glands

No atypia

MIXED ENDOMETRIAL-ENDOCERVICAL POLYP
ATYPICAL POLYPOID ADENOMYOMA
Sessile or pedunculated lesion

Irregular atypical glands with enlarged nuclei, thick nuclear membranes, and prominent nucleoli, in a cellular stroma with smooth muscle bundles (≤2–3 stromal mitoses/10 HPF)

Commonly see squamous metaplasia

Tumors of the Endometrium

ENDOMETRIAL CARCINOMA
Most common invasive gynecologic malignancy in the U.S.

80% occur in postmenopausal women

Major risk factors: excessive estrogen stimulation, obesity, diabetes, hypertension, infertility

Non-neoplastic endometrium often hyperplastic

80% are adenocarcinomas

Positive for keratin, vimentin, IgA, ±CEA

Extension into cervix occurs in 10%

Invasion of myometrium corresponds to grade

Lymph node metastases to pelvic and periaortic lymph nodes (LNs)

HISTOLOGICAL GRADING

Grade I   Highly differentiated adenocarcinoma (≤5% solid)

Grade II   Moderately differentiated with 6–50% solid areas

Grade III >50% solid or entirely undifferentiated

Note: significant nuclear atypia raises grade by I

50%, 35%, and 15% of adenocarcinomas are grade I, II, and III, respectively

NUCLEAR GRADING

Using the four criteria:

- Prominent nucleoli
- Irregular nuclear contour
- Clumped chromatin
- Nuclear size 3–4× normal

Grade I   Fewer than two

Grade II   Any two

Grade III Three or four

STAGING (FIGO; EQUIVALENT TO AJCC):

I: Confined to corpus

    Ia: Limited to endometrium

    Ib: Invasion ≤50% thickness

    Ic: Invasion >50% thickness

II: Corpus and cervix but not outside uterus

    IIa: Endocervical gland involvement only

    IIb: Cervical stromal invasion

III: Outside uterus, but not outside true pelvis

    IIIa: Serosa or positive cytology

    IIIb: Vaginal metastases

    IIIc: Pelvic or periaortic LN involvement

IV: Outside true pelvis or to bladder or rectum

    IVa: Adjacent organs (bladder or bowel)

    IVb: Distant organs

Morphologic Variants

VILLOGLANDULAR

Well-differentiated villiform variant of endometrioid carcinoma

Don't confuse with papillary serous

SECRETORY

Rare; *not* a variant of clear cell carcinoma

Neoplastic glands with subnuclear vacuolization and secretory pattern in adjacent, uninvolved endometrium

Lack of polarization distinguishes this lesion from hyperplasia with secretory changes

Very low grade; good prognosis

CILIATED CELL

Very rare

Solid areas and nucleoli distinguish from ciliated metaplasia

Very low grade; good prognosis

ADENOACANTHOMA

Squamous metaplasia (benign) in an endometrioid adenocarcinoma

Do *not* include squamous areas in determining FIGO grade

Slightly better prognosis than endometrioid, not otherwise specied (NOS)

ADENOSQUAMOUS

Both endometrioid and squamous components are malignant

Probably somewhat worse prognosis than endometrioid, NOS

GLASSY CELL CARCINOMA

Variant of adenosquamous carcinoma

Pink cytoplasm, complicated nuclei with nucleoli

Aggressive; poor prognosis

SEROUS ADENOCARCINOMA

AKA: papillary serous, uterine papillary serous carcinoma (UPSC)

Does not always have papillae, so renamed simply "serous"

Generally small, short papillae lined by highly atypical cells with hobnailing; necrosis; psammoma bodies in 30%

Lymphatic and myometrial invasion common

Don't grade—prognosis is uniformly dismal

Spread mimics ovarian carcinoma: omentum, peritoneum, colon, ascites

If isolated focus in a polyp without vascular invasion, still equally bad

Probably a multifocal disease

Not very responsive to either chemotherapy or radiation

CLEAR CELL

1–5% of all endometrial carcinomas; usually older patients

No association with diethylstilbestrol exposure

Small papillae lined by hobnailed cells with clear cytoplasm

Stroma usually hyalinized

Tubular, tubulocystic, or solid patterns focally; often all three

Hyaline globules are characteristically seen

Very poor prognosis; however, if stage I, survival slightly better than serous carcinoma; stage II or higher very bad

Closely related to serous carcinoma; the two often occur together

MUCINOUS

Usually need >25% of cells to have intracellular mucin to make this diagnosis

No significant difference in prognosis relative to endometrioid

SQUAMOUS CELL CARCINOMA

Pure epidermoid carcinoma is rare

MIXED

UNDIFFERENTIATED

Small cell (oat cell); poor prognosis

ENDOMETRIAL STROMAL TUMORS

Occur in middle-aged women (~45 yr)

Present with vaginal bleeding, pelvic pain

Soft, yellow to orange, foci of hyalinization

When <4 cm, usually don't recur; when larger or extend outside uterus, may be lethal; can metastasize

STROMAL NODULES (<25%)

Well-circumscribed, pushing margins, no invasion

Often protrude into endometrial cavity

Benign; do not recur, do not metastasize

LOW-GRADE STROMAL SARCOMAS

AKA: endolymphatic stromal myosis

Cut surface shows wormlike protrusions of tumor

Histologically similar to stromal nodule, but infiltrates myometrium, invades and permeates lymphatic vessels, broad ligament

<10 mitoses/10 HPF

50% of patients present with stage I disease

20% recur, but may not be for many years

HIGH-GRADE STROMAL SARCOMA

Patients generally over 50 yr old

Soft mass fills uterine cavity and invades myometrium

Similar to low grade but usually has larger pleomorphic cells and must have >10 mitoses/10 HPF

Poor prognosis: frequently recur; often multiple metastases

Other Variants
STROMOMYOMA
AKA: combined smooth muscle–stromal tumor
Rare; reproductive age women
More than one third of the tumor is smooth muscle
Benign
UTERINE TUMORS RESEMBLING OVARIAN SEX-CORD TUMORS
Nests, cords, tubules or islands of epithelioid cells
Benign vs. low grade vs. high grade determined by pushing vs. infiltrative margins and < or > 10 mitoses/10 HPF
EXTRAUTERINE ENDOMETRIAL STROMAL SARCOMA
Presumably arises in endometriosis
Same histology as uterine counterpart

Mixed Mesodermal Tumors

UTERINE ADENOFIBROMA
AKA: papillary adenofibroma, adenomyomatosis
Occurs in postmenopausal women
Benign counterpart of Müllerian adenosarcoma (both epithelium and stroma are benign)
Lobulated or papillary; superficial; does not invade myometrium
Fewer than 4 mitoses/10 HPF

MÜLLERIAN ADENOSARCOMA
Elderly individuals (median age 58)
Low-grade variant of malignant mixed müllerian tumor (MMMT)
Bulky, polypoid lesion filling endometrial cavity
Benign-appearing epithelium (similar to phylloides tumor of breast), often appearing as large irregular glands with more worrisome stroma
Very cellular stroma that condenses around glands; ≥4 mitoses/10 HPF

MALIGNANT MIXED MÜLLERIAN (MESODERMAL) TUMOR
Rare; practically always in postmenopausal (median age 68)
~10% of cases have history of prior radiation exposure
Present as large polypoid growth, usually arising from the posterior uterine fundus
Foci of necrosis and hemorrhage
Both carcinomatous and sarcomatous elements
Restriction to inner half of myometrium only hope of cure
On rare occasions, may arise in extrauterine site (ovary, tube, peritoneum)
Overall 5 yr survival ~20–30%
HOMOLOGOUS VARIETY
Malignant stroma formed by round cells resembling endometrial stroma or spindle cells resembling leiomyosarcoma or fibrosarcoma
HETEROLOGOUS VARIETY
Often more bulky than homologous
Malignant stroma forms skeletal muscle (most common), cartilage, bone, fat

Rarely see skin appendages, glia, or thyroid (unlike teratoma)
Slightly worse prognosis

Tumors of the Myometrium

LEIOMYOMA
Present in 20% of women 30–50 yr old and in 40% of women over 50 yr
Much more common in blacks (usually multiple)
When multiple, more likely to all be benign
Benignancy or malignancy determined by mitotic rate and cellularity (see table on next page); note: for proper mitotic count, must section and fix rapidly or cells undergoing mitosis will complete telophase and falsely depress the count
Tumor is sensitive to compromise of vascular supply: secondary changes present in 65%: hyaline degeneration (63%), myxomatous degeneration (19%), calcification (8%)
Can be infiltrated by lymphocytes: inflammatory pseudotumor
CELLULAR LEIOMYOMA
More cellular than surrounding myometrium, no atypical features, <5 mitoses/10 HPF
In pregnancy or women on oral contraceptives, may undergo central hemorrhage ("hemorrhagic cellular leiomyoma"); most are subserosal; one third rupture into peritoneum
ATYPICAL LEIOMYOMA
AKA: bizarre, symplastic, pleomorphic
Variation in cell size and shape, hyperchromatic nuclei, multinucleated cells, but normal number of mitoses
LEIOMYOLIPOMA
Mature adipose tissue intermixed with smooth muscle
LEIOMYOBLASTOMA
AKA: epithelioid, clear cell, or plexiform leiomyoma
Tend to be solitary
Rounded, polygonal cells (rather than spindled), often with clear cytoplasm (glycogen), growing in nests or compartments separated by hyalinized stroma
Usually blends into more mature smooth muscle at periphery
INTRAVENOUS LEIOMYOMATOSIS
Rare; wide age range
Coiled, lobulated, well-defined myometrial mass with "wormlike" growths into the uterine veins in the broad ligament; may extend up the inferior vena cava to the right atrium
Histology is that of a normal leiomyoma
DIFFUSE LEIOMYOMATOSIS
Involvement of nearly the entire myometrium by innumerable <1 cm poorly defined leiomyomata
Associated with pregnancy or oral contraceptives
Involute when hormone source removed
BENIGN METASTASIZING LEIOMYOMA
Patients usually 20–40 yr old, usually black women, usually following a hysterectomy or myomectomy
Multiple smooth muscle tumors in lung, peritoneum, LNs
Diagnosis of exclusion
May actually be a very low-grade leiomyosarcoma

Mitoses/10 HPF

	<2	2–5	6–10	11–15	>15
Atypical or epithelioid	B	U	M	M	M
Cellular	B	B	U	M	M
Normal (typical)	B	B	Leiomyoma with ↑ # mitoses		U

B = benign (leiomyoma); U = uncertain malignant potential;
M = malignant (leiomyosarcoma)

LEIOMYOSARCOMA
Median age: 54 yr
Rare; only 1/800 leiomyomata
In general do not arise from pre-existing leiomyomata
Diagnosis based on mitotic activity and cellularity (see chart)
Hypercellular; 67% are solitary, 25% have infiltrating margins, 10% show vascular invasion
5 yr survival 40–50% if limited to uterus; 20% overall
MYXOID LEIOMYOSARCOMA
Gelatinous appearance; appears well defined grossly
Invasive with spindled muscle cells in a myxoid matrix
Behave malignantly, regardless of mitotic count
MALIGNANT LEIOMYOBLASTOMA
AKA: clear cell (epithelioid) leiomyosarcoma
Rare; frequently infiltrating margin, necrosis
Mitotic rate still key distinguishing feature

ADENOMATOID TUMOR
AKA: adenomatoid mesothelioma
Median age 42; *benign*
Usually solitary, subserosal proliferation of mesothelial-lined capillary-like spaces intermixed with smooth muscle
Similar lesions may occur in fallopian tubes, ovary, omentum

Gestational Trophoblastic Disease

IMPLANTATION SITE CHANGES
Gold standard is chorionic villi
In absence of this, immunohistochemically confirmed intermediate trophoblasts surrounding hyalinized vessels are presumptive evidence of intrauterine gestation
ARIAS-STELLA REACTION
Seen with both intrauterine and ectopic pregnancies
Cellular stratification, enlarged cells, bizarre large hyperchromatic nuclei
IMMUNOHISTOCHEMISTRY

	Keratin	HPL	HCG
Cytotrophoblasts	++	−	−
Intermediate trophoblasts	++	++	+
Syncytiotrophoblasts	++	+	++

HPL = human placental lactogen; HCG = human chorionic gonadotropin.

PLACENTA ACCRETA
Placental villi adhere to underlying myometrium
Placenta increta: villi invade into myometrium
Placenta percreta: villi invade through myometrium

EXAGGERATED PLACENTAL SITE
AKA: syncytial endometritis
Extensive *syncytiotrophoblastic* invasion of endometrium and mesentery
Rare if any mitoses

PLACENTAL SITE NODULE
AKA: placental site plaque
Nodules of *intermediate trophoblasts* in a hyalinized stroma

PARTIAL HYDATIDIFORM MOLE
25–40% of all moles
Fetus often present, almost always anomalous
Vesicular changes in some of the villi with edema, irregular scalloped contours, trophoblast inclusions, trophoblast hyperplasia
Similar histology can also be seen in trisomies of chromosomes 13 or 18
Most are triploid (58% XXY, 40% XXX, 2% XYY); some are tetraploid; result from fertilization of normal egg with two sperm; 2 : 1 paternal : maternal chromosomes
4–10% have persistent trophoblastic disease, usually intrauterine; much less likely to invade than complete mole

COMPLETE HYDATIDIFORM MOLE
Vesicular hydropic swelling of all of the villi, trophoblast hyperplasia, usually with absence of any identifiable embryo; "bunch of grapes"
Large, bizarre mass fills and distends uterus
Total weight often >200 g
Significant degree of trophoblast hyperplasia
>90% are diploid; 85–90% are XX, 10–15% are XY
All of the chromosomes are paternal; results from fertilization of an egg that has lost its chromosomes by either one or two sperm (if one, duplicates itself)
Patients who have had a mole have increased risk for a 2nd
Villi usually lack identifiable vessels
Note: similar histology with trophoblast hyperplasia and small sheets of trophoblasts is normal at 5 wk gestation; key is numerous nucleated RBCs (hence fetus, hence not complete mole)
10–30% will have persistent trophoblastic disease: persistent complete mole (10–15%), invasive mole (10–20%), or choriocarcinoma (2–3%)

INVASIVE MOLE
AKA: chorioadenoma destruens
Mole, usually complete mole, in which the *villi* penetrate the myometrium or the vessels of the myometrium
Occurs in 16% of all moles
Serosa usually intact
Vascular invasion may lead to embolization of villi
Treatment: chemotherapy

PLACENTAL SITE TROPHOBLASTIC TUMOR
AKA: atypical choriocarcinoma; trophoblastic pseudotumor
75% follow a normal pregnancy
Grossly: well-localized, but ill-defined myometrial mass
Histology: consists of intermediate trophoblasts; some syncytiotrophoblasts may be present as well
Locally invasive but usually self-limited
10% metastasize widely and are fatal

CHORIOCARCINOMA
Highly malignant neoplasm
Dual cell population: cytotrophoblasts and syncytiotrophoblasts; do not see intermediate trophoblasts and *never* see villi
Most commonly occurs following a complete mole (50%); 25% occur following an abortion; 22% follow normal pregnancy
Hemorrhagic tumor masses that are nodular and well defined; vascular invasion common
Metastasize early: lung (50%), vagina (35%), bone, brain, liver, kidney, bowel
Immunoreactive for HCG and keratin
Exquisitely sensitive to chemotherapy: has improved survival from <20% to nearly 100%

OTHER TUMORS
CHORANGIOMA
Hemangiomas of placenta
Common: found in 1/100 placentas
Usually well circumscribed; degenerative changes common
Larger lesions (>5 cm) can be associated with hydramnios, hemorrhage, premature delivery, premature placental separation
CHORANGIOSIS
Diffuse increase in vascularity (increased number of vascular channels per villus)
May be associated with neonatal morbidity

CERVIX

REACTIVE CHANGES
SQUAMOUS METAPLASIA
Begins basally
Cells acquire nucleoli and polygonal appearance on cytology
May involve glands, giving appearance of invasion
In essence, causes retreat of transitional zone into cervix
NABOTHIAN CYSTS
Blockage of endocervical glands
Usually secondary to inflammation
ENDOCERVICAL POLYPS
Probably chronic inflammatory or hamartomatous in nature
Edematous, inflamed, fibrotic stroma with dilated glands
May have multinucleated giant cells in stroma
HERPES SIMPLEX INFECTION
Intense, nonspecific inflammation with ulceration
Only rarely are diagnostic multinucleated cells with inclusions seen in biopsy
HUMAN PAPILLOMA VIRUS
Condyloma acuminatum, flat condyloma, papilloma
Most commonly HPV-6 and HPV-11, also HPV-16
Simple koilocytic changes (binucleate cell with surrounding halo and denser peripheral cytoplasm) without disruption or expansion of the basal cell layer (latter indicates dysplasia)
CHLAMYDIA TRACHOMATIS
Most common venereal disease
Chronic nonspecific inflammation, reactive epithelial atypia, occasionally prominent lymphoid follicles

CERVICAL ECTROPION
Presence of glandular epithelium in ectocervix
Strong correlation with in utero exposure to diethylstilbestrol (DES)
MICROGLANDULAR HYPERPLASIA
Seen with oral contraceptive use, sometimes pregnancy; usually younger women
Complex proliferation of tightly packed small glands with flat epithelial cells and little if any atypia, often with squamous metaplasia
CEA negative (unlike endocervical adenocarcinoma)
Atypical variant exists with predominantly solid sheet–like growth pattern
DIFFUSE LAMINAR ENDOCERVICAL HYPERPLASIA
Proliferation of endocervical glands, typically with inflammatory infiltrate
Very well-demarcated lower extent
Benign
DECIDUAL REACTION
Often multiple, yellow or red elevations, friable
ENDOMETRIOSIS
MESONEPHRIC (GARTNER'S DUCT) RESTS
Usually lateral wall, deep to the endocervical glands
Single cell layer, usually cuboidal
Clear cells, but no hobnailing

CERVICAL DYSPLASIA
Enlargement of cells, increased nuclear:cytoplasmic ratio, irregular nuclear borders, chromatin clumping, and *loss of basal polarity*
Most often occurs at the transition zone between the columnar endocervical mucosa and the squamous ectocervical mucosa
Graded as mild, moderate, severe based on degree of atypia
Cervical intraepithelial neoplasia (CIN) graded as I, II, or III based on the degree of dysplasia and the thickness of involvement (<1/3; 1/3–2/3; >2/3)
When full-thickness changes without any differentiation at any level, carcinoma in situ
Of mild to moderate lesions, 62% will regress, 22% will persist, and 16% will progress
Of severe dysplasia, invasive carcinoma will develop in 11% within 3 yr, 22% in 5 yr, and 33% in 9 yr
HPV types 6 and 11 correlate with low-grade lesions; types 16, 18, 31, 33, and 35 with high risk for progression to carcinoma

CERVICAL EPIDERMOID CARCINOMA
Most common malignancy of gynecologic tract
Second most common cause of cancer death in U.S. women
Usually older age groups, but increasing frequency <40 yr
Single most important risk factor is age at first intercourse
Almost certainly human papilloma virus (HPV) related
May be bulky (exophytic) or infiltrative (or both)
Major subtypes include: large cell nonkeratinizing (65%), keratinizing (25%), small cell (probably worst prognosis), basaloid, verrucous
Microinvasion suggested by the presence of desmoplastic stromal reaction with metachromatic staining
Keratin and CEA immunoreactive
Microinvasive carcinoma carries a 1% risk of LN metastases
Endometrial extension decreases prognosis 10–20%

LN metastases: first paracervical, hypogastric, obturator, external iliac; then sacral, common iliac, aortic, inguinal

Distant metastases to lungs (9%) and bones (4%)

FIGO STAGING (SAME AS AJCC)

0: Carcinoma in situ (CIS)

I: Confined to cervix and/or uterus

    Ia1: Minimal microscopic microinvasion

    Ia2: Invasion <5 mm (some use 3 mm) over area of <7 mm

    Ib: Invasion >5 mm (some use 3 mm) into cervical stroma

II: Beyond cervix, but not pelvic wall or lower third of vagina

    IIa: No parametrial involvement

    IIb: Obvious parametrial involvement

III: To pelvic wall, lower third of vagina, rectum, hydronephrosis

    IIIa: No extension to pelvic wall

    IIIb: Pelvic wall and/or hydronephrosis

IV: Beyond true pelvis or mucosa of bladder or rectum

    IVa: Adjacent organs

    IVb: Distant organs

Note: Regional LN involvement (N1) makes lesion at least stage IIIB, regardless of size or local extent of primary

PROGNOSIS

5 yr survival: stage I, 80–90%; II, 75%; III, 35%; IV, 10–15%

ADENOCARCINOMA

5–15% of all carcinomas of the cervix

Association with long-term use of oral contraceptives; also with HPV 16 and 18

Alcian blue, mucicarmine, and CEA reactive material found intracellularly in almost all cells, unlike endometrial adenocarcinoma, in which reaction is only focal and superficial

Most are well differentiated and mucin producing

Dysplasia, atypical hyperplasia, CIS, malignant cells in more than one gland, and microinvasion (budding and branching with stromal reaction and inflammation) can all be seen

In general, overall prognosis is worse than for epidermoid carcinoma

Variants

~50% of endocervical adenocarcinomas show typical mucinous endocervical glandular appearance

Another ~25% appear endometrial or intestinal

Remaining ~25% are divided among the following

MINIMAL DEVIATION ADENOCARCINOMA (ADENOMA MALIGNUM)

1% of adenocarcinomas; very well differentiated

Architectural features of malignancy, but cytologically "benign"

Can only be diagnosed by location deep in cervix

VILLOGLANDULAR CARCINOMA

Papillary carcinoma occurring in young women (~30 yr old)

Surface papillary growth pattern

Good prognosis

ADENOSQUAMOUS (MIXED) CARCINOMA (~15%)

Particularly common during pregnancy (~20% of cases)

Squamous component often well differentiated

Worse prognosis than pure squamous cell carcinoma

GLASSY CELL CARCINOMA (<5%)

Many consider this a variant of adenosquamous carcinoma

Younger age group (mean 41 yr); often during pregnancy

Ground glass or granular cytoplasm, prominent eosinophilic and PAS+ cell rim, large nuclei, prominent nucleoli

Solid nests of cells, numerous mitoses, prominent inflammatory infiltrate, often rich in eosinophils

Poor prognosis

BASALOID

Older women; very good prognosis

ADENOID CYSTIC CARCINOMA

Generally elderly multigravid black women

Similar in appearance to salivary gland counterpart

Very poor prognosis

CLEAR CELL CARCINOMA

Müllerian derivation

Most common cervical carcinoma in young women; 50% of cases are related to in utero DES exposure

Usually exophytic growth pattern

Large cells, abundant clear cytoplasm, hobnailing

85% are stage I or II at presentation

Relatively good prognosis

MESONEPHRIC CARCINOMA

Rare

Clear cells, but no hobnailing

Occur deep in cervix, almost always lateral walls

NEUROENDOCRINE CARCINOMA

Spectrum from carcinoid-like to small cell carcinoma

Frequently immunoreactive for NSE, chromogranin

Even carcinoid-like tumors are more aggressive here than similar tumors elsewhere; small cell very aggressive

VAGINA

CONGENITAL AND ACQUIRED MALFORMATIONS

TUBAL FIMBRIA

May become entrapped in vaginal scar tissue following vaginal hysterectomy

ENDOMETRIOSIS

VAGINAL ADENOSIS

Any Müllerian-type glandular epithelium in the vagina, usually occurring in the upper third of the vagina

Usually become clinically detectable only after puberty

May be subdivided into *mucinous* (endocervical), *tubo-ovarian,* and mixed types

Accompanying chronic inflammation and squamous metaplasia are common, occasionally replacing most of the adenosis

Oral contraceptives can induce microglandular hyperplasia within these lesions

Seen in nearly 100% of patients exposed to DES in utero prior to the 8th wk of gestation

CYSTS

Epithelial inclusion cysts

Müllerian cyst: simple lining of endocervical type cells

Gartner's duct (mesonephric) cysts: cuboidal, no mucin

VAGINAL (FIBROEPITHELIAL) POLYPS

May have atypical cells in stroma

Do not call botryoid rhabdomyosarcoma without well-formed cambium layer or invasion

MICROGLANDULAR HYPERPLASIA
(See Cervix, earlier)

BENIGN NEOPLASMS
Papillomas
Tubulovillous adenoma
Leiomyoma
Rhabdomyoma (always in adults)

MALIGNANT NEOPLASMS
VAGINAL INTRAEPITHELIAL NEOPLASM (VAIN I–III)
EPIDERMOID CARCINOMA
Most carcinomas represent extension of cervical carcinoma
95% primary carcinomas are conventional squamous cell
Can also see verrucous, small cell variants
Staging (FIGO and AJCC)
  T1   Confined to vagina
  T2   Invades paravaginal tissues
  T3   Extends to pelvic wall
  T4   Invades mucosa of bladder/rectum or beyond pelvis
  N1   Pelvic LN metastases for upper two thirds of vagina
       Unilateral inguinal LNs for lower one third of vagina
  N2   Bilateral inguinal LNs

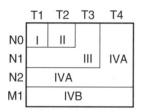

	T1	T2	T3	T4
N0	I	II		
N1			III	IVA
N2	IVA			
M1	IVB			

CLEAR CELL (MESONEPHROID) CARCINOMA
Seen in children or young adults; average age 17 yr
Anterior or lateral wall of upper vagina
Two thirds of patients have history of in utero exposure to DES
Tubules and cysts lined by clear cells alternating with more solid and papillary areas
Hobnail-shaped cells protrude into glandular lumen
Usually are *not* mucin positive
Few mitoses, clear cytoplasm due to glycogen
BOTRYOID RHABDOMYOSARCOMA
AKA: sarcoma botryoides
Special type of embryonal rhabdomyosarcoma
90% in girls <5 yr; 66% <2 yr
Polypoid invasive tumor, usually anterior vaginal wall
Grossly appears as "bunch of grapes"
Proliferation of myxomatous stroma with undifferentiated round or spindle cells, some with bright-red cytoplasm
Tumor cells crowd around vessels and beneath the squamous epithelium ("cambium layer" of Nicholson)
Foci of neoplastic cartilage may be present (older patients)
Extensive local spread; most do not metastasize
MALIGNANT MELANOMA
ENDODERMAL SINUS TUMOR
LEIOMYOSARCOMA
MALIGNANT FIBROUS HISTIOCYTOMA
EPITHELIOID SARCOMA

VULVA

CYSTIC LESIONS
EPIDERMOID CYST
PILONIDAL CYST
Most commonly clitoral area
SKENE'S DUCT CYST
AKA: paraurethral cyst
HYMENAL CYST
Newborns
MUCINOUS CYST OF THE VESTIBULE
ENDOMETRIOSIS
BARTHOLIN'S GLAND CYST/ABSCESS
Results from obstruction and/or chronic bacterial infection, esp. gonorrhea
Lining (transitional or squamous) may be destroyed

INFLAMMATORY LESIONS
SYPHILIS
Plasma cells, lymphocytes, histiocytes underlying an ulcer containing neutrophils and necrotic debris
Endarteritis common
GRANULOMA INGUINALE
Chronic infection by *Calymmatobacterium granulomatis* (gram-negative encapsulated bacillus)
Dense dermal infiltrate of histiocytes and plasma cells with islands of necrosis (small abscesses) and overlying pseudoepitheliomatous hyperplasia
Donovan bodies: small, round, encapsulated bodies inside cytoplasm of histiocytes (best seen on Giemsa or Warthin-Starry)
CROHN'S DISEASE
May be contiguous with rectal lesions or independent
LYMPHOGRANULOMA VENEREUM
Chlamydia trachomatis infection of lymphatic vessels
Small ulcer at contact site, involvement of inguinal lymph nodes by stellate abscess with epithelioid histiocytes
HIDRADENITIS SUPPURATIVA
Chronic inflammation of the apocrine glands following duct occlusion by keratin plugs
Perifolliculitis, abscesses, sinus tracts
Usually polymicrobial

VULVAR DYSTROPHIES
Postmenopausal atrophy of vulvar skin and subcutaneous tissue, producing thickened white skin clinically, often with severe pruritus
KERATOSIS AND CHRONIC INFLAMMATION
Clinically referred to as *leukoplakia*
Squamous hyperplasia, thick keratin layer, acanthosis, prominent stratum granulosum, dermal inflammation
Foci of atypia or dysplasia not uncommon
LICHEN SCLEROSUS ET ATROPHICUS
May occur anywhere on skin, most commonly vulva
Clinically referred to as *kraurosis*
White or ivory angulated macules or papules
Hyperkeratosis with epithelial atrophy; edema and sclerotic homogenization of upper dermis (loss of elastin); underlying dense lymphocytic infiltrate may be present
Telangiectatic vessels common

BENIGN NEOPLASMS
CONDYLOMA
HPV, usually type 6 or 11

Condyloma acuminatum: soft elevated mass(es) composed of papillary arrangement of well-differentiated squamous epithelium overlying connective tissue cores
Flat condyloma: not exophytic; slightly more common
In both, see koilocytosis and lymphocytic infiltration of stroma
Not specifically part of sequence including dysplasia and carcinoma, but often coexists with dysplastic areas

MELANOCYTIC NEVI
Particularly on the labia majora
Almost always intradermal or compound

HIDRADENOMA PAPILLIFERUM (PAPILLARY HIDRADENOMA)
Small, well-circumscribed subcutaneous nodule
Papillary and glandular patterns with stratification and some degree of pleomorphism
May arise from apocrine sweat glands of vulva, or perhaps ectopic breast

ANGIOMYOFIBROBLASTOMA
Small, well-circumscribed proliferation of vessels and a myxoid stroma
May be an early form of aggressive angiomyxoma
Does not recur after excision

ECTOPIC MAMMARY TISSUE
Occurs along the primitive milk line (extends from axilla to groin in embryo)
Can undergo any changes seen in normal breast tissue, from lactational changes to benign and malignant tumors

OTHER BENIGN LESIONS
Syringoma
Chondroid syringoma

BOWENOID PAPULOSIS
Usually multiple pigmented papules on vulva of young patients, resembling warts or nevi
Histologic appearance very similar to Bowen's disease, but some normal organization persists
Some pathologists consider this a clinical diagnosis only, with the corresponding pathologic diagnosis being vulvar intraepithelial neoplasia (VIN)
May spontaneously regress

MALIGNANT NEOPLASMS
VULVAR INTRAEPITHELIAL NEOPLASIA
Intraepithelial dysplasia with a progression of atypia and disorder from basal third (VIN I) to full thickness (VIN III)
HPV (esp. types 16 and 18) present in >90% cases
This lesion is more likely to progress to invasive carcinoma, and in fact may invade even before full thickness dysplasia is attained (note: only ~5% progress)

BOWEN'S DISEASE
AKA: carcinoma in situ
Some pathologists include these with VIN III
Slightly elevated, plaquelike, red; may involve perineum
Full-thickness involvement of epidermis by large dyskeratotic cells and abnormal mitoses, with acanthosis and parakeratosis, hyperchromatic nuclei

Only 10% become invasive (more if immunosuppressed)
Strong association with HPV-16

SQUAMOUS CELL CARCINOMA
Usually arises on labia minora
Grows slowly, but eventually ulcerates and spreads widely
Usually very well differentiated
Microinvasive: <1 mm of invasion; <1% have LN metastases
FIGO (AJCC) Staging
  T1   Confined to vulva, ≤2 cm
  T2   Confined to vulva, >2 cm
  T3   Invades lower urethra, vagina, or anus
  T4   Invades bladder mucosa, upper urethral, or rectal mucosa, or fixed to bone
  N1   Unilateral regional LNs
  N2   Bilateral regional LNs
  M1   Distant metastases (includes pelvic LNs)

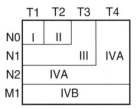

	T1	T2	T3	T4
N0	I	II		
N1			III	IVA
N2	IVA			
M1	IVB			

VERRUCOUS CARCINOMA
Typical warty appearance, generally large, locally infiltrative with pushing margin, does not metastasize

BASAL CELL CARCINOMA
Chiefly labia majora
May recur; does not metastasize

PAGET'S DISEASE
Crusting, elevated, scaling, erythematous rash
Epidermis contains large, pale-clear cells, tending to lie along the basal layer, occasionally forming clusters or glands; often involves appendages
Tumor cells are PAS+ and immunoreactive for CEA, EMA, and Cam-5.2
Usually *not* associated with underlying invasive component (unlike mammary Paget's disease)

MALIGNANT MELANOMA
Most common non-epidermoid malignancy of vulva (5–10%)
Need to distinguish from Paget's disease

AGGRESSIVE ANGIOMYXOMA
Soft tissue tumor, which may simulate Bartholin's gland cyst
Gelatinous and ill-defined mass of hypocellular myxoid stroma with vessels having dilated lumina; no mitoses, no atypia
Most patients are in teens to 20s
Recurrences common

BARTHOLIN'S GLAND CARCINOMA
Can be squamous, adenocarcinoma, adenoid cystic carcinoma, transitional cell carcinoma, etc.

21
BREAST

Normal Anatomy/Physiology
Gland = large duct system + terminal duct-lobule unit (latter responsible for fibrocystic disease and most carcinomas)

Lactiferous (collecting) ducts empty into nipple; one per lobe; ~20 lobes per breast

Lactiferous sinus: fusiform dilatation beneath nipple

Terminal duct-lobule unit (TDLU) surrounded by specialized myxoid-appearing hormone-responsive stroma; absent elastic fibers

Two cell layers:
- Epithelium: keratin, EMA, milk fat globule membrane antigen, alpha lactalbumin positive
- Myoepithelial cells: actin, other keratins, weak S-100

Nipple contains sebaceous glands, smooth muscle bundles

Marked hyperplastic changes in pregnancy; isolated lobules can undergo similar changes without pregnancy, cause unknown

Ectopia: within axillary nodes and along "milk line" (axilla to inguinal region)

INFLAMMATORY AND RELATED DISORDERS
DUCT ECTASIA
AKA: varicocele; comedo-, periductal-, or stale milk-mastitis

May produce nipple retraction or inversion; discharge in 20%

Large duct dilatation containing necrobiotic material; wall is thickened by fibrosis

If material escapes into tissue, florid inflammatory response

Calcification common; on mammogram, appears as tubular and/or annular shadows

FAT NECROSIS
Can produce skin retraction, simulating carcinoma

Foamy macrophages infiltrating partially necrotic fat

Seen in ruptured ectatic ducts or fibrocystic disease, and following trauma (often superficial subcutaneous tissue)

CALCIFICATIONS
Calcium oxalate: birefringent; faint, almost always benign

Calcium phosphate: blue, sharp; may be benign or malignant

OTHERS
Abscess

Granulomatous mastitis: TB, foreign body reaction (e.g., silicone), sarcoidosis

Breast infarct

"Mondor's disease" (thrombophlebitis of breast and chest wall)

FIBROCYSTIC DISEASE
AKA: cystic mastopathy, Schimmelbusch's disease, mammary dysplasia, chronic cystic mastitis . . .

Preferred term: *fibrocystic changes;* not necessarily premalignant

Usually 25–45 yr old; white

Usually bilateral, but may be asymmetrical

Long-term contraceptive use may decrease incidence

Disease of the terminal duct–lobule unit

Features/histologic appearance include:
- Stromal fibrosis: probably secondary to cyst rupture, mild to dense hyalinization
- Formation of cysts: microscopic to grossly visible, cloudy yellow or clear fluid, "blue dome cysts," typically clustered, flattening or loss of epithelium, thick fibrous wall
- Chronic inflammation: secondary to cyst rupture
- Fibroadenomatoid change: stromal proliferation and slit-like spaces
- Apocrine metaplasia: eosinophilic, snout cells, PAS+, prominent nucleoli
- Epithelial hyperplasia: (see later)

ADENOSIS
"Any hyperplastic process that primarily involves the glandular component of the breast"

Term generally used to refer to multifocal or diffuse process (unlike adenoma, which is usually solitary and localized)

SCLEROSING ADENOSIS
Average age 30 yr; typically confused with carcinoma

Most important feature of benign status is preservation of lobular architecture seen at low power, despite the absolute increase in the number of glands

More cellular centrally than peripherally

Two cell layers; dense stroma; no mitoses; no necrosis

Can see apocrine metaplasia, perineural "permeation"

Smooth muscle actin or collagen IV immunostain can help distinguish from carcinoma; often reveals more extensive proliferation of myoepithelial cells than is evident on H&E

May become involved by lobular carcinoma in situ

RADIAL SCAR
AKA: sclerosing duct lesion, nonencapsulated sclerosing lesion, indurative mastopathy, infiltrating epitheliosis, benign sclerosing ductal proliferation

Adenosis, epithelial hyperplasia, and sclerosis that mimics carcinoma mammographically, grossly, and often histologically

Stellate shaped; central area shows sclerosing adenosis-like lesion with fibrosis and elastosis; as move further out from center, ducts show cystic dilatation and often increased epithelial hyperplasia

Entirely benign; relative cancer risk greater only with atypical hyperplasia

When larger than 1 cm, often referred to as *complex sclerosing lesion*

BLUNT DUCT ADENOSIS
Dilatation of small ducts with blunting of the ends, hyperplasia of both luminal and basal epithelium, and an increase

191

in the associated surrounding specialized connective tissue

NODULAR ADENOSIS
Combination of blunt duct adenosis and sclerosing adenosis

Get increased cellularity without significant sclerosis

MICROGLANDULAR ADENOSIS
Irregular distribution in fat or fibrous tissue of small, uniform ducts with open lumina containing eosinophilic secretions

No associated sclerosis or stromal reaction

Myoepithelial layer may be absent!

Thick basement membrane present

Differential diagnosis: tubular carcinoma

ADENOMYOEPITHELIAL (APOCRINE) ADENOSIS
Microglandular adenosis in which the glands enlarge, undergo apocrine metaplasia, and have prominent myoepithelial cell layer

ATYPICAL APOCRINE SCLEROSING LESION
Sclerosing adenosis with apocrine metaplasia and thus large nucleoli

VIRGINAL HYPERTROPHY
AKA: gigantomastia

Unilateral or bilateral

Proliferation of ducts and stroma with little to no lobular involvement

Histologically, very similar to gynecomastia

ADENOMA
Generally refers to a focal, usually solitary proliferation of predominantly the epithelial component of the breast

In some cases, it is unclear whether these are true neoplasms or localized hyperplasias

LACTATING ADENOMA
Solitary or multiple movable masses, during pregnancy

Localized hyperplasia—may occur in ectopic breast tissue

Gray-tan cut surface, well circumscribed; necrosis and lymphocytic infiltrate common

TUBULAR ADENOMA
Present in young adults

Solitary, well-circumscribed, firm, tan-yellow mass

Closely packed regular small tubules, decreased numbers of myoepithelial cells, minimal stroma

INTRADUCTAL PAPILLOMA
Can arise in large or small ducts; average age 48

Bloody nipple discharge common; solitary in 90%

Usually <3 cm (unlike papillary carcinoma, which is larger)

Complex, cellular, arborescent

Features favoring benign: well-developed fibrovascular cores, myoepithelial cell layer, normochromatic oval nuclei, minimal mitoses, apocrine metaplasia, lack of cribriform or trabecular pattern

May see hemorrhagic infarct, squamous metaplasia, focal necrosis, pseudoinfiltration at base

Intracystic papilloma (papillary cystadenoma): variant within a large cystic (tension) duct

Single papilloma has no association with higher cancer rates

Multiple papillomas (papillomatosis) more likely to recur and associated with increased risk of malignancy

NIPPLE ADENOMA
AKA: florid papillomatosis of nipple ducts, erosive adenomatosis

Usually 30s–40s; unilateral, bloody or serous discharge

Proliferation of epithelial and myoepithelial cells, often extending into the epidermis

Three patterns: sclerosing papillomatosis, papillomatosis without sclerosis, and adenosis

Use criteria for papilloma to distinguish from malignancy

FIBROADENOMA
Most common benign "tumor" of breast

Probably not neoplasm but rather localized nodular hyperplasia of both stromal and glandular tissue

Typically young adults (20–35 yr)

Enlarge during pregnancy, regress with age

Usually single; multiple in 20%

Sharply demarcated, firm, <3 cm, with solid grayish white cut surface with a bulging, whorl-like pattern and slitlike spaces

Stroma usually loose with acid mucopolysaccharides

Elastic tissue absent; presumably derived from the terminal duct–lobule unit

Two microscopic types, of no particular significance:
- Intracanalicular: stroma invaginates glands, appears to be within them
- Pericanalicular: oval glandular configuration maintained

HISTOLOGIC VARIATIONS
Hemorrhagic infarction (more common in pregnancy)

Degenerative changes: hyalinization, calcification, ossification

Stromal changes: high cellularity, dense fibrosis, prominent myxoid change

Apocrine metaplasia (15%), squamous metaplasia (rare)

Sclerosing adenosis (10%)

Lactational change

Fibroadenomatosis: merges with surrounding fibrocystic disease

Stromal multinucleated giant cells

Hamartoma (choristoma): presence of adipose tissue, smooth muscle, or cartilage in the stroma

JUVENILE (GIANT, MASSIVE, FETAL, CELLULAR) FIBROADENOMA
Young age, large (>10 cm), hypercellular stroma; may be bilateral, often in blacks

MALIGNANT TRANSFORMATION
Occurs in 0.1%

Most are lobular carcinoma in situ

If limited to fibroadenoma, excellent prognosis

Sarcomatous transformation even more rare

HYPERPLASIA, DUCTAL AND LOBULAR
AKA: papillomatosis, epitheliosis

	Grading Scheme	Relative Risk for Invasive Cancer
I	No or mild hyperplasia	1
II	Moderate or florid hyperplasia	1.5–2
III	Atypical ductal or lobular	4–5
IV	In situ ductal or lobular carcinoma	8–10

FEATURES OF BENIGN HYPERPLASIA
Elongated clefts separate intraluminal mass from basal cells

Streaming alignment of nuclei and cells, creating irregular, nonrigid bridges

Indistinct cytoplasmic borders

Acidophilic, finely granular cytoplasm (vs. pale, homogeneous)

Apocrine metaplasia, complete or incomplete

Presence of myoepithelial cells

Oval, normochromatic (vs. round, hyperchromatic) nuclei with slight overlap and small, single nucleolus; only few mitoses

Foamy macrophages in lumen and associated with epithelium

Intraluminal or stromal (vs. basal) calcifications; no psammoma bodies

No necrosis

ATYPICAL HYPERPLASIA, DUCTAL AND LOBULAR

Hyperplasia, seen usually in a background of fibrocystic changes, which show some but not all of the features of in situ carcinoma

Breast Carcinoma

GENERAL

Most common malignant tumor among women

Affects 1/9 women

Accounts for 20% of cancer deaths in women

RISK FACTORS

Geographic (U.S. > Japan)

First degree relative with breast cancer increases risk 2–3×; familial breast carcinoma linked to a gene at 17q21 (brca-1)

Risk increases with age

Early menarche, late menopause, nulliparity

Removal of ovaries before age 35 reduces risk to one third

Women who have their 1st child before 18 yr of age have one-third risk of women who have 1st child after age 30

Exogenous estrogen may increase risk, esp. in presence of fibrocystic disease; contraceptive use shows no change in risk

Increased risk with exposure to radiation

Obesity

Atypical epithelial hyperplasia

Risk of carcinoma in contralateral breast of patients with invasive carcinoma is 5× risk of general population, reaching 25–50% for lobular carcinoma in situ

High lipid diet; moderate ethyl alcohol consumption

Multicentricity more common in lobular vs. ductal

DIAGNOSIS

40% of mammographically detectable cancers not palpable; 20% of palpable cancers not detected by mammography

Clinical evaluation of axillary nodes is wrong 30% of the time

Mammography can detect tumors 1–2 cm in size

Only 20% of mammographically "suspicious" lesions are carcinoma

Magnetic resonance imaging (MRI) cannot detect microcalcifications

50% occur in upper outer quadrant, 20% central/subareolar, 10% in each of the other three quadrants

90% of carcinomas are ductal

MOLECULAR BIOLOGY

p53 (17p13) mutations are the most common alterations seen in both familial and sporadic breast carcinoma

neu (erb-B2, Her-2; 17q11-12) often amplified; 2nd most common change

brca-1 (17q21) is third most common mutation; see decreased level of expression (hence it is a putative tumor suppressor gene); mutations seen in 5% of breast cancers, but in 40% of breast cancers from patients in families with two or more breast cancers

Amplification of c-ras and c-myc has also been seen, as have mutations in Rb

SPREAD

Direct spread, lymphatic, hematogenous

Can "recur" months, years, or decades after initial therapy

11% of cancers grossly <1 cm had tumor outside 2 cm margin

Two thirds of patients have lymph node (LN) metastases at time of diagnosis

1% of patients with apparently "intraductal" carcinoma will have LN metastases

Nodes: axilla (40–50%), internal mammary (22%), supraclavicular (20%; zero if no axillary nodes)

Enlarged axillary LN in adult female with no known primary will be breast cancer or malignant melanoma in >90%; caution: breast cancer can be S-100+

Metastases: bone, lung, pleura, liver, adrenal, CNS; invasive lobular also goes to stomach, bowel, spleen, heart

GRADING

Histologic: I–III based on score for each of percent tubule formation, nuclear pleomorphism, and mitotic count; histologic grade only used for infiltrating ductal carcinoma

Nuclear: I–III based on pleomorphism and mitoses

STAGING

T0		No primary
T1		≤2 cm
	T1a	≤0.5 cm
	T1b	0.5–1 cm
	T1c	1–2 cm
T2		2–5 cm
T3		>5 cm
T4		Any size with
	T4a	Extension to chest wall
	T4b	Edema or ulceration of the skin
	T4c	a and b
	T4d	Inflammatory carcinoma
N0		None
N1		Moveable ipsilateral axillary nodes
	N1a	All LN metastases <0.2 cm
	N1b	LN metastasis >0.2 cm
	i	1–3 LNs, all <2 cm
	ii	≥4 LNs, all <2 cm
	iii	Beyond LN capsule, <2 cm
	iv	Any LN >2 cm
N2		Fixed ipsilateral axillary nodes
N3		Ipsilateral internal mammary nodes positive

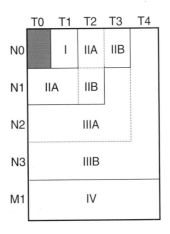

	T0	T1	T2	T3	T4
N0		I	IIA	IIB	
N1		IIA	IIB		
N2			IIIA		
N3			IIIB		
M1			IV		

THERAPY

Surgery

Radiation
- Post-op adjunct, primary therapy, or treatment for local recurrence
- Bizarre nuclear changes, extensive tumor necrosis

Hormonal
- Effectiveness of antiestrogen therapy is well correlated with presence of estrogen and/or progesterone receptors in nuclei of the tumor cells (~2/3 of all breast tumors are ER/PR+, including most lobular carcinomas and ~50% of ductal carcinomas, esp. mucinous; medullary and comedocarcinoma are usually negative)
- Castration (30–40% respond), adrenalectomy (30–40%), hypophysectomy (40–50%), medical antiestrogen
- Results in prominent, sometimes focal fibrosis, hyalinization, degenerative changes (tumor cell vacuolization, necrosis)

Chemotherapy
- Improve survival in metastatic disease, improve cure post-op in patients with positive nodes

PROGNOSIS

Overall 5 yr survival: 60% for LN–; 34% for LN+ (therefore, 50% reduction in survival with LN involvement)

Favorable
- Age <50 yr
- Early diagnosis (88% 5 yr survival if detected before development of symptoms)
- Small size (<1 cm); for node-negative disease, recurrence rate is half the rate when the primary is 1–2 cm
- Tubular, cribriform, medullary, pure mucinous, papillary, juvenile, adenoid cystic
- Pushing vs. infiltrating margin
- Absence of inflammatory response (!), except medullary

Unfavorable
- Carcinoma manifesting during pregnancy (15–35% 5 yr survival)
- *Presence of invasion/proportion of invasive component*
- *High nuclear or histologic grade*
- Number of LNs: 0, <4, ≥4; 5 yr survival: 80%, 50%, 21% (in premenopausal women, two LNs significantly decreases survival; also, at any age, single LN >2 cm equivalent to ≥3 small positive LNs)
- Signet ring, inflammatory, comedocarcinoma
- Tumor necrosis
- Vascular invasion
- Local recurrence
- Skin or nipple invasion
- Aneuploid tumor
- High S-phase
- Extensive intraductal carcinoma

No effect (or unclear effect) on prognosis
- Oral contraceptives
- CEA positivity
- *erb*-B2 status?
- Site in breast
- Paget's disease
- Cathepsin D status?
- Degree of sinus histiocytosis in nodes?
- Estrogen/progesterone receptor status: meaningful if strongly negative or strongly positive; intermediate levels do not correlate with outcome

DUCTAL CARCINOMA IN SITU (DCIS)

COMEDOCARCINOMA

May reach large size; palpable; >60% are larger than 2 cm

>50% are centrally located

One third are multifocal; 10% are bilateral

Solid inward growth of large, high-grade pleomorphic tumor cells, mitoses, central necrosis ± calcification

Myoepithelial cells may be present

Stroma: concentric fibrosis; mild to moderate chronic inflammation 20–50% recurrence rate after local excision (vs. <5% for other intraductal lesions)

Even if no invasion is identified, can have LN metastases

SOLID

Solid filling of duct with uniform cells, larger than lobular carcinoma in situ (LCIS) but smaller than comedocarcinoma, with sharp cytoplasmic borders and no necrosis

Neuroendocrine variant with mixture of spindled cells and round cells filling the duct

CRIBRIFORM

Round, regular glands within the monomorphous epithelial proliferation; "rigid" trabeculae; no nuclear atypia

PAPILLARY CARCINOMA

Most papillary breast lesions are benign (see earlier)

Features of malignancy: older patient, uniformity of cells, no myoepithelial cells, nuclear hyperchromasia, mitoses, lack of apocrine metaplasia, minimal stroma, eosinophilic look

Intracystic variant: occurs within large cyst

MICROPAPILLARY

Elongated epithelial projections into lumen without connective tissue support, ± cavity at base, bulbous expansion at tip; no nuclear atypia

CYSTIC HYPERSECRETORY

Cystic formations, abundant secretory material, single cell type, cribriform spaces (not as regular as in cribriform carcinoma)

CLINGING

One or two layers of malignant cells lining large, empty lumen with occasional individual cell necrosis

LOBULAR CANCERIZATION

Presence within a lobule of cytologically ductal carcinoma

INFILTRATING DUCTAL CARCINOMA

CLASSIC

AKA: ordinary, not otherwise specified (NOS); "breast cancer"

75% of all invasive ductal carcinomas

Yellowish gray, gritty, stellate, necrosis, hemorrhage, cystic degeneration, "chalky streaks" (duct or vessel elastosis), calcifications in 60%

Tremendous variability in microscopic appearance

Invasion of lymphatics (33%), perineural space (28%), blood vessels (5%)

Immunohistochemistry: + low molecular weight (MW) keratin, EMA, milk fat globule; lactalbumin and CEA positive in 70%, 10–45% S-100 positive

May be positive for high MW keratin if squamous metaplasia

TUBULAR CARCINOMA

Mean age 50 yr

Characteristically small (mean diameter 1 cm)

Well-differentiated glands, no necrosis, no mitoses, mild pleomorphism (simulates radial scar, microglandular adenosis)

Haphazard arrangement of glands in stroma, infiltration of fat, open lumina, basophilic secretion, apocrine-type apical cytoplasm, formation of trabecular bars

Two thirds have intraductal carcinoma, micropapillary or cribriform

56% multicentric, 10% metastasize

Excellent prognosis (<5% recur in 7 yr) if pure

CRIBRIFORM CARCINOMA

Often seen with tubular carcinoma

Well differentiated, low nuclear grade, excellent prognosis

MUCINOUS CARCINOMA

AKA: mucoid, colloid, gelatinous

Usually in postmenopausal women

Well circumscribed; crepitant, currant-jelly mass

Small clusters of tumor cells (solid or acinar) floating in sea of mucin (neutral or acid; almost entirely extracellular)

Approximately one quarter show features of endocrine differentiation

When pure, only 2–4% have LN metastases; good prognosis

May recur many years later (e.g., 12 yr!)

Some consider this an in situ lesion—only mucin is invasive

JUVENILE (SECRETORY)

Seen primarily in children, also in adults

Well circumscribed, small, pushing margins, central hyalinization

Tubuloalveolar, focally papillary growth pattern; cells with vacuolated cytoplasm, eosinophilic PAS+ secretion

100% 5 yr survival

MEDULLARY CARCINOMA

More common in women <50 yr; particularly in Japanese

~1% of breast carcinomas

Well circumscribed, may become large (5–10 cm)

Homogeneous gray cut surface with small foci of hemorrhage or necrosis

Pushing borders, diffuse growth pattern, no glandular differentiation, cytologically high grade (large pleomorphic cells, large nucleoli, many mitoses), indistinct cell borders, spindle cell metaplasia; minimal fibrosis (tend to be soft)

Prominent lymphoplasmacytic infiltrate at periphery (T cells; IgA), often with germinal centers

Axillary metastases usually few in number

Slightly better survival vs. classic (84% vs. 63% 10 yr survival)

Prognosis better for tumors smaller than 3 cm

INVASIVE PAPILLARY

Rare; most papillary carcinomas are in situ

Pushing growth pattern, excellent prognosis

APOCRINE

Very rare (<1% of breast cancers)

Large cells, abundant acidophilic, granular PAS+ cytoplasm

CARCINOID

AKA: invasive ductal carcinoma with endocrine differentiation

Carcinoid syndrome not present clinically

Solid nests of cells, ribbons, rosettes, fibrous stroma

Prognosis same as for classic type

Dense-core secretory granules present

METAPLASTIC

Well circumscribed

Predominantly sarcomatoid appearance (any sarcoma), usually vimentin positive, may maintain epithelial markers

25% metastasize

More aggressive than classic; tumor size most important

Subtypes:

- Epidermoid: rare; elderly women; extensive squamous metaplasia
- Spindle cell carcinoma
- Acantholytic epidermoid: poorly cohesive; pseudoglandular
- Adenosquamous

INFLAMMATORY CARCINOMA

Clinically, breast frequently red and warm with edema of skin

Undifferentiated carcinoma with extensive dermal lymphatic invasion

Ominous prognosis; perhaps should be considered "inoperable"

PAGET'S DISEASE

Crusted lesion of the nipple with underlying intraductal carcinoma, ± invasion

Large clear cells within epidermis, concentrated along basal layer; may form small glandular structures

Underlying tumor always ductal; may be focally continuous with skin

30–40% have metastases at time of diagnosis

EMA, milk fat globule, CEA, low MW keratin +; S-100 −

Origin of the cells is still unclear

LOBULAR CARCINOMA IN SITU (LCIS)

AKA: lobular neoplasia

Generally is a disease of premenopausal women

Multicentric in 70%, bilateral in 30–40%

Generally not identifiable grossly

Filling and distention of lobules by uniform, round, loosely cohesive small cells with low nuclear grade (round normochromatic nuclei, minimal mitoses, minimal necrosis, minimal atypia)

Three quarters will show scattered positivity for mucin

Myoepithelial cells generally still present

Can occur within fibroadenomas or sclerosing adenosis

Risk of invasive carcinoma 25–30% (10× control population); invasive component may be of ductal or lobular type and may occur in either breast; thus, LCIS is a fundamentally different disease from ductal carcinoma in situ (DCIS): it is a marker for overall increased risk; this is why some pathologists prefer the term *lobular neoplasia*

Close follow-up usually sufficient

INVASIVE LOBULAR CARCINOMA

CLASSIC TYPE

May by diagnosed without lobular carcinoma in situ

Often multicentric; 20% are bilateral

Small, relatively round uniform cells growing singly in an Indian file pattern, often concentric around lobules with in situ lobular

Dense, fibrous stroma with periductal and perivenous elastosis

Prognosis slightly better than for classic infiltrating ductal

SIGNET RING

Must have classic signet ring cells with intracytoplasmic mucin

May coexist with mucinous, classic invasive lobular carcinoma or invasive ductal

Poor prognosis

OTHERS

Different growth pattern; still small cells, low nuclear grade

- Alveolar: sharply outlined groups separated by fibrous septa
- Tubulolobular: typical invasive lobular carcinoma merging with small, "closed" tubules

SWEAT-GLAND TYPE CARCINOMAS

BENIGN

Eccrine spiradenoma (sharply circumscribed lobules, small lumens, basaloid cells)

Papillary clear cell hidradenoma (pedunculated, intracystic, papillary; two epithelial cell types: clear and granular)

Benign mixed tumor (pleomorphic adenoma, chondroid syringoma; adenomyoepithelioma with heterologous stroma [myxoid or chondroid])

ADENOID CYSTIC CARCINOMA
Most common of this rare group

Often confused with much more common intraductal cribriform carcinoma

Two types of cavity formations: true glands, and eosinophilic "cylinders" containing PAS+ basement membrane material (collagen IV)

May show foci of sebaceous differentiation

Relatively good prognosis: LN metastases in 6%; pulmonary metastases in 12%

OTHER MALIGNANT
Mucoepidermoid carcinoma

Apocrine carcinoma

MYOEPITHELIAL MALIGNANCIES
ADENOMYOEPITHELIOMA
Small (~1 cm in diameter), firm, well circumscribed

Polygonal cells, optically clear cytoplasm, arranged in nests

Some cells spindled, hence tumor is biphasic

No instances of metastases

CLEAR CELL CARCINOMA
Glycogen-rich large clear cells—not biphasic

True carcinoma: prognosis same as invasive ductal carcinoma

SPINDLE CELL MYOEPITHELIOMA
Nonencapsulated, cellular, fascicular growth pattern

Other Tumors of the Breast

PHYLLOIDES TUMOR
Despite its alternate name (cystosarcoma phylloides), most of these lesions are benign, but often locally aggressive

Median age 45; very rare below 25 yr

Round, firm, well circumscribed, with solid gray-white cut surface containing cleftlike spaces; may have hemorrhage, necrosis

Many are very large, but some remain <5 cm

Benign glandular elements with very cellular stroma ranging from predominantly periductal fibroblastic appearance with foci of mature adipose tissue (benign end of spectrum) to marked nuclear atypia and mitoses extending even distant from glands

Can have metaplastic cartilage, bone, rarely skeletal muscle, or can take on the appearance of any malignant sarcoma; overgrowth of glands can be seen

Stromal cells have progesterone but not estrogen receptors

Indicators of malignancy: >10 mitoses/10 HPF, marked atypia, stromal overgrowth relative to glands, infiltrating margin, necrosis, hemorrhage

Better differentiated tumors have tendency for local recurrence, but rarely metastasize

Cytologically malignant tumors have 3–12% incidence of metastases (usually lung or bones; rarely axillary nodes)

VASCULAR TUMORS
PSEUDOANGIOMATOUS HYPERPLASIA
Clinically and grossly simulate fibroadenoma

Benign lesion

ANGIOSARCOMA
Characteristically young women

Highly malignant to very benign appearing

Key is "freely anastomosing vascular channels"

Prognosis poor: 33% 5 yr survival

HEMANGIOMA
ANGIOLIPOMA

MISCELLANEOUS "TUMORS"
STROMAL SARCOMA
Lack the epithelial component of phylloides tumor

Usually fibrosarcoma-like; may be very anaplastic

GRANULAR CELL TUMOR
May simulate invasive carcinoma

Usually small, but may be up to 10 cm; benign

FIBROMATOSIS
NODULAR FASCIITIS
MALIGNANT LYMPHOMA
May be primary

Right breast more common than left; 25% bilateral

Soft, grayish white, no associated skin retraction

Almost always diffuse non-Hodgkin's, most common is large cell; nearly all are B cell—mucosal associated lymphoid tissue (MALT) lesions

Don't confuse with pseudolymphoma: reactive, germinal centers

GRANULOCYTIC SARCOMA
Look for eosinophilic myelocytes or metamyelocytes

MALE BREAST DISEASE

GYNECOMASTIA
Often result of increased estrogens or decreased androgens

After age 25, may be caused by hormonally active tumors

Usually centered below the nipple (unlike more eccentric carcinoma)

Unilateral (left breast more common) or bilateral

Oval, disc-shaped mass, elastic consistency, well circumscribed

Proliferation of ducts and surrounding edematous stroma; no glands

Stromal fibrosis increases with age of lesion

OTHER BENIGN LESIONS
Duct ectasia, sclerosing adenosis

Nipple adenoma

Myofibroblastoma

CARCINOMA
1% of breast cancers in U.S. occur in males (10% in Egypt)

Increased incidence in Klinefelter's syndrome

Probably some relation with gynecomastia—not clear

Usually elderly male; nipple discharge usually indicates carcinoma

Paget's disease/skin involvement common

All types seen; invasive lobular is most uncommon

40% 10 yr survival (79% and 11% for node negative and positive)

22
ENDOCRINE ORGANS

MULTIPLE ENDOCRINE NEOPLASIAS (MEN)
Autosomal dominant syndromes with high degree of penetrance

Hyperplasias almost always precede neoplasia, esp. in the thyroid (C cells) and adrenal medulla

MEN TYPE I
AKA: Werner's syndrome

Mapped to chromosome 11q13
- Pituitary adenoma
- Parathyroid gland (chief cell hyperplasia)
- Pancreas (50% G-cell tumors, 30% beta cell, 12% vasoactive intestinal peptide [VIP] cell)

Other: adrenal cortex adenoma; nodular hyperplasia of thyroid; carcinoid tumors of lung, thymus, GI tract; lipomas; Ménétrier's disease; Zollinger-Ellison syndrome with peptic ulceration and hypersecretion

MEN TYPE II (IIA)
AKA: Sipple's syndrome

Mapped to chromosome 10q11.2 (RET gene)
- C-cell hyperplasia/medullary carcinoma of thyroid
- Pheochromocytoma of adrenal medulla
- Parathyroid chief cell hyperplasia

Occasionally also seen adrenal cortical tumors

MEN TYPE III (IIB)
AKA: Gorlin's syndrome

90% of patients have mutation in codon 918 of RET gene or chromosome 10q11.2
- Medullary carcinoma of thyroid
- Adrenal pheochromocytoma
- Mucosal neuromas (ganglioneuromas) of corneal nerves, lips, GI tract (main distinguishing factor from MEN IIa)

Also skeletal abnormalities, marfanoid habitus

Occasionally adrenal cortical tumors, parathyroid tumors

PANCREATIC ISLETS, TESTIS, AND OVARY
(Endocrine lesions of these organs are discussed in their respective outlines)

THYROID

NORMAL ANATOMY
Averages 15–25 g in adult, but varies significantly with sex and iodide intake

Two lateral lobes connected by isthmus; a pyramidal lobe may protrude superiorly from isthmus

FOLLICULAR CELLS
Follicles vary in size: average 200 μm

Single layer of cuboidal to columnar cells

Some cells have abundant mitochondria: acidophilic; referred to as Hürthle cells or Askanazy cells

Immunoreactive for thyroglobulin, T3, T4, low molecular weight keratin, EMA, vimentin

Thyroglobulin (650 kD) synthesized and stored extracellularly as "colloid"; calcium oxalate crystals can be seen in the colloid in ~50% of patients

Tyrosyl residues iodinated to monoiodotyrosine (MIT) and diiodotyrosine (DIT); MIT and DIT couple to form T3 or T4

In response to thyroid stimulating hormone (TSH), T3 and T4 pinocytosed and released

Both T3 and T4 are bound by thyronine binding protein; T4 binds tighter, less is available; therefore, T3 is more active

PARAFOLLICULAR (C) CELLS
Between and within follicles, especially upper and middle portions of lateral lobes; neural crest derived

Immunoreactive for calcitonin, CEA (CEA more prominent in hyperplasia or neoplasia)

Secrete calcitonin (directly inhibits osteoclasts) in response to high serum calcium

EMBRYOLOGY
Develops as tubular invagination (thyroglossal duct) from base of the tongue called the *foramen cecum*

Grows downward in front of trachea and thyroid cartilage

Distal end becomes adult gland, proximal part regresses by the 5th–7th wk of gestation

Joined by tissue derived from the 4th and 5th pharyngeal pouches, which contributes the parafollicular cells

Hyoid bone forms from second branchial arch

THYROGLOSSAL DUCT CYST
Localized persistence of duct, usually in region of hyoid bone

May become clinically evident at any age

Pseudostratified ciliated or squamous epithelium lined, with mucous glands and follicles in stroma with inflammation

Papillary carcinoma may form: excellent prognosis; can preserve main thyroid gland

Surgical excision must include the middle third of the hyoid bone or the lesions will likely recur

HETEROTOPIA
Approximately 10% incidence, most subclinical

Most common sites are base of tongue (50%), anterior tongue, larynx, mediastinum, heart

In 70% of patients with grossly evident lingual thyroid, main gland is absent

CLINICAL SYNDROMES
GOITER
Any enlargement of the thyroid gland

May be nodular or diffuse, hyperfunctioning or hypofunctioning

197

HYPERTHYROIDISM
Warm skin, exophthalmos, tachycardia, muscle atrophy
Causes: Graves' disease, toxic multinodular goiter, adenoma
Less common causes: acute/subacute thyroiditis, functioning carcinoma, pituitary adenoma, struma ovarii, choriocarcinoma
Treatment: propylthiouracil blocks iodide to iodine conversion, preventing thyroid hormone synthesis; get decrease in T3/T4, increase in TSH, glandular hyperplasia, and hypervascularity
Before surgery (1–2 wk), give iodide: gland becomes firmer and less vascularized

HYPOTHYROIDISM
Cretinism: hypothyroidism present during development and infancy, resulting in physical and mental retardation
Myxedema: hypothyroidism in older child/adult: lethargy, cold intolerance, apathy, edema, dry skin
Causes: surgical/radiation ablation, agenesis, Hashimoto's, hypopituitarism

Thyroiditis

ACUTE THYROIDITIS
Usually infectious; associated with upper airway infections
Streptococcus hemolyticus, Staphylococcus aureus, Pneumococcus
Suppurative and nonsuppurative forms; may have abscess formation
May also be fungal or viral

GRANULOMATOUS THYROIDITIS
DE QUERVAIN'S THYROIDITIS
AKA: subacute thyroiditis, giant cell thyroiditis
Typically young women with sore throat, odynophagia
Associated with HLA-B35
Initially, elevated T3 and T4, suppression of iodine uptake
Later, may become hypothyroid
Involvement of entire gland, but often asymmetrical
Gland typically 2× normal size; fibrosis limited to gland
Inflammation, foreign body giant cells, granulomas; giant cells engulf colloid
Etiology unknown—may be viral
PALPATION THYROIDITIS
AKA: multifocal granulomatous thyroiditis
Common, clinically insignificant
Focal inflammation with epithelial loss from isolated or small groups of follicles; lymphocytes, histiocytes (±foamy), few giant cells scattered in small collections about gland
Caused by local trauma; seen in most removed glands
OTHER GRANULOMATOUS THYROIDITIDES
TB, mycoses, syphilis (tertiary)

AUTOIMMUNE THYROIDITIS
LYMPHOCYTIC THYROIDITIS
Common cause of goiter in children: low iodine uptake
May be focal, or present with diffuse enlargement of the gland with extensive lymphocytic infiltration and germinal centers, but no Hürthle cell change
Squamous metaplasia can be seen, as can fibrosis
HASHIMOTO'S THYROIDITIS
AKA: struma lymphomatosa
Predominantly women over 40 yr; male:female = 1:10
Associated with HLA-DR5

Probably genetic deficiency in antigen specific suppressor T cells, resulting in cytotoxic T-cell attack on follicular cells; later develop circulating antibodies (Abs) to thyroglobulin and/or TSH receptor; in most cases, ~50% of lymphocytes are B cells
Initially mild hyperthyroidism, later hypothyroidism
Diffuse, firm enlargement ± tracheal/esophageal compression, without adherence to surrounding structures
May be asymmetric or nodular
Lymphocytic infiltration with germinal centers *plus* oxyphilic (Hürthle cell) change of (>50%) follicular epithelium; polyclonal plasma cell infiltrate
Follicles become small and atrophic; may show nuclear clearing and overlapping nuclei (similar to papillary carcinoma)
Usually only mild fibrosis
Complications: lymphoma; less commonly: leukemia, papillary carcinoma, Hürthle cell tumors
Fibrosing variant: 12% of all cases; extensive fibrosis of hyaline type, limited to gland

RIEDEL'S THYROIDITIS
AKA: Riedel's struma, invasive thyroiditis
Member of group of idiopathic "inflammatory fibroscleroses," including retroperitoneal fibrosis, sclerosing cholangitis
Not really a disease of the thyroid but rather a disease of the neck that happens to involve the thyroid
Rare; adults and elderly; male:female = 1:3
Extremely firm, involves soft tissue, profound dyspnea
Asymmetrical and multifocal
Dense active proliferative fibrosis extending into surrounding soft tissues—patchy inflammation (lymphocytes and IgA plasma cells), no giant cells
Inflammation in walls of medium-sized vessels
Usually requires surgery, which can be difficult

OTHER NONPROLIFERATIVE LESIONS
Hemochromatosis
Amyloidosis
"Black thyroid": seen in patients on minocycline (tetracycline derivative); pigment deposition in apical surface of the follicular cells

Hyperplasias

DYSHORMONOGENETIC GOITER
Seen in abnormal iodination
Often small follicles with scanty colloid
Nodular and trabecular microfollicular patterns, focally papillary, moderate cellular pleomorphism
Differential diagnosis: papillary carcinoma

DIFFUSE HYPERPLASIA (GRAVES' DISEASE)
AKA: thyrotoxicosis, exophthalmic goiter, autoimmune hyperthyroidism
Typically young females (male:female = 1:5) with muscle weakness, weight loss, tachycardia, pretibial myxedema
Associated with HLA-DR3
Generally 80–90 g (threefold increase in size) with symmetric diffuse enlargement, reddish or gray, consistency of pancreatic tissue

Marked follicular hyperplasia with papillary infolding, columnar cells, clear to foamy cytoplasm, some oxyphilic cells, depleted colloid (note: hyperplastic changes may be less marked if patient treated before surgery)

Lymphocytic infiltration of stroma, occasional germinal centers, mostly T cells, mild fibrosis

Proliferating follicles may extend beyond gland into neck

Incidental papillary carcinomas found in 1–9% of cases

Treatment: propylthiouracil (results in florid hyperplasia), methimazole, subtotal thyroidectomy (if leave ~5 g on each side, will regenerate to euthyroid state)

The more lymphocytes and oxyphil cells at surgery, more likely to become hypothyroid

70% of patients have anti–TSH receptor antibody

NODULAR HYPERPLASIA
AKA: multinodular goiter, adenomatous hyperplasia
ENDEMIC GOITER
Low iodine intake leads to low levels of T3 and T4, elevated TSH levels, and hyperactive gland (parenchymatous goiter), which later undergoes cellular atrophy with storage of large amounts of colloid (diffuse or nodular colloid goiter)
SPORADIC NODULAR GOITER
Unknown pathogenesis

3–5% incidence clinically, 50% at autopsy

Some cases associated with Hashimoto's or lymphocytic thyroiditis

Clinically euthyroid

Multinodular gland, often very large, occasionally with a large, firm, dominant nodule, which may be functional

Gland often asymmetric; capsule usually intact

Hemorrhage into a nodule can cause rapid enlargement/pain

Some cases present as mediastinal mass

Range of microscopic appearances, which may vary significantly from nodule to nodule: large follicles with flattened epithelium, cellular and hyperplastic nodules, Hürthle cells, papillae, granulomatous inflammation, hemorrhage, calcification

Papillary or pseudopapillary lesions distinguished from carcinoma by lack of nuclear features, line walls of cyst

Highly atypical nuclei—exposure to radioactive iodine?
SEQUESTERED THYROID NODULE
AKA: parasitic nodule, lateral aberrant thyroid

Peripherally located thyroid nodule, disconnected from gland

Usually results from nodular hyperplasia or nodular Hashimoto's thyroiditis

Should exhibit same histology as main gland—no lymph node tissue

Differential diagnosis: metastatic papillary carcinoma, follicular variant

C-CELL HYPERPLASIA
Precursor lesion of familial medullary carcinoma

Most pronounced in central part of lateral lobes

May be diffuse or nodular

C cells within follicles and between them

Arbitrarily, >6 C cells/follicle = hyperplasia

Greater CEA reactivity than normal C cells

Epithelial Tumors

Follicular and undifferentiated may be more common with iodine deficiency, papillary with high iodine uptake

Radiation exposure usually leads to benign thyroid lesions, but also to an increased incidence of papillary carcinoma

Distinguishing benign from malignant clinically: more likely to be malignant for young or old, male, single nodule, ipsilateral adenopathy, cold nodule, solid (vs. cystic)
FINE NEEDLE ASPIRATION
Three recommended diagnoses:
- Probably benign: colloid, histiocytes, lymphocytes
- Follicular lesion: high cellularity, no nuclear features of papillary carcinoma
- Papillary carcinoma: nuclear features (grooves and pseudoinclusions), papillae, psammoma bodies
THERAPY
Nodulectomy no longer considered adequate

Lobectomy with isthmusectomy for follicular adenoma

Lobectomy or subtotal for minimally invasive follicular carcinoma and papillary carcinoma

Near-total thyroidectomy for widely invasive follicular, high-risk papillary, poorly differentiated; total thyroidectomy for medullary carcinomas

Radical neck dissection for medullary, but not papillary carcinoma

Postoperative suppression with exogenous Synthroid

Postoperative radioactive iodine usage (for treatment of metastases) is controversial
STAGING

T1	<1 cm, limited to thyroid
T2	1–4 cm, limited to thyroid
T3	>4 cm, limited to thyroid
T4	Extension beyond thyroid capsule
N0	No regional nodes
N1	Positive regional nodes:
N1a	Ipsilateral cervical nodes
N1b	Bilateral or contralateral

Follicular or papillary carcinoma

Low risk: men <40; women <50 (alternatively, anyone <45)

High risk: men ≥40, women ≥50 (alternatively, anyone ≥45)

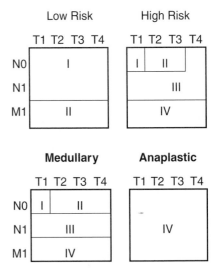

FOLLICULAR ADENOMA
Euthyroid patients; cold to slightly warm nodule, rarely hot

Usually solitary; surrounded by intact capsule; unlike uninvolved gland, compression of adjacent tissue

Variety of patterns:
- Normofollicular (simple)
- Macrofollicular (colloid)
- Microfollicular (fetal)
- Trabecular/solid (embryonal)
- Pseudopapillary structures

Mitoses rare to absent, no capsular invasion
Secondary changes: hemorrhage, edema, fibrosis, calcification, cystic degeneration, ossification
One quarter of cases show aneuploidy by flow cytometry
Treatment: lobectomy

VARIANTS
- Hürthle cell adenoma: >50% Hürthle cells
- Atypical adenoma: cellular proliferation but no capsular or vascular invasion
- Hyalinizing trabecular adenoma: well-defined, organoid trabeculae simulating paraganglioma
- Adenoma with bizarre nuclei: huge, hyperchromatic nuclei, usually in clusters
- Clear cell adenoma
- Adenolipomas: adipose metaplasia of the stroma

FOLLICULAR CARCINOMA

Uncommon (15–20% of thyroid malignancies), female predominance, older patients
Well-formed follicles, cribriform areas, trabecular formations, solid growth pattern; nuclear atypia and mitoses
Psammoma bodies absent, squamous metaplasia rare
Reactive for thyroglobulin, low MW keratin, EMA, S-100
Full-thickness capsular and/or blood vessel invasion indicates carcinoma; invasion partially into capsule doesn't
May be related to iodine deficiency

MINIMALLY INVASIVE
Grossly encapsulated with microscopic invasion in vessels within or just outside capsule; intravascular tumor nodules often covered by endothelium
Metastases in 5% with vessel invasion, 1% with only capsular invasion

WIDELY INVASIVE
Widespread infiltration of vessels and/or adjacent tissue
Metastases common

METASTASES
Blood borne: lung, bones (shoulder, sternum, skull, iliac)
Metastases often better differentiated than primary

PAPILLARY CARCINOMA

Most common thyroid malignancy: 65–60% of thyroid malignancies in adults, >90% in children
Female predominance, mean age 40 yr
Increased incidence in Hashimoto's thyroiditis or following radiation
Clinical presentation: thyroid nodule (cold) in 67%, thyroid nodule and LN in 13%, LN only in 20%
Size varies widely; may be quite small
Solid, white, firm, often infiltrating; 10% show cystic change
Well-developed branching, complex papillae with edematous or hyalinized fibrovascular cores, ± lymphocytes, hemosiderin, some follicles (irregular to tubular)
Nuclear features (may have some, none, all; focal or diffuse):
- Ground glass (optically clear) nuclei, large, overlapping (note: often absent in frozen section/cytologic material)
- Nuclear pseudoinclusions (cytoplasmic invaginations)
- Nuclear grooves

Mitoses rare; fibrosis common

Psammoma bodies present in 30–50% of cases
May see solid/trabecular pattern or squamous metaplasia (common; most common at periphery of lesion)
Multifocal in 25–75% of cases; vascular invasion in 5%
Immunoreactive for low and *high* molecular weight (MW) keratin (note: normal thyroid usually negative for high MW), thyroglobulin, EMA, vimentin, ±CEA
Associated with RET oncogene and papillary thyroid carcinoma (PTC) oncogene

VARIANTS
Follicular variant: almost entirely follicles but with nuclear features, fibrous trabeculae, psammoma bodies; behaves as conventional papillary carcinoma
Papillary microcarcinoma: 1 cm or less in diameter, usually incidental, cervical LN metastases in one third, distant metastases rare, excellent prognosis
Encapsulated variant: totally surrounded by capsule; may still have LN metastases, but no distant metastases; excellent prognosis
Diffuse sclerosing variant: diffuse involvement of one or both lobes, dense sclerosis, numerous psammoma bodies, squamous metaplasia, heavy inflammation; widespread LN metastases usually present, lung metastases common; worse prognosis than conventional papillary carcinoma; differential diagnosis: Hashimoto's thyroiditis
Tall cell variant: abundant eosinophilic cytoplasm; often lymphocytic infiltrate; worse prognosis
Columnar variant: like tall cell, but with nuclear stratification
Oxyphilic variant: see Hürthle cell carcinoma

SPREAD
Extrathyroid extension in 25%
Cervical LN involvement in ~50%; often cystic changes
Hematogenous spread less common than in other thyroid carcinomas

PROGNOSIS
Poor prognosis: >40 yr old, male, extrathyroid extension, large tumor size, nonencapsulated, multicentricity, distant metastases, aneuploidy
Anaplastic foci develop in 1%; essentially all die
Not related to prognosis: relative amounts of papillae vs. follicles, history of irradiation, fibrosis, squamous metaplasia, positive cervical LNs

MEDULLARY CARCINOMA

AKA: parafollicular cell, solid, hyaline, C-cell carcinoma
5–10% of thyroid carcinomas
Solid, firm, well circumscribed
More common in upper half of gland (more C cells)
Marked variation in cytologic appearance: round to polygonal cells with granular cytoplasm in carcinoid-like nests, trabecular, glandular, or pseudopapillary configurations; highly vascular stroma, hyalinized collagen, *amyloid,* coarse calcification, may see psammoma bodies
Most produce calcitonin; some also produce prostaglandins, histaminase, adrenocorticotropic hormone (ACTH), VIP, or serotonin, CEA
May have many neutrophils (inflammatory type)
Cells may be spindle shaped or even anaplastic
Immunoreactive for keratin, NSE, chromogranin, synaptophysin, calcitonin, CEA; negative for thyroglobulin
Spread via lymphatics and blood; metastases to LNs, lung, liver, bone
Sporadic and MEN III more prone to metastasize than MEN II
Treatment is surgical; 5 yr survival 70–80%; 10 yr ~50%

Prognosis better for young, female, familial, confined to gland, extensive amyloid

SPORADIC FORM
Accounts for 80% of cases
Adults, mean age 45, solitary, cold thyroid mass

FAMILIAL
Younger (mean age 35), often multiple and bilateral
C-cell hyperplasia in residual gland
Autosomal dominant inheritance
Belongs to MEN type II and III; also von Hippel–Lindau, neurofibromatosis
Treatment: total thyroidectomy

HÜRTHLE CELL TUMORS
More than 50% Hürthle cells
Some consider this a variant of follicular carcinoma
Usually adult females
Solid, tan, well vascularized, usually encapsulated
Usually follicular, may be trabecular/solid or papillary
Granular, acidophilic cytoplasm (filled with mitochondria)
Tumors with follicular pattern should be assessed (benign or malignant) as follicular lesions: capsular/vascular invasion; solid/trabecular areas and small cells favor carcinoma
Carcinomas tend to be aggressive: 20–40% 5 yr survival

POORLY DIFFERENTIATED CARCINOMA
AKA: insular carcinoma
Older age group, usually grossly invasive
Nesting pattern of growth, small uniform cells, necrosis
Not immunoreactive for thyroglobulin or calcitonin
May arise in well-differentiated carcinoma
60% mortality

ANAPLASTIC CARCINOMA
AKA: undifferentiated or sarcomatoid carcinoma
Rapidly growing mass, elderly, with dyspnea/dysphagia
Highly necrotic/hemorrhagic mass
Three major patterns:
• Squamoid: may even keratinize
• Spindle cell: storiform; may form bone/cartilage
• Giant Cell: usually scattered among spindle cell pattern
Usually arise within pre-existing tumor, usually papillary carcinoma
Essentially 100% mortality (mean survival 6 months), usually from local extension into neck structures

OTHER EPITHELIAL TUMORS
CLEAR CELL TUMORS
Can see clear cell change in any of the thyroid tumors
Most common in Hürthle cells (swelling of mitochondria) but can also see in papillary (glycogen accumulation)
No change in prognosis
Differential diagnosis: metastatic renal cell, parathyroid
EPIDERMOID CARCINOMA
Usually represents extensive squamous metaplasia or anaplastic carcinoma
MUCOEPIDERMOID CARCINOMA
Probably variant of papillary with mucinous and squamous metaplasia
THYMOMA
Perhaps arises from intrathyroid ectopic thymus tissue
SMALL CELL CARCINOMA
Probably poorly differentiated form of medullary carcinoma

PARAGANGLIOMA
Not primary to thyroid, but to nearby carotid body
May be confused with medullary carcinoma
S-100 positive sustentacular cells at periphery of zellballen

Non-Epithelial Neoplasms

MALIGNANT LYMPHOMA
Most common in elderly females; often arise in setting of lymphocytic or Hashimoto's thyroiditis
Often rapid enlargement
Euthyroid; one or more cold nodules
Solid, white fish flesh
Example of mucosa associated lymphoid tissue (MALT) lymphoma; most are diffuse large cell, follicular center cell origin; immunoblastic, lymphoplasmacytic are also seen
Packing of follicles with lymphocytes is a diagnostic feature; usually not seen in thyroiditis
Better prognosis if restricted to thyroid; if recurs, may recur in GI tract

PLASMACYTOMA
Local disease or manifestation of widespread myeloma
Reserve for tumors composed entirely of plasma cells

TERATOMA
Infants or children—cystic and benign
Rarely in adults—usually malignant

Metastases

Most common primary sites:

Skin (melanoma)	39%
Breast	21%
Kidney	12%
Lung	11%

PARATHYROID

NORMAL ANATOMY
Normally, four glands, each 4 × 3 × 1.5 mm, with an average aggregate weight of 120 mg (slightly higher in women)
25% of individuals have >4 glands, usually 5; 6 or <4 is rare
Chief cell: predominant cell type; centrally located nucleus, pale granular cytoplasm, ill-defined cell margins
Oxyphil cell: more cytoplasm, oncocytic, mitochondria
Clear (Wasserhelle) cells: not present in normal gland
Oxyphil cells appear soon after puberty and increase in number with age, forming islands after 40; probably derived from chief cells
Fat infiltration also begins at puberty
Follicles with "colloid" may be present; can be distinguished from thyroid by presence of glycogen in cells and absence of oxalate crystals
Parathormone: regulates calcium metabolism (in conjunction with vitamin D and calcitonin) secreted in response to low calcium; increases renal excretion of phosphate

and renal and intestinal reabsorption of calcium, and activates osteoclasts via osteoblasts (receptors are on the osteoblasts; they secrete factors that activate the osteoclasts)

EMBRYOLOGY

Upper pair arises from fourth branchial cleft; descends into neck with the thyroid; resides in middle third of posterolateral part of thyroid

Lower pair arises from third branchial cleft (initially above superior pair); descends with thymus to lie near inferior thyroid artery at lower pole of thyroid

Anomalous locations include carotid sheath, behind the esophagus, anterior mediastinum, intrathyroidal

CLINICAL SYNDROMES

Hyperparathyroidism

PRIMARY HYPERPARATHYROIDISM

Increased parathormone secretion almost always caused by adenoma or chief cell hyperplasia; carcinoma in <4%

Usually adults, can be familial, seen in MEN I and MEN IIa

Relationship exists with neck radiation and with sarcoidosis

Hypercalcemia, hypophosphatemia, duodenal peptic ulcers

• Osteitis fibrosa cystica (brown tumor, Recklinghausen's disease): expansile multilocular mass, often jaw, alternating solid and cystic areas, hemosiderin deposition, giant cells; reversible with removal of hyperfunctioning gland(s)

• Renal changes: renal stones, nephrocalcinosis

SECONDARY HYPERPARATHYROIDISM

Chronic renal disease (more common; vitamin D resistant) or intestinal malabsorption, increased serum phosphorus, decreased serum calcium; chief cell hyperplasia results

TERTIARY HYPERPARATHYROIDISM

Patients with secondary hyperparathyroidism in whom one or more parathyroid has become autonomous

Therapy for Hyperparathyroidism

Identify all four glands; if all appear normal, look for 5th, usually in the mediastinum; if can't find four, consider intrathyroid location

If one enlarged, remove (probably adenoma) and biopsy at least one other to rule out chief cell hyperplasia

For chief cell hyperplasia, subtotal parathyroidectomy (remove all of three glands, all but 30–50 mg of 4th)

Alternatively, remove all glands with autotransplantation of tissue into forearm muscle

Hypoparathyroidism

Hypocalcemia, mental changes, calcification of lens, calcification of basal ganglia (Parkinson's), cardiac conduction defects

Usually results from accidental surgical ablation

Hyperplasia/Neoplasia

CHIEF CELL HYPERPLASIA

AKA: primary nodular hyperplasia

Classically, all glands are enlarged (10 g or more!), tan to reddish, with superior glands larger than inferior glands

Pseudoadenomatous: one gland much larger than others

Parathyromatosis: numerous microscopic foci of hyperplastic parathyroid in neck; rare

Mostly chief cells, often grouped in nodules; may see fibrous septa, giant nuclei

In secondary hyperparathyroidism, can have significant variability; usually fewer giant nuclei and more oxyphil cells

Only reliable distinguishing feature from adenoma is presence of some normal parathyroid tissue in patients with adenoma

WATER-CLEAR CELL HYPERPLASIA

Rare, no familial incidence

Extreme enlargement of all glands (>100 g!), in which the superior glands are distinctly larger than the inferior glands

Optically clear cytoplasm (numerous clear vacuoles); cells vary significantly in size; giant nuclei are not seen

Associated with primary hyperparathyroidism

Entity has essentially disappeared in past few decades

ADENOMA

Male : female = 1 : 3; usually in 30s; usually too small to be palpable

75% involve inferior gland, 15% superior, 10% anomalous (of these, 70% mediastinal, 20% intrathyroid)

Encapsulated, very cellular, often with rim of compressed normal parathyroid tissue

Usually chief cells predominate, other cell types can be seen

Marked variation in nuclear size and hyperchromatic nuclei favor benign rather than malignant diagnosis

Mitoses rare

Diffuse growth usually; may be nesting, follicular, papillary

By electron microscopy (EM), may see both large amounts of glycogen and secretory vacuoles (in normal cells, only one or other)

OXYPHIL ADENOMA

Variant composed almost entirely of oxyphil cells

Most are nonfunctioning

LIPOADENOMA

AKA: lipohyperplasia, hamartoma, adenoma with myxoid stroma

Abundant mature adipose tissue; usually circumscribed

Usually functioning

PARATHYROID CARCINOMA

Typically presents with hyperparathyroidism

If nonfunctioning, more aggressive

May coexist with chief cell hyperplasia or adenoma

Very high serum calcium, palpable mass, vocal cord paralysis favor carcinoma

Trabecular arrangement of cells, dense fibrous bands, spindled tumor cells, mitotic figures, capsular invasion, vascular invasion

Treatment: removal of lesion, surrounding soft tissue, ipsilateral lobe of thyroid

Recurrence within 2 yr ominous prognostic sign

ADRENAL CORTEX

Normal

Normal adult weight 4–5 g

Derived from urogenital ridge; mesodermal in origin

Before birth: white "fetal zone": large, plump eosinophilic cells

After birth, fetal zone involutes, leaving only outermost layer, which differentiates into a 1 mm thick three-zone cortex

- Zona glomerulosa: 10–15% cortex; few lipid droplets, anastomosing network of smooth endoplasmic reticulum (SER), normal mitochondrial cristae (lamellar); mineralocorticoids, and most importantly aldosterone (major regulator of extracellular fluid volume and potassium metabolism)
- Zona fasciculata: 80% cortex; cords of cells with lipid vacuoles (grossly yellow), elaborate SER, stacks of granular endoplasmic reticulum, prominent Golgi apparatus, mitochondria have tubulovesicular cristae
- Zona reticularis: similar to fasciculata but much less lipid and therefore more eosinophilic (grossly brown)

Fasciculata and reticularis both responsible for producing glucocorticoids (e.g., cortisol) and androgens (testosterone) under control of pituitary ACTH (39 amino acid peptide derived from pro-opiomelanocortin)

Congenital Abnormalities

ECTOPIC ADRENAL

Usually in retroperitoneum, anywhere along the urogenital ridge from diaphragm to pelvis

Usually composed only of cortex

Small rests also occasionally found subcapsularly in kidney, in the hilar region of the testis or ovary, or in hernia sacs

CONGENITAL ADRENAL HYPOPLASIA

ANENCEPHALIC TYPE

Only provisional cortex; no fetal zone

Infants are anencephalic and stillborn

CYTOMEGALIC TYPE

Adrenals have combined weight <1 g

Cortex consists of large (3–5× normal) eosinophilic cells

Unknown etiology; possibly X-linked or autosomal recessive

CONGENITAL ADRENAL HYPERPLASIA

Most common congenital adrenal disorder

Actually ≥8 distinct clinical syndromes, all with congenital deficiency of a specific enzyme (autosomal recessive)

Most common is deficiency of 21-hydroxylase

Completed cortisol cannot be produced; elevated ACTH results in adrenal hyperplasia; shunting of intermediates to other pathways often results in virilization of external genitalia in girls (adrenogenital syndrome)

Hypoadrenalism

PRIMARY CHRONIC ADRENOCORTICAL INSUFFICIENCY (ADDISON'S DISEASE)

Any condition that destroys >90% of the adrenal cortex produces this clinical picture

Insidious development of weakness, fatigability, anorexia, nausea and vomiting, weight loss, hypotension, hyperpigmentation (from elevated pro-opiomelanocortin peptides)

Two most common causes are idiopathic adrenitis/atrophy (probably autoimmune) and tuberculosis; others include amyloidosis, hemochromatosis, metastatic carcinoma

In general, cortex is atrophic with variable amounts of chronic inflammatory cells

Autoimmune Addison's disease divided into two types:

- Type I: at least two of: Addison's disease, hypoparathyroidism, mucocutaneous candidiasis; defect in suppressor T-cell function
- Type II (Schmidt's syndrome): Addison's disease, autoimmune thyroid disease, and/or insulin-dependent diabetes mellitus; associated with HLA-A1 and -B8

PRIMARY ACUTE ADRENOCORTICAL INSUFFICIENCY

Can develop as a crisis in patients with Addison's disease, (precipitated by stress), following too rapid withdrawal of steroids (suppressed endogenous production recovers slowly), or can result from massive hemorrhage

In neonates, can see massive hemorrhage following prolonged or difficult delivery, presumably secondary to hypoxia or trauma

WATERHOUSE-FRIDERICHSEN SYNDROME

Hemorrhagic destruction of the adrenals related to bacterial infection

Meningococcemia by far most common cause; others include pneumococci, staphylococci, *Haemophilus influenzae*

Widespread petechiae, purpura, hemorrhages throughout body, particularly skin and mucosal surfaces

Adrenals hemorrhagic and necrotic; sometimes merely sacs of blood clot

SECONDARY ADRENOCORTICAL INSUFFICIENCY

Any disorder of hypothalamus or pituitary resulting in decreased levels of ACTH

Since tropic hormones are low, do *not* see hyperpigmentation

May also be seen in setting of exogenous corticosteroids

Hyperadrenalism

CUSHING'S SYNDROME

Clinical features include impaired glucose tolerance (overt diabetes in 20%), moon facies, "buffalo hump," abdominal striae, loss of libido, vascular fragility with skin hemorrhages

PITUITARY CUSHING'S SYNDROME (60–70%)

Bilateral adrenal hyperplasia caused by an elevation of ACTH levels, usually caused by a pituitary adenoma (Cushing's disease)

Suppressible by high doses of dexamethasone

Hyperplasia is usually diffuse but sometimes nodular

ADRENAL CUSHING'S SYNDROME (20–25%)

Functioning neoplasm of adrenal cortex, usually adenoma

Low serum ACTH, symptoms not suppressible by high doses of dexamethasone

ECTOPIC CUSHING'S SYNDROME (10–15%)

ACTH or compound with similar biologic activity elaborated by a non-endocrine neoplasm, most commonly bronchogenic carcinoma (60%), malignant thymoma (15%)

Not suppressible by high doses of dexamethasone

IATROGENIC CUSHING'S SYNDROME
Patients on chronic steroids, usually transplant recipients or those with autoimmune disorders

PRIMARY HYPERALDOSTERONISM
AKA: Conn's syndrome

Hypertension, neuromuscular symptoms, renal potassium wasting, elevated aldosterone levels *in the absence of elevated renin levels*

Unlike secondary hyperaldosteronism, generally do *not* see edema with Conn's syndrome

Almost invariably caused by adrenocortical adenoma

Aldosterone secreting adenomas usually <2 cm, bright yellow, nonencapsulated, mixed cell types (see later)

ADRENAL VIRILISM
Most readily recognized in females

Caused by androgen-secreting adenomas; generally larger than adenomas associated with Cushing's syndrome, often highly pigmented

Adrenal Cortical Neoplasms

ADENOMA/CARCINOMA
Bright yellow tumors

Varying mixtures of clear and compact cells, similar to those of the normal zona fasciculata; compact cells may predominate

Adenomas generally weigh 40–60 g and measure <5 cm; carcinomas >100 g and/or >5 cm

Adenomas may be difficult to distinguish from hyperplastic nodule; if residual cortex is normal or atrophic, probably an adenoma

Carcinomas are more likely to show necrosis, broad fibrous bands, nuclear anaplasia, high nuclear:cytoplasmic ratio, high mitotic activity, vascular invasion, capsular invasion; rapidly lethal

Many adenomas and carcinomas are functional, but not all

MYELOLIPOMA
Usually asymptomatic and benign

Sharply circumscribed nonencapsulated pale-yellow cortical lesion

Fat cells admixed with myeloid cells and lymphocytes

OTHER TUMORS
Adenomatoid tumor

Ovarian thecal metaplasia

Metastatic tumors: usually from lung, breast, GI tract, thyroid, kidney

ADRENAL MEDULLA

Normal
Derived from neural crest

A component of the sympathetic paraganglia

Body's major source of epinephrine (adrenaline)

Epinephrine:norepinephrine ratio is usually 5–6:1

Tyrosine → dihydroxyphenylalanine → dopamine occurs in cytoplasm; dopamine then enters granules and is converted to norepinephrine; norepinephrine must then re-enter the cytoplasm for conversion to epinephrine, which then re-enters the secretory granules

Major breakdown products of catecholamines include metanephrine, normetanephrine, vanillylmandelic acid (VMA), and homovanillic acid (HVA)

NEUROBLASTOMA
One of the most common solid tumors of childhood (7–10% of all childhood malignancies); equal frequency with Wilms' tumor, but occurs at an earlier age

80% occur in children under 5 yr; 35% in children under 2 yr

50–80% of neuroblastomas occur in adrenal or adjacent retroperitoneal tissues; posterior mediastinum is 2nd most common location (15–20%), cervical sympathetic chain (5%)

Large tumors (6–8 cm on average), soft, white lobular cut section with focal to extensive hemorrhage, necrosis, cyst formation; dystrophic calcification common

Small cells with hyperchromatic nuclei arranged in solid sheets or in small nests separated by fibrovascular septa; Homer-Wright pseudorosettes around tangled eosinophilic fibrils

90% of tumors will produce catecholamines; urinary VMA elevated in about three quarters of cases

NSE positive; stroma contains S-100 positive Schwann cells

Often, deletion of chromosome 1p is seen

N-*myc* amplified in ~30% of tumors (often as double minutes or homogeneously staining regions; associated with translocation to tip of 1p); when present at >10 copies, associated with a poor prognosis

trk oncogene expression seen in lower stage, younger patients; good prognosis: tumors more likely to differentiate, regress, or respond to therapy

Metastases occur early and widely

Hutchinson-type neuroblastoma: extensive bony metastases, particularly to the skull and orbit, producing exophthalmos

Pepper-type syndrome: massive metastases to the liver

GANGLIONEUROBLASTOMA
>5% maturation to ganglion cells, with residual areas of immature blastoma

Two types:
- Composite: nodules of neuroblastoma in a ganglioneuroma
- Diffuse: both elements distributed throughout tumor; better prognosis than composite type

GANGLIONEUROMA
All mature elements: fibrous and Schwann cell–rich stromal background with scattered ganglion cells

Staging

Commonly Used Staging Scheme		2 Yr Survival
Stage I	Confined to structure/organ of origin	95–100%
Stage II	Beyond site of origin; don't cross midline	85–90%
Stage III	Across midline, ± LN metastases	50–60%
Stage IV	Metastatic disease, usually to skeleton	10–15%
Stage IVs	I or II with microscopic metastases to skin, liver, marrow; usually <1 yr old; good prognosis	60–65%

Clinical TNM		Pathologic TNM	
T1	Single tumor ≤5 cm	T1	Completely excised
T2	Single tumor 5–10 cm	T2	N/A
T3	Single tumor >10 cm	T3	Multicentric tumors
T4	Multicentric tumors	T3a	Residual tumor
		T3b	Microscopic
		T3c	Macroscopic
		T4	Unresected
N1	Regional LNs	N1a	Resected regional LNs
		N1b	Incomplete resection

	T1	T2	T3	T4
N0	I	II		
N1	III			IVB
M1	IVA			

	T1	T3a	T3b	T3c	T4
N0	I				
N1a	II	IIIA			
N1b	IIIB				IVB
M1	IVA				

Prognosis

Good: Better differentiated tumors; high ratio of urinary VMA:HVA; stage IVs; young age (<1 yr); extra-adrenal, aneuploidy

Bad: High levels of ferritin or NSE; N-*myc* amplification; adrenal; >5 yr old

PHEOCHROMOCYTOMA

AKA: intra-adrenal paraganglioma

Usually induces marked hypertension secondary to catecholamine production

Usually secrete more norepinephrine than epinephrine

Peak incidence in 30s–40s

When same tumor occurs outside of the adrenal medulla, it is referred to as an extra-adrenal paraganglioma; 70–90% of paragangliomas are intra-adrenal; 10–20% are bilateral

5% of the adrenal tumors are malignant; 10–50% when extra-adrenal

80–90% are sporadic; rest associated with familial syndromes (MEN IIA or IIB)

1–4000 g; average weight is 100 g

Usually well demarcated; well-vascularized fibrous trabeculae divide tumor into lobular pattern; pale gray to light brown

Hemorrhage, necrosis, cysts common

Cytologic appearance varies widely from mature chromaffin cells with abundant basophilic cytoplasm and secretory granules to marked cellular and nuclear pleomorphism

Tumor cells often grow in small clusters (zellballen) separated by thin fibrovascular stroma

Mitotic figures are rare but do not imply malignancy

Vascular invasion may be seen; does not necessarily make it malignant

Features of malignancy: capsular invasion, numerous mitoses, necrosis, solid/diffuse growth pattern without nests or with large nests, spindled cells, aneuploidy; however, diagnosis of malignancy cannot be made by histologic criteria alone

Complications include catecholamine cardiomyopathy

Metastases may occur very late in disease

EXTRA-ADRENAL PARAGANGLIOMA

Same tumor as pheochromocytoma, but occurring outside of the adrenal gland

Generally named by site:
- Chemodactoma: carotid body
- Jugulotympanic paraganglioma (glomus jugulare; glomus tympanicum)
- Vagal paraganglioma (glomus vagale)
- Mediastinal

PITUITARY

Normal

0.5 g in adult; 10–15 mm in greatest dimension

Three "lobes": anterior (adenohypophysis), intermediate, and posterior (neurohypophysis)

Anterior lobe derived from evagination of the roof of the primitive oral canal known as Rathke's pouch

Posterior lobe develops as an outpouching of the floor of the 3rd ventricle near the hypothalamus

Pharyngeal pituitary gland: ~90% of autopsies can show small amount of pituitary tissue in roof of nasopharynx; comprises <1% of total adenohypophyseal mass in body

Portal blood supply: 1st capillary bed in floor of 3rd ventricle (hypothalamus) and 2nd in anterior lobe

In general, each cell of the anterior pituitary secretes only one hormone (exception: FSH and LH made by same cells)

25–50% of anterior pituitary cells do not stain for any specific hormones or with H&E (chromophobes) and have only a few granules by EM

Acidophils: somatotrophs (30%) and mamotrophs (20%); more concentrated in lateral portions of the anterior lobe

Basophils: corticotrophs (15%), gonadotrophs (20%), and thyrotrophs (10%); more numerous in central portion of anterior lobe

Anterior pituitary hormones:

Glycoproteins: α and β subunits; αs same, βs unique

TSH	Thyrotropin (thyroid stimulating hormone)
LH	Luteinizing hormone
FSH	Follicle stimulating hormone

Nonglycosylated protein

PRL	Prolactin
ACTH	Adrenocorticotrophin
GH	Growth hormone

Hormone release from the anterior pituitary is controlled by releasing hormones from the hypothalamus

TRH	Stimulates TSH and prolactin release
GnRH	Stimulates LH and FSH release
Dopamine	Inhibits prolactin
Somatostatin	Inhibits GH and TSH

Posterior pituitary releases vasopressin (ADH) and oxytocin, which are synthesized by cell bodies in the hypothalamus and travel along axons to the posterior pituitary

During pregnancy, tumors of the pituitary often result in enlargement of the sella turcica by x-ray, computed tomography (CT), or magnetic resonance imaging (MRI); visual disturbances (bilateral homonymous hemianopsia); rarely increased intracranial pressure

HYPERPITUITARISM

Generally age 20–50; rarely (3%) associated with MEN I
Hyperpituitarism may be hypothalamic in origin; however, almost all cases are caused by a secreting tumor, almost always an adenoma:

Prolactinoma	30%	Amenorrhea, galactorrhea
Growth hormone	17%	Gigantism, acromegaly
Mixed GH, prolactin	10%	
ACTH	14%	Cushing's disease
LH and FSH	3%	
TSH	<1%	
Nonfunctional	23%	

Adenomas account for ~10% of intracranial tumors
Adenomas may be <1 cm or >10 cm
Microadenomas (<1 cm) can be found in 25–40% of patients at autopsy
Generally poorly encapsulated, if at all; may invade surrounding structures, even bone
Monomorphous population of cells in sheets, cords, nests, sometimes pseudoglandular or papillary; obliterate the normal acinar pattern; cells may show marked nuclear pleomorphism
Invasion into surrounding structures (seen in 35%) does not necessarily mean malignancy; carcinomas of the anterior pituitary are very rare; in general, to call a lesion malignant need evidence of metastasis
Occasionally, completely infarcts ("apoplexy"): clinical picture changes from hyperpituitarism to hypopituitarism

PROLACTINOMA
Male : female = 1 : 2; present with amenorrhea/galactorrhea or impotence
Cells are granular by H&E
EM shows misplaced exocytosis of granules

GROWTH HORMONE SECRETING ADENOMA
Produces acromegaly and/or gigantism, depending on whether develops before or after closure of epiphyseal plates
Most cases present in 30s; decreases life span by 10 yr
30% of patients are hypertensive
Cells are granular by H&E
EM shows "fibrous body," composed of 7–8 nm filaments and granules, near the nucleus

ADRENAL-CORTICOTROPINOMA
>80% of patients have Cushing's syndrome (disease)
80–90% are microadenomas; rarely see visual disturbances
EM shows 7 nm filaments throughout the cytoplasm
• Nelson's syndrome: adenomatous enlargement of pituitary with a carcinomatous histologic picture, including local invasion and metastases, hyperpigmentation, expansion of sella turcica; occurs in patients from whom an ACTH-secreting pituitary tumor cannot be resected and who are therefore treated with bilateral adrenalectomy

GONADOTROPINOMA
Almost always male
Present with visual impairment, impotence, loss of libido
See elevation of FSH most commonly

HYPOPITUITARISM
Generally caused by destruction of >75% of anterior lobe
Occasionally, results from hypothalamic destruction or malfunction
Usually results in pan-hypopituitarism
Clinically, sequence of detection of dysfunction is usually gonadotropins, GH (before puberty), TSH, ACTH, lastly PRL

NONSECRETORY (CHROMOPHOBE) ADENOMA
Hormone deficits develop slowly over years, so tumors generally large at time of diagnosis
Both null (clear) cell adenomas and oncocytic adenomas

SHEEHAN'S SYNDROME
AKA: postpartum pituitary necrosis
Sudden infarction following obstetric hemorrhage or shock, perhaps because enlarges with pregnancy and requires a greater blood supply
Incidence increased in patients with longstanding diabetes
Occasionally seen in nonpregnant females or in males (in setting of disseminated intravascular coagulation, sickle cell anemia)

PITUITARY INFARCTION
Can occur independent of pregnancy; seen with hypertension, diabetes, arteriosclerosis, trauma
Usually does not involve the posterior pituitary (different blood supply)
As long as about one third of gland remains viable, usually asymptomatic

LYMPHOCYTIC HYPOPHYSITIS
Rare; associated with postpartum hypopituitarism, but can be seen in men
May be autoimmune in origin
Present with amenorrhea, galactorrhea, thyroiditis
Atrophic acini separated by lymphocytes

EMPTY SELLA SYNDROME
Primary: herniation of arachnoid through defect in sellar diaphragm with increased cerebrospinal fluid (CSF) pressure and atrophy of pituitary; most commonly obese, middle age, multiparous females; often asymptomatic
Secondary: Sheehan's syndrome, apoplexy, surgery

CRANIOPHARYNGIOMA
AKA: adamantinoma or ameloblastoma
Derived from Rathke's pouch
Anastomosing epithelial islands with cysts, straw-colored fluid, giant cells, often calcifications

CROOKE'S HYALINE DEGENERATION OF THE BASOPHILS
Glassy perinuclear cytoplasm displacing the basophilic cytoplasm to the periphery
Seen in ACTH-producing cells of the pituitary in setting of Cushing's syndrome or exogenous cortisol therapy with chronically elevated cortisol levels and subsequent feedback inhibition to corticotrophs

OTHER CAUSES
Metastatic tumors
Disruption of blood supply (vasculitis, thrombosis)
Inflammatory destruction
Rathke's cleft cyst
Surgical or radiation ablation

POSTERIOR PITUITARY SYNDROMES

ADH DEFICIENCY (DIABETES INSIPIDUS)
Polyuria and excessive thirst
Neoplastic or inflammatory destruction; surgical or radiation injury, severe head injury, idiopathic

SYNDROME OF INAPPROPRIATE ADH RELEASE (SIADH)
Abnormal retention of water with expansion of extracellular fluid volume, hyponatremia, hemodilution
Usually paraneoplastic in origin

23

SKIN

INFLAMMATORY LESIONS

The numerous environmental agents to which the skin is continuously exposed and the easy accessibility of this organ to the biopsy knife have led to a tremendous number of pathologic "entities" with names ranging from the mundane to the exotic

This outline does not pretend to represent in any way a comprehensive coverage of these entities but rather more of a sampling of the diversity that exists

The reader is referred to any of a number of texts specifically on the skin for a more detailed coverage

General Terminology

Macule: Flat discoloration ≤1 cm

Patch: Flat discoloration >1 cm

Papule: Solid elevation ≤1 cm

Plaque: Flat, solid elevation >1 cm

Nodule: Round, solid, elevated lesion >1 cm

Vesicle: Small, fluid-filled blister ≤1 cm

Bulla: Fluid-filled blister >1 cm

Telangiectasia: Dilated vessels

Scale: Visible cornified cells

Crust: Serum within scale

Acanthosis: Thickening of the epidermal layer

Lichenification: Thickening of skin from chronic rubbing

Hyperkeratosis: Increased thickness of cornified layer

Parakeratosis: Hyperkeratosis and residual pyknotic nuclei

Hypergranulosis: Thick granular cell layer (slow turnover)

Hypogranulosis: Thin granular cell layer (fast turnover)

Spongiosis: Intercellular edema

Ballooning: Intracellular edema

Acantholysis: Loss of cell–cell adhesion

Vacuolar changes: Small separations above and below basement membrane

Dyskeratosis: Premature keratinization in spinous layer

Papillomatosis: Elongation of dermal papillae

Inflammatory Dermatoses

ACUTE DERMATITIS (ECZEMA)
Gross and histologic appearance varies with site and duration

Early: erythema, aggregates of tiny pruritic vesicles that rupture easily, exuding clear fluid, crusted

Chronic lesions: scaly, thickened

Spongiosis, vesicularization, exocytosis are key features

Mild acanthosis to psoriasiform epidermal hyperplasia

Parakeratosis over spongiotic foci, hyperkeratosis over chronic lesions

Superficial perivascular mixed inflammation

An important differential diagnosis is cutaneous T-cell lymphoma (CTCL)

ATOPIC DERMATITIS
Associated with asthma and hay fever (excess IgE)

Usually starts ~6 wk of age on head and neck

Progresses to flexural aspects of limbs; often symmetric

Intense pruritus, lichenification; vesiculation rare

SEBORRHEIC DERMATITIS
Infants to early teens onward

Scalp, forehead, eyebrows, eyelids, ears, cheeks, chest

Erythema and scaling

Similar to psoriasis, but spongiosis is present

NUMMULAR (DISCOID) DERMATITIS
Pruritic coin-shaped plaques on lower legs, backs of hands, forearms

Women (15–30 yr) and middle-aged males

Pronounced spongiosis

STASIS (VARICOSE) DERMATITIS
Usually medial lower ankle; impaired venous return

Ulceration with increased risk of malignancy at margins

Hemosiderin deposition, fibrosis, new blood vessels

CONTACT DERMATITIS
Allergic (e.g., poison ivy, nickel) and irritant (e.g., soaps) types (irritant does not require prior sensitization)

Distribution initially confined to areas of exposure

Lichen Simplex Chronicus
Chronic form of any of above with irritation and trauma

Epidermis undergoes a psoriasiform thickening, but with an increased thickness of the granular layer

Scarring and broadening of dermal papillae

207

PSORIASIS

Common; affects 1–2% of population; chronic relapsing
Typically ~27 yr old; elbows, knees, scalp
Plaque (sharply demarcated, scaly surface; removing scales with fingernail results in small droplets of blood: Auspitz's sign—diagnostic)
Guttate (eruptive: small lesions on trunk, proximal extremities)
Pustular (sterile 2–3 mm pustules over trunk and limbs following fever, with surrounding generalized erythema)
Parakeratosis, hyperkeratosis: cells undergoing rapid turnover with thinning or absence of granular cell layer
Flaky scale with inflammatory cells in groups in scale
Acanthosis with long rete ridges and thinning of epidermis over dermal papillae
Extravasated RBCs in dermis
Pustular variant: intraepidermal (between granular and cornified layers) vesicle with essentially all neutrophils (Munro's microabscesses)

LICHEN PLANUS

Itchy, flat-topped purple papules with white dots (fine scale)
Most common on extremities: wrist, elbow, glans penis
4th–6th decades, idiopathic, self-limited
Hyperplasia of stratum granulosum (slowed turnover)
Basal cell hydropic changes/liquefaction—eosinophilic "colloid" bodies
Saw-toothed rete ridges (irregular epidermal hyperplasia)
Tight superficial dermal *bandlike* chronic inflammation, filling papillary dermis

LICHEN PLANOPILARIS
Variant that preferentially affects epithelium of hair follicles

VESICULAR AND BULLOUS DISEASES
(See also Acute Dermatitis)

Miliaria
Caused by eccrine duct obstruction
Most commonly seen on trunk and intertriginous regions

MILIARIA CRYSTALLINA
Obstruction in stratum corneum, with subcorneal vesicles containing a few neutrophils
Tiny vesicles ("water droplets")

MILIARIA RUBRA
Obstruction in "prickle" cell layer, creating an intraepidermal spongiotic vesicle
Multiple tiny erythematous papules

Pemphigus
Rare autoimmune disorder with blistering, which results from loss of integrity of the normal intercellular attachments within the epidermis
Usually 40–60 yr old; male = female
Blisters induced by rubbing "normal" skin (Nikolsky's sign)
Histologic common denominator is acantholysis

PEMPHIGUS VULGARIS
Most common type (accounts for 80% of cases)
Mucosa and skin, esp. scalp, face, axilla, groin, trunk
Fragile blisters that readily rupture, leaving a painful, crusted, bloody erosion

Preferentially involves layer immediately above basal layer, creating a *suprabasal* cleft or bulla; remaining basal cells tombstone into lumen of blister
Antibody to adherens junction
Treatment with high-dose corticosteroids has reduced mortality

PEMPHIGUS VEGETANS
Rare form; large, moist, warty plaque studded with pustules
Similar histology to vulgaris, but with overlying epidermal hyperplasia

PEMPHIGUS FOLIACEUS
More benign form, endemic in South America
Scalp, face, trunk; mucous membranes rarely involved
More *superficial* blisters seen, selectively involving the stratum granulosum or subcorneal layer
Numerous neutrophils may be present
Antibody to desmoglian

PEMPHIGUS ERYTHEMATOSUS
Localized and less severe form of pemphigus foliaceus
Restricted to malar region of face

Other Vesicular and Bullous Diseases

GROVER'S DISEASE
AKA: transient acantholytic dermatitis
Self-limited acantholysis of unknown etiology
Intensely pruritic linear pattern of papules, vesicles, plaques, excoriations on chest, back, thighs
Suprabasal splitting—can mimic pemphigus vulgaris, Darier's, Hailey-Hailey

TOXIC EPIDERMAL NECROLYSIS
AKA: Lyell's syndrome (note: term originally used to refer to scalded skin syndrome in infants)
Probably extreme form of erythema multiforme
Widespread, tender, erythematous rash; flaccid, fluid-filled bullae that rupture
Positive Nikolsky's sign (blister on rubbing)
Some cases may be related to drug, sepsis, lymphoma
Appreciable mortality
Extreme epidermal necrosis with *subepidermal* blistering
Mild dermal perivascular monocytic infiltrate

BULLOUS PEMPHIGOID
May present at any age, usually in 70s
Typically inner thighs, flexor surfaces of arms, groin, axilla, abdomen; spares face and scalp
Large, tense bullae, some with blood, on "normal" skin
Anti–basement membrane antibody (Ab) in serum (usually IgG), resulting in a linear direct immunofluorescent pattern for Ig and complement
Subepidermal, fluid-filled blister with eosinophils and serum without acantholysis
Inflammatory cell-rich and cell-poor variants
Edema in dermis
Increased risk of other autoimmune diseases
Usually controllable by corticosteroids

DERMATITIS HERPETIFORMIS
Intensely pruritic papulovesicular eruption involving the extensor surfaces, scalp, shoulders, buttocks; 25–50 yr old
Granular deposits of IgA at dermal-epidermal junction at the tips of the dermal papillae
Subepidermal, (blister forms below the basement membrane), multilocular vesicles with neutrophils and eosinophils; dermal papillary neutrophilic microabscesses
All patients have some form of gluten-sensitive enteropathy, 65–75% fulfilling the criteria for celiac sprue

Long-term gluten-free diet can cure both the enteropathy and the skin lesions

Skin lesions respond to dapsone (enteropathy does not)

Patients (especially males) have an increased risk of developing non-Hodgkin's lymphoma

EPIDERMOLYSIS BULLOSUM ACQUISITA

Acquired predisposition to blistering following mild trauma

Onset in adulthood; *not* inflammatory

Vesicles/bullae on dorsal fingers, wrists, feet, elbows, knees

Blood or fibrin, generally in subepidermal blisters

Dermal papillae retained (no dermal edema)

Noninflammatory—responds poorly to steroids

PORPHYRIA CUTANEA TARDA

Can be autosomal dominant, but usually sporadic

Subepidermal bullae with "festooning" of the dermal papillae into the bulla

Eosinophils, hyalinized perivascular deposits in dermis

GRANULOMATOUS DISEASES

GRANULOMA ANNULARE

Dorsum of hands and arms, young females (male : female = 1 : 2)

Four types: localized, generalized (associated with diabetes), perforating (ulcerates the overlying epidermis), subcutaneous (usually occurs in children)

One to several skin-colored to red papules in an annular or arcuate pattern

Spontaneously resolve in ~2 yr, may recur

Discrete palisading granulomas, generally superficial, with a well-defined zone of disintegrating collagen and *mucin* positivity; occasional giant cells

NECROBIOSIS LIPOIDICA

Male : female = 1 : 3, most in 4th decade; 60% have diabetes mellitus

Sclerotic, round, circumscribed, slightly elevated plaque; initially red brown, then yellow with violaceous border

Predilection for lower extremities; may be symmetrical

Dermal granulomas with palisading histiocytes (arranged in tiers), plasma cells, poorly defined areas of disintegrating collagen, but *no mucin*

Widespread changes in collagen; more extensive vascular changes than with granuloma annulare

May be a primary vascular disease or a primary collagen disease with secondary vascular changes

RHEUMATOID NODULES

Develop at sites of trauma/pressure points in 30% of patients with rheumatoid arthritis

Erythematous plaques/nodules, often fixed to bone/fascia

Histology: deep dermis and subcutaneous fat

Large, multinodular granulomas in deep dermis and subcutaneous fat with palisading histiocytes, occasional giant cells, and central fibrinoid degeneration (fibrin, immunoglobulins [Igs], lipid)

SARCOID

Cutaneous involvement in 20–35%

Widespread, asymptomatic maculopapular eruption

Associated with increased incidence of pulmonary fibrosis

"Lupus pernio": chronic violaceous plaque, usually on nose

Deep (subcutis) non-necrotizing granulomata: lobular panniculitis; small lymphocytes with Langhans' giant cells

Stretched but intact overlying skin

INFLAMMATION OF HAIR FOLLICLES/ADNEXAE

ACNE VULGARIS (COMEDONES)

Cystically dilated hair follicle

May be inflamed or not inflamed

FOLLICULITIS

Papulopustules centered about hair follicles

Neutrophilic infiltrate (also lymphocytes) with dilatation and often rupture of the infundibulum of the follicle

Special stains may reveal the organism

FOLLICULAR MUCINOSIS

AKA: alopecia mucinosis

Hairless edematous plaques, usually on the head and neck of children

Mucin pools within the hair follicle infundibulum dissect and separate the keratinocytes

Eosinophils usually present in benign, childhood form

When occurs in adults, may be a precursor lesion for CTCL

ROSACEA

Crops of papules over forehead, malar areas, nose, chin

Persistent lymphedema and sebaceous hypertrophy result in rhinophyma

Etiology unknown; can follow prolonged use of topical steroid

Nonspecific perivascular inflammation with telangiectasia

Enlargement of sebaceous glands

FOCAL EPIDERMAL ATROPHY

LICHEN SCLEROSUS ET ATROPHICUS

Rare; females 45–60 yr; genital area

White or ivory angulated macules or papules

Pathogenesis unknown

Hyperkeratosis with epithelial atrophy, edema, and homogenization of upper dermis (loss of elastin)

Underlying dense lymphocytic infiltrate may be present

Telangiectatic vessels common

In postmenopausal women, progressive and unresponsive to therapy; ~5% will develop squamous cell carcinoma

BALANITIS XEROTICA OBLITERANS

Lichen sclerosus et atrophicus in men, occurring on the glans penis

Can lead to phimosis or squamous cell carcinoma

More commonly associated with extragenital lichen sclerosus et atrophicus

PANNICULITIS

ERYTHEMA NODOSUM

Commonest nodular panniculitis; often associated with infections, drug administration, inflammatory bowel disease, some malignancies, sarcoidosis, pregnancy

Male : female = 1 : 9; usually anterior and lateral lower legs

Pyrexia, malaise, joint pain

Predominantly septal inflammation; septal widening caused by edema, fibrin, and infiltration of neutrophils (later lymphocytes)

Granulomatous inflammation with giant cells may develop

ERYTHEMA INDURATUM

More chronic form of panniculitis; unknown cause, although probably vasculitis

Presents as erythematous, slightly tender nodule; often ulcerates

Necrosis and inflammation within the fat lobules; a necrotizing vasculitis of medium-sized vessels often seen

INFECTIOUS LESIONS
WART (VERRUCA VULGARIS)
Caused by human papilloma virus (HPV) types 2, 4, 7 (plantar: 1, 2; condylomata acuminata: 6, 11, 16)

Persist for months to years

"Papillary" acanthosis with parakeratosis over the tips of the exophytic component

Marked orthokeratosis with prominent granular cell layer
HERPES SIMPLEX
Cutaneous lesion appears after nerve involvement

Lesions recur, but become less florid and less frequent

Multinucleated giant cells, nuclear inclusions (ground glass, blue speckled nucleus); necrosis with vesicle formation
MOLLUSCUM CONTAGIOSUM
Self-limited poxvirus infection

Lobulated, endophytic hyperplasia → circumscribed intradermal pseudotumor

Keratinocytes contain a large intracytoplasmic inclusion
IMPETIGO
Staphylococcus infection of mild abrasions; children most commonly affected

Neutrophil-filled intraepidermal vesicles (split beneath stratum granulosum)

May progress to cellulitis, glomerulonephritis, erythema nodosum, or erythema multiforme
SYPHILIS
Genital chancre develops 20–30 days after exposure to *Treponema pallidum;* painless ulcer, resolves by itself

Secondary cutaneous lesions—head and neck common

Variable appearance

Intense perivascular infiltrate with plasma cells
CANDIDA
Tight, protective scale with neutrophils in epidermis and chronic inflammation in dermis

MISCELLANEOUS EXTERNAL AGENTS
URTICARIA (HIVES)
Most commonly 20–40 yr old

Individual lesions usually develop and fade within 24 hr; new lesions appear elsewhere

Very subtle histology: mild superficial perivascular chronic inflammation, dermal edema, dilated lymphatics
ERYTHEMA MULTIFORME
Predominantly young individuals; may be recurrent

Etiology usually unknown but can be caused by infectious agents or drugs

Groups of maculopapules, often with annular configuration, on elbows, knees, acral regions; sometimes face and trunk, mouth

Keratinocyte necrosis, spongiosis, vacuolization of basement membrane

Both epidermal and dermal involvement

Can see either intraepidermal or subepidermal bullae, or both

Inflammatory infiltrate in high papillary dermis; eosinophils; RBC extravasation

Stevens-Johnson syndrome:

    Severe form of erythema multiforme with mucosal involvement, conjunctivitis, high fever

    5% of cases are fatal

    (See also Toxic Epidermal Necrolysis)
ARTHROPOD BITE
Superficial and deep perivascular mixed chronic inflammation

Eosinophils

Edematous dermis; mild acanthosis of overlying epidermis
FIXED DRUG
Seen with trimethoprim-sulfamethoxazole, acetylsalicylic acid, tetracycline, barbiturates; recur at same site with each administration

Hydropic degeneration of basal cells; pigment incontinence
PHOTO–DRUG
Sun-exposed areas

Allergic type: eosinophils, contact dermatitis picture

Toxic type: sunburn-type picture
POLYMORPHOUS LIGHT ERUPTION
Papular, papulovesicular, plaque, or diffuse type eruptions occurring on sun-exposed skin 4–24 hr after sun exposure

Onset after puberty

Histology is nonspecific

CONGENITAL DISEASES
ICHTHYOSIS
Multiple types: most common: autosomal dominant (vulgaris)

Dryness to fine fishlike scale, involving predominantly extremities but sparing flexures

Believed to be secondary to increased adhesiveness

X-linked recessive disorder has larger coarse scales

Hyperkeratosis on normal/atrophic epidermis with thin to absent granular layer

May get keratin plugging of hair follicles
URTICARIA PIGMENTOSA
Round to oval erythematous macules to nodules that weal after slight stroking or rubbing

Lesions present at birth or appear in 1st yr; darken with time (increased melanin); usually regress within 5–6 yr

Adult form: pigmented, usually on trunk, systemic involvement common (bone marrow)

Many mast cells (± eosinophils) in dermis; associated edema
DARIER'S DISEASE
AKA: keratosis follicularis

Plaques of greasy, crusted, sometimes warty, yellow-brown papules on scalp, forehead, upper chest, back

Usually autosomal dominant; also see palmar pits, longitudinal splitting of nails

Marked hyperkeratosis, acantholysis (suprabasal clefts)

Corps ronds: dyskeratotic cells in granular layer with surrounding halo
HAILEY-HAILEY DISEASE
AKA: benign familial chronic pemphigus

Autosomal dominant, appears in early adolescence

Massive acantholysis with suprabasal vesicles/bullae on normal to erythematous skin at friction sites on neck, axilla, groin; erode and crust; adnexae are spared

Acantholysis incomplete—some connections preserved

Superinfection by *Candida* and *Staphylococcus* common

Symptoms worsened by trauma or sun
XERODERMA PIGMENTOSUM
Autosomal recessive defect in repair of thymidine dimers

Extreme photosensitivity (freckles to blistering rash)

Eventually develop widespread cutaneous tumors

Solar damage, hyperkeratosis, epidermal atrophy, pigment incontinence

TUBEROUS SCLEROSIS

Autosomal dominant, although most represent new mutation

"Adenoma sebaceum": pink papules/nodules in butterfly pattern over nose and cheeks, sparing the upper lip

Fibrovascular hamartomatous proliferation with prominent sebaceous glands; later perifollicular concentric fibrosis

"Shagreen patch": flat, raised lesion on the lower back

Periungual fibromas

LUPUS

DISCOID LUPUS

Cutaneous form of lupus erythematosus with no systemic manifestations

Generally face, ear lobes, neck, scalp

A vacuolar and interface dermatitis

Acute: lichenoid perivascular inflammation (always superficial, may also be seen deep); hydropic degeneration of basal cells; edema in papillary dermis

Chronic: hyperkeratosis with follicular plugging, epidermal atrophy, thick basement membrane

Direct immunofluorescence shows granular band of immunoglobulin and complement along the dermal-epidermal junction

LUPUS ERYTHEMATOSUS

Male : female = 1 : 9; 20s–40s; prevalent in blacks

Butterfly rash, multisystem involvement

Histology similar to discoid lupus

In patients with systemic disease, granular band of Ig and complement deposition can also be seen in clinically normal skin—can help distinguish discoid from systemic

PRIMARY VASCULAR DISEASES

(See also Vessels outline)

LEUKOCYTOCLASTIC VASCULITIS

Most common vasculitis

Polymorphic, but palpable purpura most common

Necrotizing vasculitis of small superficial vessels with fibrinoid necrosis and Ab-antigen (Ag) complexes (autoimmune)

POLYARTERITIS NODOSA

Systemic necrotizing vasculitis of medium-sized to small arteries; overlaps with leukocytoclastic vasculitis

50% 5 yr mortality

Joint, peripheral nervous system, CNS, renal involvement common

WEGENER'S GRANULOMATOSIS

Necrotizing granulomas of upper airway, glomerulonephritis, granulomatous vasculitis

Before treatment, 80% 1 yr mortality

LYMPHOCYTIC PROLIFERATIVE LESIONS

MYCOSIS FUNGOIDES

Dense lymphocytic infiltrate with epidermotropism of lymphocytes without spongiosis

Lymphocytes in epidermis ± Pautrier's microabscesses

Plasma cells

LYMPHOMATOID PAPULOSIS

Male : female = 2 : 1; usually 30s; unknown etiology

Erythematous dermal papules, hemorrhagic, necrotic, scars

Dermal and epidermal infiltrate of atypical lymphoid cells

Mostly T-helper cells; may mimic PLEVA histologically

Looks malignant, but usually benign course

GRAFT-VERSUS-HOST

Acute: basal cell hydropic degeneration, degenerate keratinocytes, exocytosis, mild dermal perivascular lymphocytic infiltrate

Chronic: lichenoid infiltrate, hyperkeratosis, hypergranulosis, basal cell hydropic degeneration

Late chronic: epidermal atrophy, abolition of ridges, loss of adnexal structures, scarring of superficial and deep dermis

MISCELLANEOUS

CALCINOSIS CUTIS

Dystrophic calcification

PRURIGO NODULARIS

Chronic, intensely pruritic nodules: globular, dark, with a warty or excoriated surface

5–75 yr at onset, lasting average of 9 yr

Compact orthokeratosis, acanthosis, pseudoepitheliomatous hyperplasia, vascular hyperplasia in dermis

ERYTHEMA ANNULARE CENTRIFUGUM

Annular erythematous bands, well circumscribed

May remain stationary or spread outward

Trunk most common, then lower limbs, arms, hands

Tight dermal perivascular mononuclear infiltrate with normal overlying epidermis

PITYRIASIS ROSEA

10–35 yr old; "rose colored scale"

Starts as herald patch, single red papule enlarges over 48 hr

After incubation period (1–2 wk), generalized eruption of pink elliptical lesions 1 cm long along skin tension lines

Focal alternating hyperkeratosis/parakeratosis; slight acanthosis; focal spongiosis and dermal edema

Superficial loose lymphohistiocytic infiltrate with extravasation of RBCs into dermis

PLEVA

Pityriasis lichenoides et varioliformis acuta (Mucha-Habermann disease)

Male : female = 3 : 1; late childhood to early adult

Pink papules on trunk and extremities that ulcerate and then heal without scarring

Acute ulceronecrotic lesions with wedge-shaped keratinocyte necrosis, spongiosis, and exocytosis of lymphocytes and RBCs

Obscured dermal-epidermal junction

Extravasated RBCs in dermis

KAWASAKI'S

AKA: mucocutaneous lymph node syndrome

PROLIFERATIVE LESIONS

Keratinocyte "Tumors"

CUTANEOUS HORN

Protuberant column of keratin

May be found over other lesions

ACROCHORDON

AKA: fibroepithelial papilloma/polyp, skin tag

Histology: normal skin, seborrheic keratosis, etc.

ACQUIRED (DIGITAL) FIBROKERATOMA
Collagenous protrusions with hyperkeratotic epidermis
Usually around interphalangeal joints

SEBORRHEIC KERATOSIS
Very common, developing in middle aged to elderly
Sharply delineated, round, tan to black, mostly on face, arms, upper trunk—never on palms or soles
Leser-Trélat sign: sudden increase in size or number, associated with internal malignancy
Full-thickness proliferation of keratinocytes with horn cysts, thick basal cell layer, hyperkeratotic
Multiple variants:
- Keratotic (papillomatous): verrucous; flat bottom
- Adenoid: thin strands of proliferating basal cells; horn cysts may not be present
- Acanthotic: rounded, smooth surface; may have marked melanocyte proliferation
- Inverted (irritated) follicular: penetrating but circumscribed lower border

PSEUDOEPITHELIOMATOUS HYPERPLASIA
Occurs at sites of trauma, chronic irritation, ulcers
Can be produced by fungal infections
Thin, elongated anastomosing ridges
Inflammatory cells, dermal vascular proliferation

LICHENOID (LICHEN PLANUS–LIKE) KERATOSIS
Asymptomatic, 0.5–2 cm, slightly verrucous or scaly
Sun exposed skin, bright red to brown
Basketweave hyperkeratosis
Similar histology to lichen planus but tends to be solitary, contains eosinophils or plasma cells, and has focal areas of parakeratosis or epithelial atypia

ACANTHOSIS NIGRICANS
Hyperkeratosis and papillomatosis
80% occur in children
When occurs in adults, usually associated with underlying malignancy, most commonly gastric

HYPERPLASTIC VULVAL DYSTROPHY
(See also Uterus and Vulva outline)
Clinical term: leukoplakia
Hyperkeratosis, irregular acanthosis, hyalinization of the papillary dermis, mild chronic inflammatory cell infiltrate
With or without atypia

KERATOACANTHOMA
Rapidly growing benign skin tumor of pilosebaceous origin, occurring on sun-exposed skin of face, back of hands, wrists, forearms; male : female = 3 : 1
Clinical stages: rapid growth (over couple of months), maturation, resolution (spontaneous regression)
Round, reddish nodule with central cup-shaped crater filled with keratin; symmetrical, well-differentiated squamous cells
Perineural invasion of small nests of squamous cells can be seen
Differentiation from squamous cell carcinoma is based on the fact that a keratoacanthoma grows rapidly, has an exophytic component, abundant glassy cells, and a mixed inflammatory cell infiltrate

CLEAR CELL ACANTHOMA
Rare, usually solitary; elderly; most commonly lower limbs
Well-demarcated lateral border with abundant glycogen
May arise from intraepidermal eccrine ducts

NONINVASIVE SQUAMOUS LESIONS
ACTINIC (SOLAR) KERATOSIS
Yellow brown, scaly lesions on sun-exposed skin (face, upper back, arms)
Stratum corneum replaced by parakeratotic scale: alternating parakeratotic/orthokeratotic horn (follicular areas spared)
Granular layer absent; focal basal cell proliferation
Chronic inflammation in papillary dermis with basophilic degeneration of collagen
Hyperplastic and atrophic variants
Only a small proportion progress to invasive squamous cell carcinoma (SCC)
BOWENOID ACTINIC KERATOSIS
Similar to, but smaller than, Bowen's disease
Occurs on sun-exposed skin
Usually not full-thickness involvement
INTRAEPIDERMAL EPITHELIOMA
Nests of enlarged, atypical keratinocytes in the epithelium, but with normal underlying basal layer
BOWENOID PAPULOSIS
Glans penis of circumcised men, vulva of women
20–40 yr old, multiple red papules; rapidly developing
Histology is very similar to Bowen's disease but more orderly background with some surface maturation
BOWEN'S DISEASE
AKA: squamous cell carcinoma in situ
Slowly enlarging, scaly, erythematous, sharply demarcated lesion occurring anywhere on skin or mucous membranes; devoid of adnexae
Middle-aged to elderly; may be associated with arsenic exposure; not related to sun exposure
Full-thickness dysplasia (carcinoma in situ) with cytoplasmic vacuolization, nuclear hyperchromasia, multinucleated keratinocytes, dyskeratosis, mitoses, parakeratosis
~5% will develop invasive squamous cell carcinoma
ERYTHROPLASIA OF QUEYRAT
Squamous cell carcinoma in situ of the glans penis
Occurs in uncircumcised men
Asymptomatic, erythematous, well defined

SQUAMOUS CELL CARCINOMA
2nd most common cutaneous malignancy (after basal cell carcinoma [BCC])
Occurs at sites of "trauma" (sun exposure, burns, chemical exposure, PUVA, renal transplantation)
Prognosis related to depth of invasion and tumor thickness
Tumors >2 cm thick: <5% lymph node (LN) metastases

Histologic Variants
Well differentiated (80%): large amount of keratin and involucrin, dermal invasion required
Spindle cell: sun exposure (lip), spindled, differential diagnosis: malignant melanoma, atypical fibroxanthoma

Acantholytic (adenoid, pseudoglandular): sun-exposed areas, desmosome defect with loss of cohesiveness and false glands

Verrucous: usually sole of foot, extremely well differentiated, ulcerates, locally invasive on a broad front to bone (metastases rare)

Clear cell: rare, primarily head and neck, males, clear cells in foci or throughout lesion; differential diagnosis: sebaceous carcinoma

STAGING

Note: same staging scheme used for all carcinomas of the skin (including those arising from appendages); melanomas and lesions of the eyelids are specifically excluded

T1 Tumor ≤2 cm   N1 Regional LNs
T2 2–5 cm   M1 Distant metastases
T3 >5 cm
T4 Invades muscle, bone, cartilage

	T1	T2	T3	T4
N0	I	II		
N1	III			
M1	IV			

BASAL CELL CARCINOMA

Most common cutaneous malignancy

Predominantly sun-exposed skin, in proportion to number of pilosebaceous units; slow and indolent growth

Prevalent in transplant patients

Synchronous and metachronous tumors common

Proliferation of basal cells with peripheral palisading, separation artifact, stromal mucin, incomplete differentiation toward adnexal (usually pilar) structures

Mitotic rate unrelated to prognosis

Immunohistochemistry: keratin+, EMA−, CEA−

If untreated, may invade subcutaneous fat; only one third of incompletely excised lesions recur

Metastases rare (<.002%); if does metastasize, usually fatal within 1 yr

Multiple Variants

SUPERFICIAL
Arises in skin with thin epidermis and fine hairs
Chiefly lateral growth; high recurrence rate

LOCALIZED—ULCERATIVE
75% of lesions—nonhealing ulcer
Telangiectatic vessels

LOCALIZED—CYSTIC
Lobulated, smooth, pearly nodule

DIFFUSE SCLEROSING TYPE (MORPHEAFORM)
Poorly defined margins
Extent often far beyond clinical appearance
Loss of peripheral palisading, dense stroma
Tend to be more aggressive

BASOSQUAMOUS (METATYPICAL)
Atypical squamous cells—more aggressive

CLEAR CELL
Clear vacuoles—occasional signet ring cells

BASAL CELL NEVUS SYNDROME
AKA: Gorlin's syndrome
Multiple BCCs, starting at an early age
Autosomal dominant
Jaw cysts, skeletal abnormalities, falx cerebri calcification, palmar pits

FIBROEPITHELIAL TUMOR OF PINKUS
Back, abdomen, and thigh; look like skin tags
Two to three cell thick basaloid epithelial strands anastomosing to compartmentalize fibrous stroma

PAGET'S DISEASE
Most common extramammary sites: vulva, penis, scrotum, anus, axillae, umbilicus, eyelids
Mammary Paget's: associated with underlying carcinoma
Paget cells cluster; pink cytoplasm, vesicular nuclei
Large cells, PAS+, pseudoglandular
CEA positive; usually keratin and S-100 negative

Appendage "Tumors"

CUTANEOUS CYSTS

EPIDERMAL INCLUSION CYSTS
Pilosebaceous units or implantation trauma
Unilocular, granular cell layer present

MILIA
Subepidermal blisters or plugged eccrine ducts
Miniature epidermoid cysts

TRICHOLEMMAL (PILAR) CYSTS
Scalp, yellowish, intradermal swellings
No granular cell layer, cholesterol clefts

PROLIFERATING TRICHOLEMMAL CYSTS
Slow growing, large tumor on scalp of elderly female
Lobulated intradermal mass of squamous epithelium
Peripheral palisading, thick refractile basement membrane
Mitoses limited to basal layer

HAIR FOLLICLE LESIONS

PILAR SHEATH ACANTHOMA
Upper lip, solitary, central pore with keratinaceous material
Multiloculated lobulated tumor masses radiating into surrounding dense stroma

TRICHILEMMOMA
Small warty or smooth papule on face of older adults
Proliferation of outer root sheath with uniform small cells forming one or more lobules arising from epidermis
Peripheral palisading; thickened basal membrane

PILOMATRICOMA
Slowly growing, firm, chalky nodule, usually on face
Biphasic population of basaloid and ghost cells (hair matrix differentiation); 75% show calcification

TRICHOFOLLICULOMA
Dome shaped; central pore with silky white threadlike hairs
Dilated hair follicle with numerous secondary (mature and immature) follicles arising from its stratified squamous wall

TRICHOEPITHELIOMA
Small, flesh-colored nodule
Lobules of basaloid cells and keratinocytes disconnected from the epidermis; peripheral palisading; horn cysts; cellular fibrotic stroma surrounding lobules is part of tumor
Differential diagnosis: basal cell carcinoma

PILOLEIOMYOMA
Small, firm, intradermal nodules
Groups or linear arrays on trunk or extremities

SEBACEOUS GLANDS

NEVUS SEBACEUS (OF JADASSOHN)
Single, round, usually head/neck, yellow, flat; becomes warty

Acanthotic, abortive hair papillae, ectopic apocrine glands in 50%
Prone to evolve into BCC

SEBACEOUS HYPERPLASIA
Face of older adults; yellowish dome-shaped papule
Hyperplastic glands high in dermis, drain into central duct

SEBACEOUS ADENOMA
Rare—yellow papule, looks like BCCs
Individual lobules, collagenous pseudo-capsules, peripheral small germinative cells with round to oval vesicular nuclei and eosinophilic cytoplasm

SEBACEOUS CARCINOMA
Aggressive periocular variant and relatively nonaggressive extraocular form
Irregular lobular pattern in upper dermis with basophilic sebaceous cells containing small granular nuclei with eosinophilic nucleoli

ECCRINE GLANDS

SYRINGOMA
Multiple symmetrically distributed small papules on lower eyelids that appear at puberty; female predominance
Intraepidermal eccrine sweat duct tumor (acrosyringium)
Interconnecting eccrine strands + ducts in a fibrous stroma
Small ducts with two rows of cells
Lumens, lined by cuticle, with eosinophilic granular material

ECCRINE ACROSPIROMA
AKA: eccrine hidradenoma, clear cell hidradenoma
Arises from distal excretory duct of the eccrine gland
Superficial dermal nodules with monomorphic cuboidal cells with a basophilic cytoplasm mixed with clear cells

ECCRINE POROMA
This may be a specialized form of eccrine acrospiroma
Solitary, slightly red, scaly nodule, usually sole, sides of foot
Tumor of upper dermal eccrine duct (outer acrosyringium)
Tumor replaces epidermis (sharp demarcation) and grows down into dermis; monomorphic, cuboidal cells; occasionally with duct differentiation
Malignant form: rare, marked nuclear pleomorphism

CYLINDROMA
99% head, neck, scalp; female : male = 9 : 1; slow growing, red
Multiple lobules in a *jigsaw pattern* in upper dermis, no connection to epidermis
Each lobule: *thick PAS+ basement membrane,* basal cells (hyperchromatic nuclei), and central cells (vesicular nuclei)

ECCRINE SPIRADENOMA
Solitary intradermal lesion, blue overlying skin: *painful*
Basophilic nests of tumor cells in dermis: peripheral small cells with round hyperchromatic nuclei surrounding large cells with vesicular nuclei and eosinophilic nucleoli
Rich vascular supply

CHONDROID SYRINGOMA (BENIGN MIXED TUMOR OF THE SKIN)
Firm, lobulated nodules in dermis or fat; solitary, asymptomatic, usually head and neck
Multilobulated, well-circumscribed mass with nests or cords of polygonal cells with basophilic nuclei and lots of eosinophilic cytoplasm
Stroma has a pseudocartilaginous appearance

ECCRINE CARCINOMA
Classic, syringoid, microcystic adnexal, mucinous, and adenoid cystic variants

APOCRINE GLANDS

APOCRINE NEVUS (SYRINGOCYSTADENOMA PAPILLIFERUM)
Solitary, usually scalp, gray to brown papillary, moist
Double-layered "apocrine" epithelium lining glandular spaces and papillae; fibrovascular core, typically with plasma cells

TUBULAR APOCRINE ADENOMA
Dermal nodule, long duration, may be large; scalp, axilla
Poorly circumscribed dermal tumor within foci of ductular communication with the epidermis
Lobular masses of tubular structures
Columnar epithelium, myoepithelial layer, apocrine secretion

HIDRADENOMA
Females only—asymptomatic nodule in genital/perianal region
Well-demarcated dermal nodule composed of papillary fronds with columnar cells and underlying myoepithelial cells
Fibrous pseudocapsule common

MERKEL'S CELL CARCINOMA
Highly aggressive, firm, raised, painless nodule
Occurs on sun-damaged skin: head and neck (44%), leg, arm, buttock
Epidermis: normal, tumor, squamous cell carcinoma not uncommon
Predominantly dermal tumor with trabecular growth pattern, dissection of collagen by small basophilic cells with small eccentric nucleolus, nuclear molding
EM: 100–150 nm neurosecretory granules, paranuclear filament whorls
Recurrence common (36%), metastasizes (28%)
50% 2 yr mortality

AGGRESSIVE DIGITAL PAPILLARY ADENOCARCINOMA
Appendage tumor seen almost exclusively on the digits
Papillary projections into cystic spaces and tubular structures intermixed with more solid, poorly differentiated areas with necrosis
Tends to metastasize to lungs

Fibrous Proliferation

HYPERPLASTIC SCAR
Increased amount of collagen, in thin fibers

KELOID
Exuberant scars, predominantly in blacks
Large eosinophilic collagen fibers; unusually large fibroblasts

FIBROMATOSIS
Juvenile hyalin type, Dupuytren's type
Round, plump spindle cells in collagenous stroma with hyalinization

NODULAR FASCIITIS
Reactive, unknown etiology, usually limbs
Rapidly growing subcutaneous nodule—painful
Plump spindle cells in loose myxoid and collagenous stroma
Numerous thin-walled vessels with prominent endothelium
Sparse chronic inflammation

MORPHEA (LOCALIZED SCLERODERMA)
White, indurated area(s)
Sclerotic hyalinized thickening of the dermis; epidermis normal
Superficial and deep perivascular infiltrate
Sclerosis extends into fibrous septa of deeper adipose tissue

DERMATOFIBROMA (FIBROUS HISTIOCYTOMA)
Middle adult life: trunk, proximal extremities
Firm cutaneous nodule, reddish brown, slowly growing, painless
Interlacing fascicles of slender spindle cells with foamy histiocytes, giant cells, vessels, hemosiderin, chronic inflammation
Infiltrative margins; superficial; overlying pseudoepitheliomatous hyperplasia separated from the underlying lesion by a thick zone of normal dermis (Grenz zone)
FIBROCARTILAGINOUS TYPE ("TYPICAL")
Plump capillaries, fibroblasts, foamy histiocytes
Cellular (histiocytoma) and angiosiderotic (sclerosing hemangioma) variants
PLEOMORPHIC TYPE ("ATYPICAL")

ATYPICAL FIBROXANTHOMA
Firm, often ulcerated nodule on sun exposed head and neck (60s–70s) or limbs (30s–40s)
Predominantly dermal—may involve superficial fat
Marked pleomorphism: "too bad to be malignant"
Should *not* see storiform pattern, necrosis, myxoid change
Proliferation of factor XIIIa positive histiocytes

DERMATOFIBROSARCOMA PROTUBERANS
Multinodular, reddish-blue nodule, 20s–30s, usually trunk
Deep dermis to subcutis (dermatofibroma more superficial)
Well-differentiated spindle cells in storiform pattern, interlacing bundles—basket weave
Moderate mitotic activity, abundant reticulin
Pigmented and myxoid variants exist
Local recurrence 33%, metastases rare

GIANT CELL TUMOR OF TENDON SHEATH
Slow growing, painless nodule of hands, feet, usually fingers
Fibrous pseudocapsule, lobulated; pleomorphic histiocytes, giant cells, hemosiderin; collagenous stroma with cholesterol clefts
Local recurrence (15%), no malignant potential

NEURILEMOMA (SCHWANNOMA)
Solitary, painless mass, head, neck, limbs
Encapsulated, biphasic
Antoni A: tightly packed spindle cells, tapering elongated wavy nuclei; nuclear palisading (Verocay bodies)
Antoni B: irregularly scattered spindle or stellate cells in abundant loose myxoid stroma; small blood vessels with hyalinized walls

NEUROFIBROMA
Generally young individuals; any site; solitary or multiple (von Recklinghausen's)
Irregular, spindle-shaped cells in loose matrix within superficial dermis; no capsule, no mitotic activity

Mast cells
Variants: myxoid, plexiform, epithelioid, pacinian

MELANOCYTIC LESIONS

Melanocytes
Neuroectodermally derived cells
Stain with silver stains (melanin), S-100, vimentin, dihydroxyphenylalanine (DOPA) reaction
Negative for keratin, neurofilament, glial fibrillary acidic protein
Melanoblast: immature form
Melanophage: macrophages that have phagocytosed pigment (pigment incontinence)
Color depends on melanin location: epidermis, brown; superficial dermis (clumped), black; deep dermis, blue

BENIGN DISORDERS OF PIGMENTATION
FRECKLES (EPHELIS)
Reactive to sunlight, 1–10 mm, irregular borders
Increased melanin deposition, melanocyte hypertrophy, normal or decreased numbers of melanocytes
MELASMA
"Mask of pregnancy"; can also occur outside of pregnancy
Increased pigmentation but normal number of melanocytes
VITILIGO
Hypopigmentation, often irregular, hyperpigmented border
Complete absence of melanocytes (unlike albinism, in which melanocytes are present but don't make melanin)
LENTIGO (LENTIGO SIMPLEX, NEVUS SPILUS)
Usually seen in children; unresponsive to sunlight
5–10 mm, tan-brown with smooth, well-demarcated borders
Melanocyte hyperplasia and hyperpigmentation of basal epidermis, with elongation of rete ridges but generally without melanocyte nesting

NEVI (MELANOCYTIC, NEVOCELLULAR)
Any localized benign abnormality of melanocytes
Most appear at 2–6 yr of age, nearly all by age 20
Nevus cells and melanocytes are derived from the same lineage (neural crest) but show different biologic behavior and may in fact be different cells
JUNCTIONAL
Flat or slightly elevated, nonhairy, fawn colored
Melanocytic nests (theques) on epidermal side of dermal-epidermal junction
May give rise to malignant melanomas
INTRADERMAL
Papillary, pedunculated, or flat; often hairy
Small nests or bundles of melanocytes in papillary dermis (if deeper, think congenital)
Not circumscribed, but surrounded by basement membrane
Degree of pigmentation varies
Lower half of lesion less cellular, spindled, neuroid
Almost never give rise to melanoma
COMPOUND
Junctional plus intradermal features
Junctional component tends to decrease with age (except on palms, soles)

A prominent junctional component indicates "activity": activation occurs from sunlight, pregnancy, recurrence following excision, melanoma elsewhere

BLUE NEVUS
Usually head, neck, upper extremity
Abundant melanin pigment
Band of uninvolved dermis between epidermis and lesion

CELLULAR BLUE NEVUS
Usually buttock, lower back, back of hands or feet
Large, intensely pigmented, very cellular, pushing margins, dermal sclerosis, elongated dendritic processes with fine melanin granules
No junctional activity or inflammation
25% are congenital
Usually benign

SPITZ NEVUS (SPINDLE CELL AND/OR EPITHELIOID CELL NEVUS)
50% occur before puberty, but can occur at any age
Pink red papule on face, prepubertal
Compound (70%), intradermal (20%), junctional (10%)
Generally scanty pigment (except pigmented variant)
Symmetrical, sharp lateral demarcation, mature with depth (become more neural looking)
Overlying epidermal hyperplasia, telangiectasia
Intraepidermal hyaline globules (Kamino bodies)
Almost always benign

GIANT CONGENITAL PIGMENTED NEVI
Bathing-trunk distribution
Large, coarse skin with folds, often satellite lesions
Histology: deep lesions
Before surgery, need to expand skin because need to cover a large defect to achieve resection; nevertheless, still usually requires multiple surgeries
~50% of patients show an extra chromosome 7 when grown in culture (may all be an artifact of cell culture); similar change seen in some smaller congenital nevi
Figures for risk of malignant transformation range from 2% to 40%

BULKY PERINEAL NEUROCYTOMA
Congenital, large, polypoid or pedunculated, hyperpigmented mass in the genital area, often obscuring the genitals
Histology is that of a benign congenital nevus; often have cystic structures lined by nevus cells
Large numbers of small neuratized bodies (look like Meissner's corpuscles)
HMB-45 positivity extends deep into lesions and includes the cystic structures but not the neural structures
S-100 positivity in all structures
Probably an uncommon variant of giant congenital pigmented nevus
May have aggressive histology in newborn; however, malignant transformation is rare before 6 months of age

DEEP PENETRATING NEVUS
10–30 yr old, usually face or upper trunk
Darkly pigmented, dome-shaped nodule
Nests of nevus cells with scattered melanocytes that fill the dermis; may infiltrate erector pili muscles
May extend through the dermis into the subcutis
Benign lesion; does not recur or metastasize

OTHER NEVI
Halo: surrounded by unpigmented skin, secondary to regression
Balloon: large, foamy melanocytes
Congenital (non-giant): involve reticular dermis, subcutaneous tissue, and skin adnexae

Dysplastic Nevus
Familial—predisposed to melanoma
Some atypical melanocytes
Lymphocytic infiltrate in papillary dermis
Bridging of rete ridges by melanocyte nests
Junctional component extends beyond intradermal
Eosinophilic concentric/lamellar fibrin deposition
Believed by some to be precursor for malignant melanoma

LENTIGO MALIGNA (HUTCHINSON'S FRECKLE)
AKA: malignant melanoma in situ
Sun-exposed areas, most common on cheek of elderly
Tan to black; solar elastosis; individual (± nesting) atypical junctional melanocytes; minimal transepidermal migration; often involves adnexae
Slow growing, 30–40% invade if untreated (premalignant)

MALIGNANT MELANOMA
Most associated with sunlight, especially in red-haired whites
Almost always have junctional component; therefore, if intradermal, probably metastatic
~20% are believed to arise from a pre-existing nevus
Markedly varied histologic appearance, often with some areas of nesting
Nucleoli commonly present and large; nuclear pseudoinclusions composed of cytoplasm very common

TYPES
• Lentigo maligna melanoma
    Arises from lentigo maligna
    Atypical cells present in dermis (vertical growth phase)
    Better prognosis than other types
• Superficial spreading melanoma
    Most common form
    Blue with admixed tan and brown (early)
    White, pink, blue = areas of regression
• Nodular melanoma
    Younger age group—usually shorter duration
    Elevated lesion
• Acral-lentiginous
    Intraepidermal with hyperplastic epidermis
• Desmoplastic

GROWTH PHASE
Radial: restricted to epidermis, or individual cells, or small, regular nests in the dermis
Vertical: large or atypical nests in dermis

FEATURES OF MALIGNANCY
Large, high mitotic rate, poorly circumscribed/low cohesiveness in nests, lateral extension of individual cells (trailing off), extension within adnexal epithelium, variation in size/shape, lack of maturation, prominent nucleoli, fine dusty melanin granules, melanocyte necrosis (if not related to ulceration), lymphocytes in tumor

REGRESSION
Primary can spontaneously regress (metastases do not)
Clinically: white, often with a bluish hue
Irregularities along dermal-epidermal junction, focal necrotic cells, bandlike lymphocytic infiltrate, melanophages, subepidermal fibrosis, atrophy of rete ridges
For two lesions of the same size, regression is a bad prognostic sign, because it indicates lesion was once larger

STAGING

Tis In situ (Clark Level I)
T1   ≤.75 mm thick; invades papillary dermis (Clark Level II)
T2   .75–1.5 mm; fills papillary dermis (Clark Level III)
T3   1.5–4 mm thick; into reticular dermis (Clark Level IV)
    T3a   1.5–3 mm
    T3b   3–4 mm
T4   >4 mm thick; into subcutaneous tissue (Clark Level V)
    T4a   No satellite lesion
    T4b   Satellites within 2 cm
N1   Regional LN metastasis ≤3 cm

N2   Regional LN metastasis >3 cm or in transit metastasis

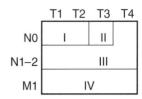

Breslow level: measure depth in millimeters from overlying stratum granulosum or ulcer bed to deepest extension *in the primary tumor*

24

CENTRAL NERVOUS SYSTEM

NORMAL ANATOMY

Brain

The cerebrum is divided, on each side, into the frontal, parietal, occipital, and temporal lobes

Sylvian fissure: marks the upper border of the temporal lobes; separates from parietal lobes

Rolando fissure (central sulcus) separates the frontal from parietal lobes, and is bounded by the precentral motor cortex and the postcentral sensory cortex

Convolutions are termed *gyri* for the cerebrum, *folia* for the cerebellum

Cranial nerves 1 and 2 are CNS extensions and are myelinated by oligodendrocytes; the other 10 cranial nerves are "peripheral" and are myelinated by Schwann cells

Perikarya: neuronal cell bodies

Stria of Gennari: prominent horizontal layer of myelinated fibers in the visual cortex

Bergmann glia: elongated astrocytes of the cerebellum

Rosenthal fibers: intracytoplasmic hyaline structure, sometimes corkscrew shaped, found in pilocytic astrocytes

Corpora amylacea: argyrophilic and PAS$^+$ polyglucosan globules in the terminal processes of astrocytes

CEREBROSPINAL FLUID (CSF)

CSF produced in the choroid plexus, which projects into the lateral, 3rd, and 4th ventricles

Lateral ventricles connect to 3rd ventricle via the foramina of Monro, which then connects to the 4th ventricle via the aqueduct of Sylvius

There is no lymphatic system in the brain to drain excess fluid; therefore, the brain is very sensitive to edema

Hydrocephalus: increase in the volume of the ventricles and thus of the CSF

MENINGES

Dura mater (pachymeninx): mostly collagenous; reduplicated in the midline to form the falx cerebri and rostral to the cerebellum to form the tentorium cerebelli; contain branches of the middle meningeal artery

Arachnoid: delicate weblike membrane

Pia mater: lies along surface of brain, tightly adherent to it

CELLS

Neurons: large nuclei, prominent nucleolus; neurofilaments

Astrocytes: large, vesicular nuclei; cytoplasm usually not evident unless becomes reactive; markedly GFAP positive

Oligodendrocytes: small, round nuclei, usually with surrounding halo (artifact), giving a fried egg appearance

Microglia: elongated cigar-shaped nuclei

Ependyma: epithelial layer lining ventricles; S-100 positive; GFAP negative

Spinal Cord

Dorsal portion predominantly sensory

Ventral portion predominantly motor

Central canal becomes discontinuous by puberty

Tapered at caudal end to form the filum terminale, a fibrous extension containing nests of glia and ependymal cells; adipose tissue may be present in 10% of individuals

EMBRYOLOGY

Arises in the midline of the developing embryo as the primitive neural groove, which bulges up and fuses in the mid-dorsal region (neural tube); this tube fuses rostral to caudal

Cylindrical neural tube develops focal constrictions to form four segments:

- Prosencephalon (forebrain)
    - Diencephalon: thalamus and hypothalamus
    - Telencephalon: lateral ventricles and cortex
- Mesencephalon (midbrain): aqueduct of Sylvius
- Rhombencephalon (hindbrain)
    - Metencephalon: pons and cerebellum
    - Myelencephalon: medulla
- Spinal cord

INFLAMMATORY/NON-NEOPLASTIC DISORDERS

DEVELOPMENTAL DEFECTS

ECTOPIA

Nodular, mature; predominantly astrocytic

Most common site: nasal "glioma"

Can also see neural tissue in occipital bone

Other tissue may also be ectopic to the CNS:
  Thyroid tissue in sellar region
  Salivary gland in cerebellopontine angle

Neural Tube Defects

Any failure of closure of midline structures over the neural tube: ranges from occult spina bifida to craniorachischisis (completely open neural tube)

ANENCEPHALY

1/1000 live births

ENCEPHALOCELE

1/8000 live births

Usually occipital

SPINA BIFIDA

1/800 live births; female > male

Occult spina bifida is present in 1–25% of the population

70% are lumbosacral; cervical-occipital is 2nd most common site

Associated malformations include hydrocephalus (25%) and Arnold-Chiari malformation (elongation of the brainstem and cerebellum)

Classification of defect is based upon where the defect is and what is contained in the resulting "sac"
• Meningocele
• Meningomyelocele
• Syringomyelocele
• Lipomeningomyelocele
• Myelocele
• Encephalocele
91% have motor disability
50–70% have urinary or anal sphincter involvement
35% of patients survive

CEREBROVASCULAR DISEASE
Accounts for ~50% of patients on neurology service
Mostly a disease of the elderly (>60 yr old)
CEREBROVASCULAR ACCIDENT
Causes:

Atherosclerosis	40–60%
Embolism	15–40%
Intracerebral hemorrhage	10–15%
Subarachnoid hemorrhage	10–15%
Others	5–20%

Brain has an absolute requirement for oxygen; following cessation of blood flow:

11 sec	Unconscious
40 sec	EEG flat
3 min	Glucose gone; irreversible
5–7 min	Tissue ATP gone

Different cell types show different sensitivities to ischemia; in order: neurons, oligodendrocytes, astrocytes, microglial cells, vessels
Different regions of the brain show different sensitivities to global ischemia; in order: hippocampus (Sommer sector [CA-I], CA-II spared), external pyramidal layer (layer 3) of the neocortex, Purkinje cells of the cerebellum, inferior olivary neurons, subthalamic nucleus
Histologic evidence of neuronal anoxic/ischemic injury: acidophilic degeneration, glassy cytoplasm, loss of Nissl substance, hyperchromatic nuclei, shrinkage of neuron with increase in perineuronal space
INFARCT
May be hemorrhagic or anemic, depending upon whether or not blood flow is re-established

Gross
6 hr	No changes
8–48 hr	Swelling
>48 hr	Mushy, friable
2nd wk	Liquefaction
≥3 wk	Cavitation (1 ml/3 months)

Microscopic
8–12 hr	Classic ischemic changes
12–48 hr	Macrophages appear
48 hr	Macrophages become foamy
3rd day	Astrocytes proliferate, become gemistocytic; nuclei enlarge
7th day	Capillary walls thicken
>30 days	Only astrocytes remain

HEMATOMA
EPIDURAL (EXTRADURAL) HEMATOMA
Between the skull and the dura

Localized; usually large angle edges
Bleeding is from torn meningeal arteries, usually associated with a skull fracture
Patient typically recovers from initial unconsciousness, but over the next few hours regresses into a deepening coma
High pressure bleed; must be surgically drained
SUBDURAL HEMATOMA
Between the dura and arachnoid space
Sharp angle borders as extends outward over a larger area
Bleeding from bridging veins; occurs at sites where brain is able to move (often contrecoup)
Slower, low pressure bleed: patient shows a gradual decline in level of consciousness over days to weeks
May be self-contained; clot eventually reabsorbed leaving a yellow-stained "membrane"
SUBARACHNOID HEMORRHAGES
Generally *not* related to trauma but rather to vascular insult: hypertension, aneurysm, embolus, infarct
(See later)

VASCULAR/HEMORRHAGIC DISEASES
HYPERTENSIVE HEMORRHAGE
>60% occur in the basal ganglia
Other common locations include thalamus, pons, and midbrain
DURÉT HEMORRHAGE
Secondary brainstem hemorrhage, usually caused by supratentorial mass
Results in punctate hemorrhages throughout the tectum of the pons
Basilar artery is anchored at the tentorium; as the brainstem is forced downward by a mass lesion, pulls on the penetrating arteries, inducing ischemia; when restore blood flow, get multiple small hemorrhages into the brainstem
SACCULAR (BERRY) ANEURYSM
(See also Vessels outline)
Most commonly at branch point between anterior and middle cerebral arteries; caused by a defect in the vessel wall
Aneurysms are present in 5% of adults (25% are multiple, 20% are bilateral)
Only 12/100,000 rupture per yr; 30% mortality within the first 24 hr; 60% within the first 30 days
ARTERIOVENOUS MALFORMATION
1.5% of intracranial "tumors"
Most common location is distribution of the middle cerebral artery
Presentation: hemorrhage (86%), seizure (8%), headache (6%)
Irregular thickening of the vessel walls; elastin stain shows duplication or triplication of the internal elastic lamina alternating with areas lacking any elastic lamina

INFECTIOUS LESIONS
Major routes of infection:
• Direct extension from neighboring structures
• Retrograde extension from other neural structures
• Hematogenous dissemination
• Inoculation following trauma or iatrogenic
MENINGITIS
Inflammation predominantly limited to the meninges

Acute pyogenic: *E. coli* (neonates), *H. influenzae* (children), *N. meningitidis* (adolescents), pneumococcus (very young and very old)
Acute lymphocytic: usually viral
Chronic: TB, syphilis, cryptococcus

CEREBRITIS
Focal inflammation of the brain parenchyma
Usually bacterial, less commonly fungal or parasitic
Some pathologists do not distinguish this from encephalitis

BRAIN ABSCESS
Arise in necrosis resulting from cerebritis or encephalitis, often 1–2 wk following infarction
Most commonly streptococci, *E. coli, Staphylococcus aureus* (trauma), *Bacteroides,* fungi (especially in immunocompromised)

ENCEPHALITIS
Diffuse inflammation, often involving the meninges as well (meningoencephalitis)
Usually viral or rickettsial
- Herpes simplex: temporal or frontal lobes; early lesions mimic ischemia; later perivascular chronic inflammation, focal necrosis, hemorrhage
- Postinfectious: following varicella or influenza; prominent demyelination
- Herpes zoster: predominantly unilateral vasculopathy causing contralateral hemiparesis
- Subacute sclerosing panencephalitis: measles virus
- AIDS: markedly varied histologic picture, including encephalitis, leukoencephalopathy, vacuolar myelopathy, toxoplasmosis, *Candida,* cryptococcus
- Transmissible subacute spongiform encephalopathy: i.e., Creutzfeldt-Jakob disease; see later under Dementia

PROGRESSIVE MULTIFOCAL LEUKOENCEPHALOPATHY
Multifocal destruction of oligodendrocytes, resulting in demyelination with minimal inflammation and minimal damage to axons
Caused by DNA papovavirus, usually JC virus
Occurs in setting of underlying disease: AIDS, chronic lymphocytic leukemia (CLL), carcinoma, TB, systemic lupus erythematosus, status post transplant
Ground-glass oligodendroglial nuclei (filled with virions), large pleomorphic astrocytes, perivascular chronic inflammation

DEMENTIAS
ALZHEIMER'S DISEASE
Accounts for 50% of dementia in pure form, 70–75% in combination with other forms
Marked atrophy, esp. of the frontal lobes
Cell loss, senile plaques, neurofibrillary tangles, granulovacuolar degeneration, amyloid angiopathy
Hirano body: eosinophilic, football-shaped structure; part of normal aging, but more numerous in Alzheimer's disease
Note: neurofibrillary tangles are also seen with postneoplastic parkinsonism, progressive supranuclear palsy, and Down syndrome

MULTI-INFARCT DEMENTIA
Pure multi-infarct dementia accounts for only 15% of all dementias, but probably plays a significant role in 30%

PICK'S DISEASE
Rare; peak incidence at 60 yr of age, male = female; familial cases are autosomal dominant
Profound dementia that shows a time course similar to Alzheimer's disease
Sharply demarcated focal atrophy of the anterior frontal and temporal lobes
Pick bodies: subtle, swollen, filamentous, eosinophilic bodies in the cytoplasm of neurons

CREUTZFELDT-JAKOB DISEASE
AKA: transmissible subacute spongiform encephalopathy
Related to "kuru" and the sheep model "scrapie"
Rapidly progressive dementia, ataxia, myoclonus; specific clinical picture depends upon which portions of the brain are involved
85% of cases are sporadic; 10–15% are familial (autosomal dominant); 5% are iatrogenic
CSF usually normal
EEG shows characteristic changes in two thirds of patients: generalized bilateral short interval periodic sharp wave complexes
Vacuolar spongiform degeneration of the neuronal processes (neuropil) with neuronal loss and glial proliferation
Amyloid plaques composed of prion protein (PrP) seen
Infectious agent is not clearly molecularly defined; the term *prion* for "proteinaceous infectious agent" has been coined by advocates of the theory that nucleic acid is not needed for transmissibility; others favoring a more traditional agent refer to it as a "slow virus"
Prion protein gene localized on chromosome 20p; the gene product in normal individuals is 33–35 kD and is completely digested by proteinase K; in affected patients, the gene product (PrP 33–35sc) is degraded only to a 27–30 kD protein by proteinase K digestion, and this smaller protein can polymerize into rods with amyloid features; in the disease, this product is what accumulates in and around neurons
Mutations in the prion protein gene have been linked to familial forms of this disease
Formalin does not inactivate infectivity; however, treating formalin fixed material with >90% formic acid does inactivate it
Always fatal, usually within 6 months

PARKINSONISM
Expressionless facies, pill-rolling tremor, rigidity, slowed voluntary movements
Can be caused by a number of agents, including adverse drug reactions and postencephalitic
PARKINSON'S DISEASE
Idiopathic form of Parkinsonism
Prevalence: 1–2/1000; most common in 50–60 yr old range
Lewy bodies: round, concentrically laminated, pale eosinophilic cytoplasmic inclusion
Loss of pigmented neurons from the substantia nigra, with pigment in macrophages and a reactive astrocytosis

MULTIPLE SCLEROSIS
Onset usually in 20s–40s; slightly more common in women
Relapsing episodes of paresthesias, visual disturbances, incoordination
Genetic susceptibility: 25% concordance among monozygotic twins
May have an infectious etiology (viral?)
Multiple subtypes: Charcot (classic), Marburg (acute), Schilder (diffuse sclerosis), Balo (concentric), Devic (neuromyelitis optica)

Tan-gray plaques of demyelination in the white matter, typically just off the lateral angle of the ventricles

PRIMARILY MOTOR DISORDERS

AMYOTROPHIC LATERAL SCLEROSIS (ALS)
Disease linked to chromosome 21; 10% of cases are autosomal dominant

Lower motor neuron and upper motor neuron loss; little if any sensory deficits

Weakness of the extremities (pyramidal tract involvement), muscle atrophy (hands first), labioglossolaryngeal paralysis (bulbar disturbances)

On exam, see fasciculations (rapid fine repetitive spontaneous movements of a part of a muscle; manifestation of denervation hypersensitivity, i.e., upper motor neuron lesion), exaggerated deep tendon reflexes

Histology: pyknosis, swelling, and loss of motor neurons; demyelination in the white matter

Median survival: 3 yr (1.5 yr with bulbar involvement)

HUNTINGTON'S DISEASE
Autosomal dominant inheritance (chromosome 4p16.3) with complete penetrance

Symptoms appear at ~35–40 yr of age; progress ~10–15 yr to death

Chorea, psychiatric changes (promiscuousness, violence, sociopathic behavior, depression); later confusion, memory deficits, dementia

Juvenile form: rigidity, seizures, dementia

Marked primary atrophy of the caudate nuclei bilaterally; may involve the putamen

Large neurons remain, but all of the small ones are gone

Gene encodes a 348 kD protein of unknown function

Terminal CAG repeats in the gene; the more repeats, the earlier the presentation

WERDNIG-HOFFMAN DISEASE
Autosomal recessive

"Floppy infant syndrome"

Rapidly progressive muscle weakness secondary to loss of lower motor neurons from anterior horns of the spinal cord

LEUKODYSTROPHIES
Abnormalities of myelin metabolism leading to ineffective myelination and subsequent demyelination

Most are autosomal recessive enzyme defects

METACHROMATIC LEUKODYSTROPHY
Deficiency of cerebroside sulfatase

Leads to accumulation of sulfatides in and around neurons

Progressive motor impairment

KRABBE'S DISEASE
AKA: globoid cell leukodystrophy

Onset usually by 6 months of age: rigidity, decreased alertness; fatal by age 2

Deficiency of galactocerebroside B galactosidase

Demyelination, plus multinucleated histiocytes (globoid cells) around blood vessels

ADRENOLEUKODYSTROPHY
X-linked recessive

Accumulation of long-chain fatty acids

Patients have a concurrent adrenal insufficiency

Juvenile form: boys ~10 yr old; large plaques of demyelination; fatal within 3 yr

Adult form: slowly developing spastic paralysis, cerebellar ataxia, peripheral neuropathy

TUMORS OF THE CENTRAL NERVOUS SYSTEM

General
15% CNS tumors are in the spinal cord, 85% in the brain

Metastatic tumors are usually extradural

Account for 2% of all cancer deaths, but ~20% of cancer deaths before age 15 (second only to leukemias)

Most are idiopathic; radio waves from cellular phones have been implicated by some

CNS tumors seen with von Recklinghausen's, von Hippel-Lindau, Turcot's familial polyposis, tuberous sclerosis, and the multiple nevoid basal cell carcinoma syndromes

70% of intracranial tumors are supratentorial in adults (most commonly astrocytomas [40–50%], metastases, meningiomas [~15%]), but 70% are infratentorial in children (most commonly astrocytoma [45%], medulloblastoma [40%], ependymoma, and craniopharyngioma)

Even benign tumors can be lethal; lethality more commonly caused by compression and herniation rather than actual destruction of brain tissue by the tumor itself

Rarely metastasize out of CNS

Gliomas

Most common type—account for 50% of all CNS tumors

GLIOBLASTOMA MULTIFORME
Account for more than half of the gliomas

Originally used to represent grade IV (or III) astrocytoma, but often so poorly differentiated that no astrocytic features persist

Most commonly occur in cerebrum, usually >40 yr of age

Key distinguishing feature from lower grade lesions is necrosis

Other characteristic histologic features include peripheral pseudopalisading of tumor cells around necrosis, multinucleated giant cells, gemistocytes, glomeruloid endothelial cell proliferation, infiltrative growth pattern

Tend to evolve toward small cell malignancy

Median survival decreases with patient age, but is very poor (without treatment, median survival ~2 wk)

(See discussion of grading under Astrocytoma)

GLIOSARCOMA
Rare tumor; occurs in ~2% of glioblastomas

Glioblastoma with sarcomatous changes, most commonly arising from fibroblasts of the hyperplastic blood vessels

Sarcomatous component most commonly malignant fibrous histiocytoma–like

ASTROCYTOMA
Account for 20% of gliomas

Unencapsulated; infiltrate surrounding parenchyma; margins can be very difficult to define, even microscopically

With time, astrocytomas tend to progress in grade

GRADING
Three- and four-tiered grading systems exist; in general, grades I and II of a four-tiered system are grouped into grade I in the three-tiered system

Three tiered (World Health Organization): astrocytoma, anaplastic astrocytoma, glioblastoma

Four tiered: astrocytoma, cellular astrocytoma, anaplastic astrocytoma, glioblastoma

Prognosis correlates well with grade (median survival with radiation therapy):

Grade	Overall	<50 yr	>50 yr
I	[50% survive]	—	—
II	4 yr	5.5 yr	0.5 yr
III	1.6 yr	2.5 yr	0.7 yr
IV	0.7 yr	1 yr	0.5 yr

Frequency of mitoses, vascular proliferation, and cellular atypia increase with grade; necrosis needed to advance to highest grade

STAGING

	Supratentorial		Infratentorial
T1	≤5 cm, unilateral	T1	≤3 cm, unilateral
T2	>5 cm, unilateral	T2	>3 cm, unilateral
T3	Invades ventricular system		
T4	Crosses midline or invades infra- (supra-) tentorially		

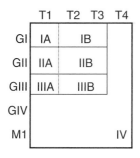

Special Types

CEREBELLAR ASTROCYTOMA
Cells are fibrillary and fusiform, resembling reactive astrocytes

Better prognosis than cerebral astrocytomas

JUVENILE PILOCYTIC ASTROCYTOMA
Occur usually in children surrounding the 3rd ventricle or within the cerebellum

Slow growing, usually well circumscribed

Tight clustering of astrocytes around blood vessels, with loose infiltration of tumor cells into surrounding tissue

Dual cell population: spindled, "pilocytic" cells admixed with microcystic areas

Most are low grade

Prognosis is good unless the brainstem is involved

GEMISTOCYTIC ASTROCYTOMA
Occur at an earlier age, on average

Most will progress to glioblastoma multiforme within 5 yr of presentation

Poor survival (mean = 2.5 yr)

DIFFUSE ASTROCYTOMA
AKA: gliomatosis cerebri

Diffuse enlargement without grossly or microscopically identifiable tumor margins

Perineuronal tumor cell aggregates

Relatively poor survival (though not as bad as gemistocytic astrocytoma)

SUBEPENDYMAL GIANT CELL ASTROCYTOMA
Largely intraventricular lesion seen in tuberous sclerosis

OLIGODENDROGLIOMA
Comprise ~5% of gliomas; more common in adults

Classically, monotonous proliferation of small cells with central round nuclei and a clear cytoplasm (artifact), creating a "fried egg" appearance; calcifications common

Small thin-walled vessels may separate tumor into lobules, creating a "chicken wire" appearance

Although more aggressive lesions tend to show greater cellular atypia, mitoses, vascular hyperplasia, or necrosis, there are no reliable histologic features upon which a prediction of prognosis can be made

EPENDYMOMA
Account for ~5% of gliomas

Most commonly seen in children and young adults

Most common tumor occurring in the spinal cord

Arise from ependymal cells in spinal cord (central canal, filum terminale) or the ventricular system of the brain

Grow in a perivascular pattern, with uniform elongated cells aligned perpendicular to vessels with their nuclei polarized away from the vessels; may also form small tubules or rosettes with a central lumen

EM reveals basal bodies and cilia

Seeding through CSF can occur; malignant forms can also occur

MYXOPAPILLARY EPENDYMOMA
Variant occurring in the filum terminale of the spinal cord

Papillae with core composed of a dilated vessel; grow in a myxoid stroma

Glial fibrillary acidic protein positive

Generally very good prognosis

Differential diagnosis: chordoma

SUBEPENDYMOMA
Multiple small nodules in the walls of ventricles

Almost always asymptomatic; usually an incidental finding

CHOROID PLEXUS PAPILLOMA
Constitute <2% of gliomas

Most commonly seen in children and young adults

Most commonly arise in lateral ventricles or 4th ventricle

Hemorrhagic, friable mass

MIXED GLIOMAS
Most commonly astrocytoma and oligodendroglioma

Less commonly oligodendroglioma and ependymoma

Other Primary CNS Tumors

NEURONAL AND GLIO-NEURONAL TUMORS
GANGLIONEUROMA
AKA: gangliocytoma

Tumor of differentiating neuronal cells with reactive glial stroma

GANGLIOGLIOMA
Mixture of both neoplastic neural and glial elements

CENTRAL NEUROCYTOMA
AKA: central neuroblastoma

Arise in paraventricular area, often forming an intraventricular mass; usually younger patients

Geographic clusters of small blue cells separated by perivascular zones of fibrillar stroma

Histology similar to oligodendroglioma but with fibrillar areas

Very good prognosis

MEDULLOBLASTOMA

Located in midline or lateral cerebellum, most frequently in children (5–10 yr) with a second peak in 20s

Small blue cell tumor composed of undifferentiated cells in sheets, occasionally aggregating into Homer-Wright rosettes without a lumen

N-*myc* gene product overexpressed in ~30% (gene is *not* amplified); associated with a poorer prognosis

Malignant; 5 yr survival is 40%

DESMOPLASTIC MEDULLOBLASTOMA

Invade the meninges and induce a fibroblastic proliferation

MENINGIOMAS

Account for ~20% of all CNS tumors (10–15% of intracranial tumors, 25% of spinal cord tumors)

Usually occur in adults, most commonly in women

Usually attached to the dura, encapsulated, pushing margins

Tumor cells are spindled but plump and at least focally arranged in circular whirls, which may calcify and form psammoma bodies

Tumor cells are EMA and vimentin positive

Three major histologic divisions: syncytial (meningotheliomatous), fibroblastic, transitional (includes psammomatous)

Most recurrences caused by incomplete excision

Angioblastic and papillary variants have worst prognosis

ATYPICAL MENINGIOMA

Cellular lesion with numerous mitoses and micronecrosis

MALIGNANT MENINGIOMA

Malignant cytology and presence of cerebral invasion

TUMORS OF ANCILLARY STRUCTURES

SCHWANNOMA (NEURILEMOMA)

Accounts for 10% of intracranial tumors, 25% of spinal cord tumors

Arise from cranial and spinal nerve roots, predominantly sensory nerves: thoracic for spinal cord, cranial nerves VIII (acoustic) and V (trigeminal) for head

Encapsulated eccentric enlargement of nerve root with cellular areas (Antoni A) alternating with more myxoid areas (Antoni B); reticular fibers surround each individual tumor cell

NEUROFIBROMA

Rare except for patients with von Recklinghausen's disease

Diffuse, concentric enlargement of the nerve; enlargement often extends into nerve branches (plexiform neurofibroma)

CRANIOPHARYNGIOMA

2–3% of CNS tumors; most commonly child or young adult

Circumscribed, slow-growing tumors arising at base of brain; generally do not invade brain, but reactive astrocytic proliferation often present

Epithelial in origin: clusters of squamous cells in pituitary stalk (Rathke's pouch remnant)

Thick brown fluid, keratin and cholesterol in cysts surrounded by and containing nests of epithelial cells that are columnar at periphery and more squamoid toward center; calcifications common

Rupture of cysts or escape of contents induces a vigorous inflammatory response

Benign tumor, but survival (overall ~70%) related to ability to completely remove surgically; will usually recur if not completely excised

HEMANGIOBLASTOMA

2–3% of CNS tumors; most commonly 20–50 yr of age, esp. in association with von Hippel-Lindau syndrome

Cerebellum most common site; also seen in spinal cord

Thin-walled vessels anastomosing within a "stroma" composed of plump oval to polygonal cells of uncertain histogenesis

Good prognosis

PITUITARY ADENOMA

(See Endocrine outline)

HEMATOPOIETIC TUMORS

Lymphomas may be primary to the CNS; 1% of CNS tumors; 1% of non-Hodgkin's lymphomas; increased incidence in setting of immunosuppression

Usually B cell, most commonly diffuse large cell type

PINEAL GLAND TUMORS

GERM CELL TUMORS

Most commonly in males near pineal gland or base of brain

Seminoma (dysgerminoma) most common type

Used to be referred to as *pinealomas*

PINEALOMA

Rare

Tumor of pineal parenchymal cell

METASTASES

~20% of all CNS tumors; usually multiple

Most common primary sites: lung, breast

Favored metastatic site for some less common tumors: renal cell carcinoma, choriocarcinoma, melanoma

APPENDIX
SYNDROMES AND BODIES

Syndromes

Addison's disease: primary chronic adrenocortical insufficiency, with weakness, fatigability, anorexia, weight loss, and hypotension

Adrenogenital: group of disorders caused by adrenocortical hyperplasia: masculinization in women; feminization in men; precocious puberty in children

Agammaglobulinemia of Bruton: X-linked primary immunodeficiency syndrome with defective B-cell maturation and near-total absence of immunoglobulins (Igs) in serum

Alagille: autosomal dominant; jaundice caused by progressive loss of bile ducts, vertebral anomalies, hypogonadism, pulmonic stenosis

Albright's: polyostotic fibrous dysplasia with skin pigmentation, endocrine dysfunction, and precocious puberty

Arthus reaction: localized form of type III (immune complex mediated) hypersensitivity reaction

Ataxia-telangiectasia: autosomal recessive cerebellar ataxia and telangiectasias resulting from defective repair of x-ray damage, leading to chromosome instability; patients prone to develop lymphoma, leukemia, gastric carcinoma

Beckwith-Wiedemann: macroglossia, omphalocele, hemihypertrophy, and/or visceromegaly; also see adrenal cytomegaly and islet hyperplasia; cancer develops in 5%, usually Wilms' tumor; association with 11p15 duplication

Bloom's: Spontaneous chromatid breakage; leukemia, GI carcinoma

Caplan's: development of pulmonary rheumatoid nodules in a background of progressive massive fibrosis

Carcinoid: combination of symptoms produced by serotonin release from carcinoid tumors that have metastasized to the liver: mottled blushing, angiomas of the skin, acquired pulmonary and tricuspid stenosis, diarrhea, bronchial spasm, mental aberration

Caroli's disease: communicating cavernous biliary ectasia; may be seen in conjunction with congenital hepatic fibrosis

Chédiak-Higashi: several defects in leukocytes, including impaired chemotaxis; autosomal recessive

Churg-Strauss: variant of polyarteritis nodosum associated with bronchial asthma, pulmonary vessel involvement, and granulomatous inflammation

Conn's: primary hyperaldosteronism caused by an adrenocortical adenoma

Cowden's: multiple non–Peutz-Jegher's colonic hamartomatous polyps with facial trichilemmomas and oral mucosal papillomas

CREST: calcinosis, Raynaud's phenomenon, esophageal dysmotility, sclerodactyly, telangiectasia: a limited form of scleroderma

Cri du chat: chromosome 5p-; see Congenital Disorders

Crigler-Najjar: impaired conjugation of bilirubin by the liver, leading to an unconjugated hyperbilirubinemia

Cronkhite-Canada: gastrointestinal polyposis, alopecia, hyperpigmentation, and dystrophic changes in fingernails and toenails

Cushing's: increased adrenocortical secretion of cortisol caused by elevated ACTH levels; moon facies, acne, abdominal striae, hypertension, amenorrhea, and hirsutism; when associated with pituitary adenoma, called Cushing's disease

DiGeorge's: selective T-cell immunodeficiency resulting from failure of development of the 3rd and 4th pharyngeal pouches (thymus, parathyroids, C cells of thyroid)

DiGuglielmo's: erythromyeloblastic leukemia (M6 AML)

Down: trisomy 21

Dubin-Johnson: autosomal recessive defect in bile canalicular transport, producing a conjugated hyperbilirubinemia and a black liver

Edwards': trisomy 18

Ehlers-Danlos: heterogeneous group of disorders of collagen synthesis/structure

Eisenmenger's: right ventricular hypertrophy and pulmonary hypertension caused by a left-to-right shunt that results in reversal of the flow through the shunt (right to left)

Fabry's disease: X-linked lysosomal storage disease (sphingolipidosis)

Fanconi's anemia: autosomal recessive chromosomal breakage; associated findings: renal hypoplasia, absent or hypoplastic thumbs or radii, hyperpigmentation of skin, microcephaly; patients at risk for acute nonlymphocytic leukemia, squamous cell carcinoma, hepatoma

Fitz-Hugh-Curtis: stabbing right upper quadrant pain secondary to perihepatitis caused by spread of untreated gonorrheal cervicitis into the peritoneum

Gardner's: autosomal dominant; colonic polyposis, osteomas, keratinous cysts of the skin, soft tissue fibromatosis; high risk of colon cancer

225

Gaucher's disease: autosomal recessive lysosomal storage disease (sphingolipidosis)

Gilbert's: constitutional hepatic dysfunction; decreased uptake of bilirubin by the liver; produces unconjugated hyperbilirubinemia

Goodpasture's: anti–basement membrane antibody mediated destruction of glomerular and pulmonary basement membranes, leading to a rapidly progressive glomerulonephritis and a necrotizing, hemorrhagic pneumonia

Gorham's disease (AKA: massive osteolysis): reabsorption of whole or multiple bones and filling of residual spaces with heavily vascularized fibrous tissue

Hansen's disease: leprosy

HELLP: combination of hemolysis, elevated liver function tests, and low platelets; seen in severe toxemia of pregnancy

Horton's disease: temporal (giant cell) arteritis

Hunter's: type II mucopolysaccharidosis; X-linked recessive

Hurler's: type I mucopolysaccharidosis

Kartagener's: congenital absence of cilia leading to situs inversus, chronic sinusitis, bronchiectasis

Kasabach-Merritt: thrombocytopenia complicating a giant hemangioma

Klinefelter's: XXY

Krabbe's disease (AKA: globoid cell leukodystrophy): lysosomal storage disease (sphingolipidosis)

Löffler's: eosinophilic pneumonia with granulomas; usually self-limited

Maffucci's (AKA: dyschondroplasia with vascular hamartomas): multiple hemangiomas and enchondromas

Marfan's: autosomal dominant defect in connective tissue integrity

McArdle's: type V glycogenosis

Menkes': X-linked recessive disorder of intestinal copper absorption, needed by lysyl-oxidase, resulting in changes in aortic collagen and elastin

Mikulicz's: originally used to refer to what is now called Sjögren's syndrome, now used to refer to any swelling of the salivary gland and lacrimal gland

Milroy's disease: resembles lymphedema praecox but present from birth and inherited as Mendelian trait

Morquio's: type IV mucopolysaccharidosis

Nelson's: adenomatous enlargement of the pituitary with a carcinomatous histologic picture occurring in patients with unresectable pituitary tumor treated with bilateral adrenalectomy

Nezelof's: absent thymus and cell mediated immunity (like DiGeorge's) but with normal parathyroids

Niemann-Pick disease: autosomal recessive lysosomal storage disease with zebra bodies

Ollier's disease: multiple unilateral enchondromas; often associated with ovarian sex cord–stromal tumors

Osler-Weber-Rendu: autosomal dominant hereditary hemorrhagic telangiectasias of the face and oral mucosa

Parinaud's (AKA: oculoglandular syndrome): swelling of the eye, jaw, and high cervical lymph nodes

Peutz-Jeghers: autosomal dominant; multiple gastrointestinal hamartomatous polyps, melanotic mucosal and cutaneous pigmentation around the lips, mouth, face, genitalia, palmar surfaces of hands

Plummer-Vinson: microcytic hypochromic anemia, atrophic glossitis, esophageal webs

Pompe's disease: glycogenosis II, a lysosomal storage disease

Pott's disease: tuberculous spondylitis

Ramsay Hunt: involvement of the geniculate ganglion by herpes zoster, resulting in facial paralysis

Raynaud's disease: Raynaud's phenomenon occurring in the absence of an anatomic lesion in the vessel walls

Raynaud's phenomenon: pain and color changes in the skin, usually of distal extremities, in response to cold

Reiter's: triad of conjunctivitis, urethritis, and arthritis

Reye's: fatty degeneration of the liver and encephalopathy seen in children treated with aspirin for a viral illness

Sanfilippo's: type III mucopolysaccharidosis

Schmidt's: type II autoimmune Addison's disease

Sheehan's: postpartum pituitary infarction and necrosis

Sicca: Sjögren's syndrome occurring without another autoimmune disorder (like rheumatoid arthritis)

Stein-Leventhal: polycystic ovaries, amenorrhea, and sterility

Stevens-Johnson: severe form of erythema multiforme with mucosal involvement, conjunctivitis, high fever

Sturge-Weber: port wine stain of face in distribution of trigeminal nerve associated with ipsilateral vascular malformations of the leptomeninges and/or the retina

Tay-Sachs disease: lysosomal storage disease (sphingolipidosis)

Trousseau's: migratory thrombophlebitis seen in patients with a malignancy; first described for pancreatic carcinoma

Turcot's: autosomal recessive; colonic adenomatous polyps and glioblastomas of the CNS

Turner's: XO

Vanishing bile duct: irreversible loss of bile ducts caused by a destructive cholangitis within 100 days following liver transplantation

von Gierke's: type I glycogenosis

von Hippel-Lindau: cavernous hemangioblastomas of cerebellum or brainstem, hemangiomas and cysts of pancreas, liver, kidneys; autosomal dominant

von Recklinghausen's disease: autosomal dominant disorder with multiple plexiform neurofibromas, café-au-lait macules, and Lisch nodules

Waterhouse-Friderichsen: hemorrhagic destruction of the adrenals, usually secondary to meningococcemia

Werdnig-Hoffman disease: infantile spinal muscular atrophy; autosomal recessive congenital hypotonia caused by absence/loss of lower motor neurons from the anterior horns of the spinal cord

Wiskott-Aldrich: X-linked recessive immunodeficiency of T cells associated with thrombocytopenia and eczema

Zollinger-Ellison: gastric hyperplasia secondary to a gastrin secreting tumor

Bodies

Acidophil bodies: see Councilman bodies

Adria cell: cardiac myocyte that has lost its cross-striations and myofilaments secondary to Adriamycin (doxorubicin) toxicity

Aschoff bodies: foci of fibrinoid necrosis within the myocardium of a patient with acute rheumatic fever

Asteroid bodies: acidophilic, stellate inclusions in giant cells in sarcoidosis and berylliosis

Auer rods: red rod–shaped lysosomes (abnormal) seen in malignant cells of predominantly M3 acute myelogenous leukemia

Barr bodies: inactivated X chromosome—dark staining mass in contact with the nuclear membrane

Birbeck granules: "tennis racket"–shaped granules in cytoplasm of Langerhans' cells (histiocytosis X) with trilaminar "handle"

Blue-blobs: atrophy in Pap smears

Blue bodies: laminated PAS+ iron-containing bodies in alveolar macrophages of desquamative interstitial pneumonia

Call-Exner bodies: small glandlike "follicles" filled with acidophilic material often seen in ovarian granulosa cell tumors

Caterpillar cells: large multinucleated giant cells with lengthwise chromatin clumping in nucleus; appear owl-eyed on cross section; seen in heart in acute rheumatic fever

Charcot-Leyden crystals: crystals shaped like double pyramids; found in sputum of asthma patients; made by eosinophils

Councilman bodies: apoptotic, eosinophilic hepatocytes extruded into the sinuses

Corpora amylacea: argyrophilic and PAS+ polyglucosan globules in terminal processes of astrocytes

Corpora arantii: small fibrous nodules at the centers of the semilunar valve cusps along the lines of closure

Cowdry type A inclusion: acidophilic intranuclear inclusion separated from the nuclear membrane by an artifactual cleft—typical of herpes-infected cells

Curschmann's spirals: twisted mass of mucus seen in sputum of patients with asthma

Donovan's body: intracellular bacillus (*Calymmatobacterium donovani*) seen in histiocytes in the genital skin of patients affected with granuloma inguinale

Dutcher bodies: "intranuclear" inclusions of immunoglobulin in plasmacytoid cells

Faggot cells: malignant promyelocytes of M3 AML containing numerous Auer rods, like "sticks in a fireplace"

Gandy-Gamna bodies: calcium and hemosiderin deposits in the spleen: seen in setting of increased hemolysis

Glomus bodies: regulated arteriovenous anastomoses in the skin that play a role in thermoregulation

Guarnieri's bodies: epidermal cells with eosinophilic cytoplasmic inclusions in skin of patients with smallpox

Hassall's corpuscles: concentric aggregates of keratinized epithelial cells and keratin in the medulla of the thymus

Heinz bodies: clumps of precipitated oxidized hemoglobin in the cytoplasm of red cells

Hematoxylin bodies: see LE bodies

Hirano body: eosinophilic, football-shaped inclusion seen in neurons of the brain; part of normal aging, but more numerous in Alzheimer's disease

Hutchinson's teeth: inflammatory destruction of the teeth seen in tertiary syphilis

Kamino bodies: intraepidermal hyaline globules seen in a Spitz nevus

Kayser-Fleischer rings: rings of discoloration on cornea of patients with Wilson's disease

Koplik's spots: spotty lesions that blister and ulcerate deep in the cheek mucosa; diagnostic for measles

Lambl's excrescences: small fibrin vegetations overlying sites of endothelial damage on flow side of cardiac valves

LE bodies (AKA: hematoxylin bodies): nuclei of damaged cells with bound anti-nuclear antibodies that become homogeneous and lose chromatin pattern; when phagocytosed, form LE cells

Lewy bodies: round, concentrically laminated, pale eosinophilic cytoplasmic inclusions seen in neurons in Parkinson's disease

Libman-Sacks nodules: non-bacterial verrucous cardiac valve leaflet vegetations seen in SLE

Lipofuscin granules: polymers of lipid complexed with proteins; responsible for brown atrophy

Lisch nodules: pigmented iris hamartomas seen in patients with type I neurofibromatosis

Loose bodies: fragments of bone or cartilage that become detached into the joint space; may continue to grow by surface apposition; centers eventually necrose and calcify

MacCallum's plaques: maplike thickening of the endocardium over myocardial lesions in acute rheumatic fever

Mallory bodies: alcoholic hyalin-eosinophilic intracytoplasmic inclusions in hepatocytes: intermediate filaments, predominantly prekeratin

Michaelis-Gutmann bodies: partially digested bacteria (calcified) in stroma and in cells; seen in malakoplakia

Negri bodies: bullet-shaped cytoplasmic inclusions in neurons (esp. Purkinje cells); pathognomonic for rabies infection

Nemaline bodies: Z-bands seen by electron microscopy in degenerative skeletal muscle diseases

Neurofibrillary tangles: microtubule-associated proteins and neurofilaments, seen in Alzheimer's disease

Physaliferous cells: very large tumor cells with bubbly vacuolated cytoplasm (some glycogen) and vesicular nuclei, seen in chordomas

Reinke's crystalloids: crystals found in Leydig cells of testes: hexagonal prisms, tapered ends, moderately electron dense

Rokitansky's protuberance: central area of an ovarian mature cystic teratoma containing bone and well-formed teeth

Rosenthal fibers: intracytoplasmic hyaline structure, sometimes corkscrew shaped, found in pilocytic astrocytes

Russell bodies: cytoplasmic immunoglobulin inclusions in plasma cells or plasmacytoid cells

Schaumann bodies: concentrically laminated inclusions (up to 50 μm) in giant cells seen in sarcoidosis? and berylliosis

Schiller-Duval bodies: endodermal sinuses: glomeruloid structures seen in yolk sac tumors

Smudge cell: cell with a large, ovoid nucleus filled with a granular amphophilic to deeply basophilic mass and an indistinct nuclear membrane; seen in adenovirus-infected cells

Soldier's plaque: white thickening of the epicardium from a healed pericarditis

Sulfur granules: yellow foci of *Actinomyces*

Sucquet-Hoyer canals: shunts of glomus bodies, involved in thermal regulation

Verocay bodies: palisades of nuclei at the end of a fibrillar bundle in a schwannoma (neurilemoma)

Warthin-Finkeldey cells: multinucleated giant cells with eosinophilic nuclear and cytoplasmic inclusions found in lymphoid organs of patients with measles

Weibel-Palade bodies: rod-shaped cytoplasmic organelles in endothelial cells containing von Willebrand factor

Zebra bodies: palisaded lamellated membranous cytoplasmic bodies seen by electron microscopy in macrophages of patients with Niemann-Pick disease, Tay-Sachs disease, or any of the mucopolysaccharidoses

Zellballen: clusters of tumor cells surrounded by a thin fibrovascular stroma, seen in pheochromocytoma and extraadrenal paragangliomas

REFERENCES

This following is a list of the major sources used in compiling these outlines. Additional sources, such as individual lectures, journal articles, etc., have been omitted. The reader is encouraged to consult these references for additional information, photographs, or simply for a prose discussion of any of the topics covered in these outlines. The references used are by no means the only texts available on this subject. After all, pathology is pathology, and what makes one text different from another is the selection of material, the organization of that material, and the style of the presentation. The reader may find any of a number of other excellent works preferable. The selections here represent the bias imposed by my personal collection of texts and the references readily available to me during my training. I particularly recommend the Robbins text for its discussion of non-neoplastic pathology and have found the Ackerman text invaluable for tumor pathology.

General Texts

Cotran, R., Kumar, V., and Robbins, S. *Robbins Pathologic Basis of Disease,* 4th edition (1989). W.B. Saunders Company, Philadelphia.

Kissane, J., editor. *Anderson's Pathology,* 9th edition (1990). C.V. Mosby Company, St.Louis.

Rosai, J. *Ackerman's Surgical Pathology,* 7th edition (1989). C.V. Mosby Company, St. Louis.

Sternberg, S., editor. *Diagnostic Surgical Pathology,* 2nd edition (1994). Raven Press, New York.

Specialized Texts

Alberts, B., Bray, D., Lewis, J., Raff, M., Roberts, K., and Watson, J. *Molecular Biology of the Cell,* 2nd edition (1989). Garland Publishing, New York.

Beahrs, O., Henson, D., Hutter, R., and Kennedy, B., editors. The American Joint Committee on Cancer's *Manual for Staging of Cancer,* 4th edition (1992). J.B. Lippincott Company, Philadelphia.

Enzinger, F., and Weiss, S. *Soft Tissue Tumors,* 2nd edition (1988). C.V. Mosby Company, St. Louis.

Jaffee, E. *Surgical Pathology of the Lymph Nodes and Related Organs.* Major Problems in Pathology, 2nd edition, Volume 16 (1995). W.B. Saunders Company, Philadelphia.

Jawetz, E., Melnick, J., and Adelberg, E. *Review of Medical Microbiology,* 17th edition (1987). Appleton and Lange, Norwalk, CT.

Katzenstein, A., and Askin, F. *Surgical Pathology of Non-Neoplastic Lung Disease.* Major Problems in Pathology, 2nd edition, Volume 13 (1990). W.B. Saunders Company, Philadelphia.

Knowles, D., editor. *Neoplastic Hematopathology* (1992). Williams & Wilkins, Baltimore.

McKee, P. *Pathology of the Skin with Clinical Correlations* (1989). J. B. Lippincott Company, Philadelphia.

Moore, K. *The Developing Human: Clinically Oriented Embryology,* 3rd edition (1982). W. B. Saunders Company, Philadelphia.